Chariot of Sadhana

Yoga of the Inner Teacher

Chariot of Sadhana

Yoga of the Inner Teacher

Martin and Marian Jerry

Mahamandaleshvara Swami Veda Bharati

Foreword by David Frawley

Unlimited Publishing
Bloomington, Indiana

2M Communications
Canmore, Canada

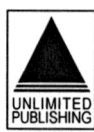

Dedicated to

Our Gurudev H.H. Sri Swami Rama

Disclaimer

This book is designed to provide information in regard to the subject matter covered. It is sold with the understanding that the publisher and authors are not rendering yogic, medical, psychological or other professional services. We are not endorsing any of the referenced resources.

It is not the purpose of this book to reprint all the information that is otherwise available to readers, but to complement, amplify and supplement other texts. For more information, please see the references.

Every effort has been made to make this book as complete and as accurate as possible; however, despite our best efforts there may be errors. Therefore, this text should be used only as a general guide and not as the ultimate source of information. Furthermore, this book contains information only up to publication date.

We are concerned that the teachings of the Himalayan Tradition of Yoga be presented and preserved as purely and accurately as possible. In the interests of the mutual advantage of a dialogue between East and West we have also included material from modern psychology which is distinct from Himalayan Yoga, but which can be used along with it as a useful complement.

While all of the suggestions in this book may be helpful in part or in whole to some individuals, none of them are guaranteed to make the connection with the Inner Teacher or to open the intuition. This is not a mechanical process. They are simply suggestions to help the process get started. They may be helpful to some people but not to others. The reader should consult an experienced teacher of Himalayan Yoga for guidance before practicing any of the methods or meditations discussed in this book.

The authors and publishers shall have neither liability nor responsibility to any person or entity with respect to any loss or damage caused or alleged to be caused directly or indirectly by the information contained in this book.

Contents

Preface

The Yoga Tradition – more specifically called "Yoga *Dharma*" or Yoga as a spiritual path – is a vast system of spiritual knowledge, teaching us the inner truth of life, consciousness, the universe and our real nature beyond time and space, birth and death and suffering. Yoga is the great gift to humanity from the Himalayan sages since the time of the Vedic *Rishis* thousands of years ago to modern masters who travel throughout the world spreading its exalted message.

Yoga *Dharma* teaches spirituality as a science of Self-realization that can be made relevant to every individual in every culture. As such, Yoga transcends all beliefs and dogmas, though it can embrace the essential aspiration of each soul to reach the highest. Yoga is not a "name and form" tradition. It does not insist upon a particular label, but emphasizes the actual energies that we set in motion in our lives, showing us how we can direct them both to unfold our highest potential and bring the greatest benefit to the world in which we live.

Yoga in this broader sense is what is called a "*sadhana*" tradition, from the Sanskrit word *sadhana* meaning "spiritual practice," leading us step by step to Self-realization and union with God or the Supreme Reality, which are ultimately one and the same. Yoga accomplishes this great task through an integral development and harmonization of our entire being, showing us how to spiritualize our outer behavior, how to spiritualize the body and its urges, how to direct our senses inwardly, how to increase our vitality and, most importantly, how to awaken our inner intelligence that is one with the Cosmic Mind. Even Yoga *asanas* are meant to allow the practitioner to sit for long periods in meditation as part of *sadhana*. They were never regarded as an end in themselves.

Yet rather than as a *sadhana* or spiritual practice, most Yoga today is performed either as an exercise system to improve bodily flexibility or as a healing therapy to counter mainly structural problems in the spine and joints. There is nothing necessarily wrong with these approaches and Yoga has great benefit both as an exercise system and a healing methodology, but these are preliminary to what real Yoga has always been about, which is taking even the healthy and happy human being to a higher level of existence and awareness.

For all the New Age talk of new paradigms about life and the universe, our approach to Yoga remains largely Newtonian: physical, material and commercial. Few books on Yoga today approach Yoga as a *sadhana* and how it affects our minds and hearts, helping us to address the ultimate questions of life and existence.

In spite of – or perhaps because of its popularity in the West – there remains a great deal of confusion about what constitutes a real and complete Yoga practice. Often Yoga gets reduced to the mechanics of *asanas*, with some deep breathing or a quick and stereotyped approach to meditation thrown in on the side. A good Yoga practice is usually defined in terms of a good workout at a physical level. A complete practice is defined as one that addresses the entire body. Yet any serious examination of the Yoga tradition shows that real Yoga is something much more. While culturally we have embraced the outer aspects of Yoga, it is important that we go further to its inner levels that are much more significant.

Many Yoga practitioners are looking for the more spiritual, inner Yoga that they find in the older traditions and in the stories of the great masters. The problem is that they do not always have a lot to examine in the existent literature, particularly if they are not versed in the Sanskrit of traditional Yoga texts.

More serious Yoga students study the *Yoga-Sutra* of Patanjali to help them understand the greater basis of Yoga, as it is generally known to be the most authoritative traditional work on Yoga practice. There are several examinations of the *Sutras* available today but there also remains much confusion as to the real meaning and scope of the text and its short cryptic statements. Some scholars invent their own interpretations without having really examined the context of the older Yoga tradition from which the *Sutras* arose.

The *Chariot of Sadhana* is a refreshing and insightful alternative to the common mass approaches to Yoga. It is one of the most in depth and sophisticated explanations of Yoga *Dharma* today. It provides a clear and authentic presentation of traditional Yoga, including key teachings of the *Yoga-Sutra*, examined with logic, clarity and insight, faithful to the tradition, the meaning of the text and to an experiential application in *sadhana* today.

The book is one of the best new in depth studies of Yoga as a spiritual practice, an exploration of consciousness and a means of taking us to the highest Self-realization. The book follows the Yoga-Vedanta tradition, which has historically been the main Yoga tradition to come to the West through such great spiritual masters as Swami Vivekananda, Paramahansa Yogananda, Swami Rama and the many disciples of Swami Sivananda of Rishikesh, to name but a few. The book, however, like this profound tradition, takes a broad view with reference to other spiritual and religious traditions and contemporary scientific thought. It is not the work of a particular sect, but a grand synthesis of spiritual seeking that is relevant to everyone.

The *Chariot of Sadhana* is an excellent reference guide to the greater Yoga, Veda, Vedanta and Tantric traditions, revealing the underlying unity of these Himalayan teachings. It is also an important aid for any individual attempting an inner practice, regardless of the particular tradition they may have been born into.

The book is well-researched and features many relevant quotes on the most important issues of both Yoga and the spiritual life in general. More importantly, it contains many practical teachings and specific techniques that the individual can adapt, so the floodgates of our inner being can open and reveal the greater universe that lives and is aware both within and around us.

The book's explication of the role of the inner teacher, and the inner reality of the *guru*, is very important in these times in which people either superficially reject the value of a *guru* or merely worship the outer personality of the teacher and don't take up any real inner practice themselves.

For serious students of yogic spirituality, the book provides a clear analysis of the crucial issues of Yoga practice. This includes the ethical foundation of practice, the philosophy or view beyond the practice, and important details of meditation and the workings of the mind. The book provokes profound thinking and sharp examination on the part of its readers and requires a concentrated study to extract its valuable essence.

Swami Veda Bharati is one of the foremost *gurus* and teachers of Yoga and Vedanta in the world today. His translation and interpretation of the *Yoga-Sutra* is the best available in the English language. He is one of the few individuals over the last century in India who has the intuitive ability to compose new *mantras* in the ancient Vedic language. His knowledge of *Sadhana*, particularly of the role of *Kundalini Shakti*, is extraordinary. His influence is reflected in the precision, comprehensiveness and thoughtfulness present in every page of the book.

Drs. Martin and Marian Jerry write with a great deal of conviction, confidence and experience, showing how those born in the West can enter into the deeper Yoga tradition and learn to practice it, master it and teach it.

The *Chariot of Sadhana* makes an excellent textbook for deeper Yoga studies, for those who want to go beyond the bodily Yoga and the personal Yoga to the Yoga of the Infinite and Eternal. Those who study the book carefully will find all their misconceptions about Yoga dispelled and will discover a clear path forward for their own inner unfoldment. Hopefully, this book marks a new era in books on Yoga, in which philosophically astute and practically useful studies of the deeper Yoga become more available in the West. May the world of Yoga students embrace this wonderful book and learn to imbibe its wisdom!

David Frawley (Pandit Vamadeva Shastri)
Author, *Yoga and the Sacred Fire, Yoga and Ayurveda*
Director, American Institute of Vedic Studies
www.vedanet.com

Introduction

"I know WHAT to do, but I don't know HOW to do it!"

What versus how. So often we are told what to do, but we are left puzzled as to how to put that into action. To be helpful, it is often not sufficient to tell people what to do. We may need also to be able to guide them into how to actually do it. When we consulted for the World Health Organization for many years in the field of cancer control, we were often asked what to do about national cancer control programs at whole country level in the developing world. It is not difficult to know what to do in those situations, given an adequate situation analysis. The procedures are quite straightforward, and can be found in most relevant textbooks. We found that the consulting report that gave a prescription of what to do in a particular situation was often not sufficiently helpful in the long run. What were missing were detailed instructions on how to put these recommendations into action. This requires experience on the part of the consultant, and the ability to find unique ways to implement recommendations into a particular context of cultural and social development. People seem to do the HOW in unique ways.

We believe the same applies to you the reader. A good Yoga teacher will not only instruct students about what to do with their practice, but based on his or her experience in a particular tradition will also share helpful hints on how to get these recommendations to work. This process must recognize that each student has a unique personality and will put a unique twist on how he or she carries out a process.

We intend that this be a book about the HOW. The WHAT is covered in the first book of this series called *Sutras of the Inner Teacher: The Yoga of the Centre of Consciousness* (Jerry & Jerry, 2001). We will refer to and cross reference it many times throughout this text. *Sutras of the Inner Teacher* describes for the new disciple how to begin to work with the opening of the Centre of Consciousness, or the Inner Teacher of Yoga. Some aspects of what to do are fairly obvious for the experienced student of Yoga who knows the basics of the practices. But the more one moves from the gross through the subtle to the subtlest, the more difficult it becomes to describe the processes involved, the *how* of *what* to do, for doing and process shift into states of being. What actually goes on inside the mind and personality? What is the actual process for emotional purification? Can Western psychology and science provide tools to complement processes derived from the perennial wisdom to enhance their efficacy?

This text, as well as *Sutras of the Inner Teacher*, is addressed to advanced students of the Himalayan Tradition to assist at a critical stage of the unfolding of spiritual consciousness on the path. We assume some basic knowledge of Yoga as taught in the Himalayan Tradition as well as practical familiarity with practices and methods. But every reader interested in Yoga and spirituality will find something of value in both texts.

Samahita Yoga: The Yoga of the Centre of Consciousness

Samahita Yoga is the term we use to refer to the theory and practice given in this text and in *Sutras of the Inner Teacher*. We also call it the Yoga of the Centre of Consciousness. "Centre of Consciousness" and "Inner Teacher" are used as synonyms here. Our spiritual master, Sri Swami Rama, used the term "Centre of Consciousness" frequently to refer to the divine flame or core of divinity within us all. By the use of these terms we refer to the experiences, teachings and practices appropriate to a critical stage of the journey on the spiritual path. This is the point at which the master takes the prepared student as a new disciple in the Himalayan Tradition, and through initiation links him or her to the Tradition by opening an eternal inner access to the Inner Teacher. This is a momentous transition for the new disciple. We hope that this text as well as *Sutras of the Inner Teacher* can provide some practical guidance for this critical juncture.

By Centre of Consciousness, we refer to the Inner Teacher of Yoga, the Inner *Guru* or *Hiranyagarbha* in the Yoga tradition. Similar concepts include the Holy Ghost or Holy Spirit of Christianity as the teaching spirit of the universe, or the *sambhogakaya* of Buddhism (Veda Bharati, 1979a).

The Chariot of *Sadhana*

Samahita Yoga, the Yoga of the Centre of Consciousness, is based in what Swami Rama used to call the Chariot of *Sadhana*. One wheel is *abhyasa* (practice) and the other is *vairagya* (nonattachment). They must turn together for the vehicle to progress. *Abhyasa* and *vairagya* are discussed as two core practices in the first *pada* of Patanjali's *Yoga-Sutra*. The concepts are integrated with a third called *Ishvara pranidhana*. What we call *Samahita* Yoga integrates all three concepts into practice flowing from the experience of the opening of the Centre of Consciousness. This is just a different emphasis of Himalayan Yoga relative to a particular stage of the spiritual path. What we are describing is anchored in the eight-limbed Raja Yoga of Patanjali, and uses meditation as the core technique. But the practices become reinterpreted with the experience of the opening of the Centre of Consciousness which gives them new and deeper experiential meaning and significance. Moreover, the Yogas of life – Karma, Bhakti and Jnana, also integrate and become unified in the experience of the Centre of Consciousness in everyday life.

East Meets West

Sri Swami Rama was given a planetary mission by his own spiritual master.

The objective of both science and spirituality is to find the source of peace and happiness. Science asks it in the external world, spirituality in the inner world. Human needs are not just physical – they are also mental and spiritual. Science helps us meet our physical needs, and spirituality helps us meet the needs of the mind and soul. In isolation from science, spirituality shrinks into religious dogma, and in isolation from spirituality, science turns into a cold, life-defying mechanism.

You are going there to deliver a message not to the East or to the West, but to the whole world. Always remember: that message is the message of the sages. Teach only what you have practiced. Let it be scientifically verified if science has the capacity to verify it.

Pandit Rajmani Tigunait (1998a, pp 48–49)

"Science without religion is lame, religion without science is blind."

Albert Einstein

Bridging East and West, science with the perennial wisdom, was a central theme throughout Swamiji's mission. He participated extensively in the 1960s and 1970s with scientists in North America researching the voluntary control of involuntary states and the autonomic nervous system. The result was a key contribution to the establishment of the science of biofeedback. The core theme in all of Swamiji's work was the application of Yoga science to healing and medicine for the betterment of humankind.

One of the co-authors of this book is a physician-scientist and the other a clinical psychologist. Together we have spent over 30 years in laboratory and clinical research with a major interest in immunology and behavioral oncology. It is in the spirit of Swamiji's mission that we present here occasional scientific commentary as well as some leading edge Western methodology which we believe can illuminate and complement material from the perennial wisdom.

In doing so, however, we are mindful of the injunction to keep the teachings of the perennial wisdom pure. We do this here by making clear at every step exactly what comes from the teachings of the Himalayan Tradition, and what represents Western science and technology. Swamiji understood the complementary contributions that East and West could each make to the betterment of the human condition. He was not averse to using the best of both. It is from that perspective that we offer here some of both in the belief that from our own experience some of these new Western technologies can complement and facilitate traditional Yogic practices.

The Structure of the Book

Part One is a review and introduction to the concept of the Centre of Consciousness or Presence. Part Two introduces the basic structure of the book with the organizing metaphor of the chariot of *sadhana* and describes what we mean by *Samahita* Yoga. Parts Three and Four examine the two wheels of the chariot of *sadhana*: *vairagya* or nonattachment, and *abhyasa* or practice. The core method of meditation which links together the two wheels of the chariot of *sadhana* is reviewed in Part Five. Part Six introduces the roles of grace, the *guru* and the Inner Teacher.

The Himalayan Tradition is the root source of all meditative traditions in Yoga (Swami Veda Bharati, personal communication), and all forms of meditation can be found within this tradition. Meditations in the Himalayan Tradition are transmitted orally through initiation and are based in Mantra Yoga. Transmission and initiation in the Himalayan Tradition are discussed in detail elsewhere (Veda Bharati, 1981; Tigunait, 1996). The science of meditation as expounded in the perennial wisdom is a complex and very large body of knowledge. Competent teachers assign specific methods to meet the unique needs of each student, particularly in the advanced forms. Thus the meditations here on the Centre of Consciousness are not for everyone; that inner experience must be present and available. As an example of the variation we also include some discussion of the Centre of Consciousness as sound, or Nada Yoga. The Himalayan Tradition is rooted in Raja Yoga, but also includes Vedanta as well as the higher *samaya* Tantra including the solar science, Sri Vidya. The meditations here involving the Presence relate particularly to the *saccidananda* of Vedanta.

An extensive bibliography is given at the end for readers who may wish to pursue aspects of the text in more depth. Academic citations are used throughout in brackets with first author and year of publication, for example, (Smith, 1997). The full citations are then arranged alphabetically by first author and year in the bibliography.

Authorship

The book has been written by the Jerrys. But the material it contains reflects so much of the teachings of their spiritual teacher and senior disciple of Swami Rama, Swami Veda Bharati, that they are delighted that he has agreed to be a co-author in recognition of his extensive contribution to its material.

Acknowledgements

We acknowledge with gratitude the guidance and love of the late H.H. Sri Swami Rama to whom this book is dedicated. We also specially thank our co-author Swami Veda Bharati for his teaching and guidance over so many years. His constant encouragement has provided the inspiration to write. Our deep appreciation goes to Dr. David Frawley for providing the Preface. Over the years we have benefited by the influence of many students and disciples from the Himalayan Tradition. We acknowledge their inspiration and wisdom. We also specially thank those who have given us of their time and wisdom or who have acted as reviewers: Pandit H.S. Dabral, Dr. Paul Jerry, Dr. Shiv and Savitri Jugdeo, Mayanne Krech, Judy Law and Valery Petrich. Especially we acknowledge the support of our many colleagues of the Foothills Yoga Society and of other students of Yoga in Calgary, Alberta and Canada. Our deep appreciation goes to Charles King and his expert staff at Cox-King Multimedia for editing, typesetting and cover design, and to Danny Snow and the staff at Unlimited Publishing for their outstanding work and warm collegiality. To our supportive family, Paul and Leslie Jerry, and Marc and Marnie Jerry, we express our deep appreciation and love.

Part One

The Yoga of the Centre of Consciousness

1
Spirituality

Our purpose here is to explore how to work with the Centre of Consciousness in a practical way in daily life. Elsewhere we have discussed the concept and nature of the Centre of Consciousness in depth (Jerry & Jerry, 2001). To begin our journey here we need to review what we mean by the Centre of Consciousness, otherwise known as the Inner Teacher or Inner *Guru* in Yoga. In a sense, what we are really talking about here is what we mean by spirituality, for the Centre of Consciousness is a manifestation of Spirit. Let us begin our exploration by moving from the general to the specific, from the general concept of spirituality to the specific concept of the Centre of Consciousness.

What Do We Mean by "Spirituality"?

"When *I* use a word," Humpty Dumpty said, in rather a scornful tone, "it means just what I choose it to mean – neither more nor less."

"The question is," said Alice, "whether you *can* make words mean so many different things."

Lewis Carroll, *Alice through the Looking Glass*, Chapter 6.

This is a difficult area to discuss in Western society in any context. It was not that long ago in the West that both sexuality and death were forbidden topics. Now we are much more open about these basic aspects of life (some would say too open in the case of sexuality and others would say not open enough in the case of death). However, of the three, we believe that spirituality (as opposed to religion) remains difficult for Westerners to discuss. Perhaps one reason is that so few people have any direct and consistent experience of the Divine Core, the Self that lies within us all. One has nothing to go on but faith and belief. Most of us in the West have neither the philosophical preparation nor the practical tools to work directly with spirituality.

We would caution some considerable discrimination in dealing with the popular Western literature on spirituality and healing. There is much confusion, and like Humpty Dumpty, people make the word mean what they want it to. It is not to be confused with religion. It is not the emotional agony or the militant advocacy that may accompany the suffering, for example, in cancer or AIDS. Neither is it high values, "isms" or ideologies like secular humanism. Nor is it charity, or benevolent and positive feelings and emotions. It is not the psychic or the paranormal. There is particularly a great deal of misunderstanding about the *kundalini* and its awakening that at times borders on hysteria. It is not complementary medicine or energy healing. It is not altruistic acts (that sometimes can border on poor social work). Nor is it a preoccupation with personal existential issues, or empathy, or new age counseling. It is not visions, or images of goodness and light or many, many other things, which may be all fine and good in themselves, but which have their source in the personality, the ego, the small or "political self" (Alarius, 1988). They are fundamentally of the mind, psychological, perhaps sometimes ABOUT Spirit (and in that sense may try to address the spiritual), but they are not directly OF Spirit.

Yet from another point of view, everything can have a spiritual aspect because everything comes out of life and relationships.

> The highest practice is to search for Truth through one's thoughts, speech, and actions. Entire life is *sadhana* (spiritual practice).
>
> Swami Rama

One might say that what constitutes the spiritual dimension of anything, whether thought, word or action, lies in the intent behind it and the awareness with which it is carried out. Later we will discuss in detail the spiritual nature of action done with the awareness of and flowing from the awakened Centre of Consciousness. As for intentionality, it is everything in behavior at any level. Does one negotiate something with a personal agenda – an expectation, a personal benefit, a personal advantage? This comes from the ego, the "political self" (Alarius, 1988). Or is action done with altruism as selfless service with no agenda, no negotiation and with complete transparency?

The field of transpersonal psychology attempts to deal with this area (Boorstein, 1996; Cortright, 1997; Grof, 2000; Hart et al, 2000; Rothberg et al, 1998; Scotten et al, 1996; Vaughan et al, 1993). But to the perennial wisdom the term "transpersonal psychology" is an oxymoron, for the transcendent is transpersonal or beyond the personality while psychology deals with the psyche as mind and emotions, which are part of the personality.

If we are to study spirituality scientifically in healing or in any context, we must be able to define clearly, what it is we are trying to study. The dictionary does not provide us with definitive help. The entry with related words in the *New Oxford Dictionary* (1993) goes on for two pages of very fine print. On the one hand the word *spirituality* can mean ecclesiastical, referring to the church, the clergy and to things religious, and on the other it can refer to something alcoholic (spirits)! But more germane to this discussion it can refer to:

- The animating or life-giving principle in humans and animals.
- Immaterial substance as opposed to body or matter and specifically the soul. But this meaning becomes clouded by its use to refer to the immaterial intelligent or sentient part of a person as the seat of action and feeling, and confused further when it is used to refer to the mind or the emotions.
- The divine nature or essential power of God as a creative, animating or inspiring influence (e.g., the Holy Spirit).

Under the auspices of McGill University recently, a group of experts in palliative care met to try to develop a shared vocabulary to deal with spirituality and health (Freedman et al, 2002). Consensus proved difficult to obtain. However, they were unanimous in distinguishing spirituality from religion and were critical of a major study by Larson (1997) which fails to recognize this distinction. Religious activities such as churchgoing, for example, are easy to measure and often used as surrogates for spirituality. This is an issue central to the major controversy around defining spirituality in healing today. Indeed in the matter of this issue of spirituality versus religion, some take an extreme view, for example, Ken Wilber on academic religion.

> When I was a youngster, and being the mad scientist type, I used to collect insects. Central to this endeavor was the killing jar. You take an empty mayonnaise jar, put lethal carbon tetrachloride on cotton balls, and place them in the bottom of the jar. You then drop the insect – moth, butterfly, whatnot – into the jar, and it quickly dies, but without being outwardly disfigured. You then mount it, study it, display it. Academic religion is the killing jar of Spirit.
>
> Wilber (1996), p 152

The real issue here, of course, has nothing to do with religion versus spirituality. It has everything to do with the fundamental error of accepting intellectual knowledge as a substitute for the knowing of practical experience. Our spiritual preceptor, the late Sri Swami Rama, always emphasized over and over the importance of practical experience. While acknowledging the usefulness of a good map, the map is never a substitute for the actual journey.

The McGill group offers the following:

Spirit: Spirit, from the Latin *spiritus*, is the term used by some individuals to describe a constituent element of their being that is related to the sacred.

Spirituality: The term spirituality refers to spirit and the human capacity to respond to the sacred in the search for meaning in life.

Sacred: The sacred refers to that which is deemed holy, consecrated, esteemed or special by virtue of an association with ultimate reality, ultimate meaning, or God, however perceived by the individual.

We should interject here that the source of our position comes from Yoga, which we define as the science of spirituality. From this perspective, there is only one spiritual tradition on the planet. But over the millennia of human evolution, it has manifested in many different forms through the numerous spiritual movements and religions which have appeared during humankind's history. The core tradition is like a tree. One tends to see the wide diversity of its branches. When followed historically back they all merge into a common trunk. The science of Yoga in its many expressions provides the roots.

Our training is with the Tradition of the Himalayan Masters or the Shankaracharyan Tradition, acknowledging that the great sage Shankara who founded Vedanta and the Swami orders in India is part of that lineage. Records in the cave monasteries preserved even today in the remote Himalayas document an oral master-disciple tradition whose generations of sages can be traced back 5000 years. Our spiritual preceptor, H.H. Sri Swami Rama, with whom we studied in both North America and India for over 10 years, was a highly skilled adept and Yogi who was trained in the cave monasteries of the Himalayas, and to whom later was passed the full authority and knowledge of the lineage of the Himalayan Masters (Rama, 1978; Boyd, 1976; Tigunait, 1998a, 2002).

Individuals come to the study of a spiritual discipline like Yoga for one of four reasons (Niranjanananda, 1993a): physical, mental-emotional, psychic and spiritual. Most come for physical reasons that range from a search for a cure for a sore back, a stiff neck or worrisome headaches, to gymnastics and sport through to esthetics and physical culture either in the interests of holistic health or the pursuit of the body-beautiful through Hatha Yoga. This physical approach has been humorously referred to as Hollywood Yoga. A smaller group of students come for mental-emotional reasons, seeking relief through meditation and relaxation from stress or solutions to problems with relationships or even neurosis. This has been humorously referred to as Harvard Yoga, referring to Benson's pioneering studies of the relaxation response. A few come for psychic reasons. They are interested in the *chakras* and the *kundalini*. They seek *siddhis* (accomplishments or powers) like clairvoyance or special healing powers and psychic experiences. They confuse the psychic with the spiritual. All of these three stages are appropriate for different degrees of engagement with the spiritual path. However, they are byproducts, which can divert one from the final goal. Finally there are a very few who come for spiritual reasons, who seek to know the Truth that underlies it all. In addition, of those very few there are even fewer who are sincere and committed enough to succeed. It is said that there are Masters aplenty. What are needed are sincere and qualified students.

> Among thousands of human beings only a few endeavor for perfection. Of those endeavoring accomplished ones, only a few know Me in reality.
>
> *Bhagavad Gita* 7.3 (Rama, 1985).

And why is this? Why are there so few real seekers? Here is an answer from a modern sage (Kristof & Houman, 1999).

> Because such is the level of humanity. It is a question of evolution again. In reality to look for the Inner Light, is the desire of very few souls. Most are like children. They still need to play with the toys of phenomenal reality. It's simply their level of evolution. . . . A true seeker simply is, you can say, in heart and in the mind completely devoted to the task of self-discovery. A real seeker is craving the truth and will do everything to complete the Path. A true seeker must have the essential sincerity in the heart and a certain capacity in the mind. In most cases either sincerity or capacity is missing.

However, whatever path one may choose (for example, see Rama, 1982a on Choosing a Path) one should be certain that it is authentic. What is the lineage and what are the qualifications of the teacher? There is an unfortunate tendency in North America to co-opt, alter and water down authentic teachings and then copyright and market them aggressively (humorously referred to as Dot.Com Yoga because of the commercialism). Altering a superb recipe for a cake may mean that the cake does not turn out. Given the prolonged effort that must go into *sadhana* one would want to be sure that the guidance and the methods used are authentic and actually work.

So how then are we to define the object of our study? Let us begin by offering a pragmatic definition given by an Eastern sage. When he began his work in the United States at the Menninger Foundation in Topeka, Kansas, where he was studied by Elmer and Alyce Green as part of their project on voluntary control of involuntary states. Swami Rama based his entire teaching on the interconnectedness of body, breath, mind and soul. "All of the body is in the mind," he would say, "but not all of the mind is in the body." (Tigunait, 1998a). As consciousness, the soul pervades the body and mind. Body, mind and soul – yes – but why breath?

The word "spirit" actually derives from the Latin word *spiritus* which means breath. It soon came to mean also vital power or energy and eventually an intangible element that animates a material thing. The breath plays a key role in linking body and mind, and breath control (*pranayama*) in Yoga constitutes a very important aspect of spiritual training, much less the maintenance of health and longevity.

> Spiritual practices which help us awaken our inner being are called yoga, and those who have access to the deeper dimensions of their being can gain mastery over their body, breath and mind. They alone can enjoy life to the fullest. For such yogis none of their physical, biochemical, biological and psychological functions are involuntary or unconscious, for they have conscious control over every aspect of their being. This is what Swamiji called spiritual science, and according to him the techniques leading to the direct experience of these truths are spiritual practices.
>
> Tigunait (1998a), p 51.

This broader definition of spirituality will give us a practical start in our analysis. Later we shall make use of a more limited definition related to the inner experience of the opening of the Centre of Consciousness or the Inner Teacher (Jerry & Jerry, 2001). For this is the first direct experience of spirit for the student on the path. All else is to talk about spirit, but without the actual personal experience of it.

The reader should note that our purpose here is not to prescribe a "correct" definition of spirituality. Rather we wish to clarify what we mean by it for the sake of the discussion to follow.

> Man is a mixture of three ingredients: first, an animal with all the physical propensities and sense urges that one shares in common with animals; second, the rational, logical human level; and third, the dormant Divinity, the sleeping God within. The whole of the spiritual life is the gradual elimination, eradication, of the animal within, and the refinement or purification and education of the entire human nature so that it stops its movement in all other directions and starts taking on an ascending vertical direction. Once the human nature is given an upward turn, one simultaneously starts awakening the sleeping Divinity with the help of all one's spiritual practices.
>
> Swami Chidananda (1998), p iv

Spirituality, Religion and Health Starting in the late 20th century there has been a huge increase in the medical literature of studies on spirituality and religion in health and their appropriate role in the clinical setting. Prior to this time there is very little literature going back to what may have been the first of such research by Francis Galton in 1872 (Galton, 1874). He found that intercessory prayer did not seem to affect mortality among English royalty, clergy and missionaries.

The current literature is controversial (Garrison, 2005). Advocates refer to a growing literature suggesting that religiosity is linked with improved health, such as reduced all-cause mortality, disability, cancer mortality, the incidence of cardiovascular disease and how medical services are used (Koenig, 2000; Koenig et al, 2000; Post et al, 2000). A recent meta-analysis even suggests that regular religious attendance may be more cost-effective than statin drugs used to lower serum lipids (Hall, 2006)! The study found that weekly attendance at religious services added 2 to 3 life-years compared to 3 to 5 life-years for physical exercise and 2.5 to 3.5 life-years for statin drugs, and at half the cost. As a big part of personal identity, religious activities also influence how patients cope with disease and make decisions about medical treatment. Thus health-care providers should address spiritual concerns (Koenig, 2000; Lo et al, 1999; Cohen et al, 2001) with a spiritual history (Lo et al, 1999), and encouragement to use health-supportive resources from their own religious traditions (Matthews et al, 1998).

Those who criticize the link between spirituality, religion and health point out that studies are methodologically flawed and that the size of the associations between religious practice and improved health are very weak (Sloan et al, 1999). They raise ethical concerns about physicians using religious or spiritual interventions because they do not have theological expertise (Sloan et al, 2000). Indeed, supporting a patient's religious beliefs may do harm by encouraging a belief that illness is a punishment for moral shortcoming or that he or she has created his or her disease, perhaps through adverse *karma*.

Note that the arguments rapidly come down to religion versus spirituality, perhaps because religion can be measured by observable behaviors such as church going, prayer, and reading of religious texts. Spirituality is quietly set aside or subsumed under religion as a synonym. But we have seen that despite their close relationship, they are not synonymous. Indeed some of the writing seems to confuse prayer and "spirituality" with the psychic and paranormal (for example, Dossey, 1997a and b).

In this regard, Gallup polls (2005) have surveyed Americans on the paranormal five times since 1990 and most recently in 2005. 73% of Americans profess at least one of ten paranormal beliefs and 27% profess none. Among these are beliefs in psychic or spiritual healing and in the power of the human mind to heal the body or to create disease. 55% of Americans believe in placebos as examples of the healing powers of the mind. Interestingly, Christians (75%) are slightly more likely to hold some of these beliefs than non-Christians (66%).

It is generally assumed that academics and especially scientists are not religious. This is presumed to reflect the materialist paradigm that underlies science, and modern scientific or evidence-based medicine shares this stance. But a study to be completed in 2006 by Ecklund (2005) from Rice University is showing that more than half of 1600 scientists from 21 elite universities in all disciplines to some degree identify themselves as spiritual, even if not affiliated with a specific religion. Religiosity was measured as attendance at religious services and spirituality was measured by participation in yoga, meditation, reading of scriptures, and prayer. Contrary to previous findings there are now higher rates of religiosity among social scientists (who used to be called the village atheists of the academy), compared to natural scientists, with a resurgence in the study of religion in sociology and in political science. There is a clear distinction between religion and spirituality. The idea of being spiritual as opposed to religious is increasingly popular in the scientific community as it is in American culture in general. Recently geneticist Francis Collins who was director of the Human Genome Project, has written compellingly on the compatibility of science with spirituality and faith (Collins, 2006; Falk & Collins, 2004). As both a scientist and a Christian he found for himself "a richly satisfying harmony between the scientific and spiritual world views." He lectures and writes to persuade others that "belief in God can be an entirely rational choice, and that the principles of faith are, in fact, complementary with the principles of science." (Collins, 2006).

Incorporating spirituality into research is acknowledged as a major challenge. Prescribed and standard research methods used by scientists have no space for spirituality and do not work for investigating spiritual issues. Few have analyzed the relationship between health and religion from a theological perspective, and those who have consider subjecting religious beliefs to standard scientific methodologies which use a quantitative approach like attending religious services, prayer or scriptural reading, to be overly reductionistic (Shuman & Meador, 2003; Ellis, 2002). There is not a common core of faith shared among persons of different religions that can be measured. Religious beliefs and behaviors very much reflect the specific religion involved; religion cannot be studied generically. The concern of most major traditions is with worship and faith rather than with health. Considering worship and prayer as health interventions can lead to major misunderstandings. For example, people use intercessory prayer to petition for divine intervention for a particular outcome or event. Science wants to study it as an intervention like any other therapy. But theists object to labeling prayer as a kind of technology (Chibnall et al, 2001). It requires and expresses faith in a deity. To conceive of it solely for its efficacy as a treatment requires no faith, and so it is not proper prayer (Bishop, 2003).

Taking into account the specific context of a patient's religious practice and faith is also important for the theist. The prevailing view in medicine, for example, in palliative care, counsels physicians to avoid theological discussions about God, sin and suffering, and to encourage patients to pursue their own religious beliefs using multidenominational pastoral care resources in the community as needed. "Ultimately there is little agreement as to whether religious beliefs and practices are fundamentally instruments that can be used in the service of improved health, or instead are ways of being faithful to a specific set of practices and beliefs that will not necessarily provide health in exchange for worship." (Garrison, 2005). The issue is analogous to the use of Yogic practices for spiritual *sadhana*, which is their true intent, versus their use as restorative or therapeutic interventions for health, which are really a byproduct of their primary intent.

The Perennial Philosophy

Based on Spinoza, Huxley (1944) formulated the perennial wisdom, the *Philosophia Perennis*, in three statements, to which we would add a fourth:

1. There is an infinite, changeless Reality beneath the world of change.
2. This same Reality lies at the core of every human personality.
3. The purpose of life is to discover and to experience this Reality: that is, to realize God while here on earth.
4. The interior experiments for realizing this Reality constitute the science of Yoga – an unbroken oral Tradition of continuous Master-Disciple relationships for over 5,000 years. There is only one Tradition, one spiritual science, but it manifests in many forms.

The essence of the perennial wisdom lies in the very causation, nature and cure of suffering in general. Yoga is the science of spirituality. The proper study of spirituality is the practical study of this infinite, changeless, ultimate Reality which is Consciousness. It is this changeless Reality that we refer to as the Centre of Consciousness.

2

The Centre of Consciousness

Mystical Experiences in the General Population

Mystical experiences may occur in up to a third of the general population (Austin, 1999; 2006). A gallop poll (1977–78) showed that 31% of the North American adult population acknowledged sudden or dramatic religious or mystical experiences at some time in their lives. This was shown to be independent of gender, age, occupation, social condition, education or religion. The commonest experience was described as, "An other-worldly kind of union with a Divine Being." There was "the conviction of the forgiveness of sin and salvation."

Greeley (1975) found that 33 to 43% of 1,467 Americans over age 20 reported mystical experience. This was described as, "Being very close to a powerful spiritual force that seemed to lift you outside of yourself."

Abraham Maslow (White, 1972) studied the "core-religious" or "transcendent" experience. He found that more individuals have them than not, so he studied the "non-peakers" who in his opinion suppressed, denied or forgot these experiences.

Hardy (1979) found that 35% of 1,865 individuals surveyed in Great Britain replied "yes" to the question of "ever being aware of or influenced by a presence or power different from everyday selves, whether or not this is referred to as God." Positive responses were greater in the highly educated, up to 56%.

From studies like these one might conclude that up to one third of the population may experience mystical events. While one might argue about the veracity of the Gallup opinion poll, the other studies are serious attempts to answer this question. It is interesting that the mystical experiences did not necessarily occur in church or during meditation. A study by Wilson (1972) found that 31% of experiences occurred spontaneously with no formal religious context. Moreover, 45% of experiences occurred on exposure to the beauties of nature (Greeley, 1975).

A problem arising in these studies is that the language used to code the experience is not universal. Some respondents used religious language, and others used aesthetic language – descriptions based on beauty, to describe their experiences. These distinctions sometimes make comparisons of experiences difficult.

The studies showed that in most cases there were only a few, one or two, episodes of mystical experience lasting minutes and rarely longer than an hour. For most individuals the experience appeared not to enrich their lives. It caused no change in their religious orientation or their interpersonal relationships. Personal transformation was seen usually only with peak episodes. Only 1–4% of individuals were transformed by their experience. This is a surprising and puzzling observation. These experiences open the question of spiritual emergence and spiritual emergency, as well as the distinction between mystical experience and psychopathology (Nelson, 1994a; Grof & Grof, 1989).

We mention these general mystical experiences by way of contrast with the experience of the Centre of Consciousness. When we talk about the Centre of Consciousness, we are not referring to these mystical experiences described in the general population. In contrast, the experience of the Centre of Consciousness is unique, very subtle, and is stable and deeply transformative.

The Role of the *Guru*

The role of the sage in the Himalayan Tradition of Yoga is to awaken within the student the divine flame, that spark of divinity that all human beings carry within them, which the late H. H. Sri Swami Rama called the Teacher within, or the Centre of Consciousness. He described his mission thus: "I am a messenger, delivering the wisdom of the Himalayan sages of my tradition. My job is to introduce you to the Teacher within." In the Himalayan Tradition, a master is one who can give the higher spiritual initiations of *shaktipata*. It is through this descent of Divine Grace that the divinity within is awakened in the form of the *kundalini*.

Students confuse the role of the external *guru* with the Teacher within. They may ask, sometimes with great angst, whether they need an external *guru* or whether they can depend alone on the Inner Teacher. Such a question betrays a fundamental misunderstanding about the two. In reality at the level of inner consciousness, the two are identical. The *guru* is a physical manifestation of the Inner Teacher which manifests in the life of the student when that student is prepared and ready. It represents the response of divine grace to the effort of the student. When the student is ready, the master will appear. The student will not be able to avoid the encounter. But if the student is not ready, he or she can search the planet and not find the *guru*.

There are many stories of how students found their way to Swami Rama. If they were to meet him, they could not avoid him, even if it meant finding themselves standing next to him in the lineup at the bank, or literally bumping into him in the crowd in an airport waiting room. And there are other stories of those who were not meant to meet him and simply could not arrange a meeting no matter how hard they tried. The idea is not to search endlessly for a *guru* in the external world as though one were buying an automobile or a house, comparing the merits and deficiencies of each candidate in turn. Rather one should work diligently with oneself to make oneself qualified (*adhikara*) in order to invoke the Divine Grace of a *guru* who will appear at the right moment.

The Centre of Consciousness

Many terms are used in the literature to refer to the Centre of Consciousness. We summarize a few of them in the table below. The list is by no means exhaustive or complete and not all commentators use the terms the same way, which adds to the confusion. Some even use the terms Self or *Atman* in this context. Other terms are used in modern and New Age writings such as Source, Source Energy, Unified Field, All-That-Is, Center, Stillpoint, Silence, Core, Love, Ground of Being, and so on.

This collection of terms should not be considered a list of synonyms. Rather one should think of them as referring to the same "ball park" in this discussion. In everyday life, each of us carries out many functions. In the course of a day one plays many roles: professional, businessperson, parent, teacher, lover, etc. Each role may require different behaviors and different attire. The demands of each role may be so different that it may be difficult to recognize that the same person is playing these different roles. Consider the list of terms in this tabulation in the same way. Consciousness plays many roles and functions in manifestation and each of these terms tries to describe that fundamental unity of Consciousness as it manifests in different ways.

Vasudeva principle	The Indweller
Holy Ghost/Spirit (Christianity)	*Antaryamin*
(Some use the term Christ Consciousness)	Presence
The Voice for God (Course in Miracles)	Awareness
Hiranyagarbha (The Golden Womb)	*Ishvara*
The Inner Teacher	Universal Intelligence
The Inner *Guru*	The *Guru* Spirit
The Teaching Spirit of the Universe	One Becoming Many
That Which Sanctifies	*Sambhogakaya* (Buddhism)
Sutratma, Sutratma Prana	*Sakshi* – The Witness
Drashta – The Seer	

Swami Veda Bharati in his book, *God*, compares the terms referring to the Trinity in different traditions as follows (1979a, p 102):

Yoga-Vedanta	Buddhism	Christianity
Brahman	*Dharmakaya*	*God, the Father, Logos, the transcendent reality.*
Hiranyagarbha or Ishvara	*Sambhogakaya*	*Holy Ghost, the teaching spirit in the universe.*
Avatara	*Nirmanakaya*	*Son, God in history.*

What we refer to as the Centre of Consciousness here is *Hiranyagarbha* or *Ishvara* in Yoga-Vedanta or the Holy Ghost in the Christian tradition (Paramahamsa Yogananda uses the term Christ Consciousness). We use the term Centre of Consciousness because our preceptor Swami Rama used it to describe that core of the personality from which consciousness flows in various degrees and grades (referring to the sequence of *turiya*, deep sleep, dreaming and wakefulness as described in the *Mandukya Upanishad*).

Both Yogananda and Swami Rama also referred to It as the conscience. Yogananda (2004, Vol. I, p 283) describes It this way:

> Absolute standards cannot always be applied in this relative world. To adhere to truth in everyday living, man must be guided by intuitive wisdom; that alone illumines unerringly what is right and virtuous in every circumstance. The voice of conscience is the voice of God. Everyone has it, but not everyone listens to it. Those who have a trained sensitivity can detect wrong by the inner disturbance of uneasiness it engenders. Virtue is known by the vibration of harmony it creates within. Always the light of God is there, guiding through discriminative wisdom and through calm feeling. If one does not disturb feeling by emotion or discriminative intelligence by rationalized wrong behavior, he will be guided by that inner voice. To follow the light of inner wisdom-guidance is the way to true happiness, the way to be always of God, the way to disengage oneself from the coercive influence of bad habits that usurp man's decision-making power.

In Yoga-Vedanta God is understood on three levels of reality as a *Brahman-Ishvara-Avatara* triad. At the first level *Brahman* is the absolute, transpersonal and transcendental being, the One Principle, the Transcendental Reality or the Expansive One, the ultimate Reality or ground of the universe. The word derives from the Sanskrit verb root *brah* "to expand, to be expansive." (Veda Bharati, 1986). In the *Upanishads* it is presented on two levels: the Reality of which the universe is only an appearance, and as the all-inclusive ground of the universe. In Advaita Vedanta these two forms are *nirguna brahman* which is free from all limiting conditions, and *saguna brahman* which is *brahman* with qualifications or limiting conditions of the distinctions of name and form. The former is described negatively as "not this, not this" (*neti, neti*), and the latter positively as existence or being (*sat*), knowledge in the sense of awareness and consciousness (*cit*), and plenitude or bliss (*ananda*) absolute, which is also infinite (*ananta*) (Grimes, 1989).

The second level is *Hiranyagarbha* or the golden womb, God as the immanent spirit of the universe or as *Ishvara* the Lord or Personal God. This is what we refer to as the Centre of Consciousness. As *Hiranyagarbha* it is the first *guru*, the universal Presence, the first wise one known as the teaching spirit of the universe. *Hiranyagarbha*, whose grace is the source of the flow of all revelation, is the original teacher of Yoga. It is said that the first human being was an incarnation of the Golden Womb (Veda Bharati, 1986). The term also refers to *Prajapati*, the Progenitor, who is also *Brahma*, the creator who takes the universe as His body (Veda Bharati, 1986).

"*Hiranyagarbha* alone is the teacher of Yoga, and no other."

Brhad-yogi-yajnavalkya-smrti XII.5

The alternative conceptual term at this second level, *Ishvara*, refers to the personal Lord or God or *parama-atman*. It is the Divine with form (*saguna brahman*), possessing the qualities of knowledge, strength, lordship, potency, virility and splendour. In Advaita Vedanta, *Ishvara* is *brahman* as conditioned by *maya*, God immanent, and is the material and efficient cause of the universe. He is existence (*sat*), knowledge or consciousness (*cit*) and bliss (*ananda*) absolute. These are not His qualities or properties, rather He is these things. He is said to be omnipotent, omniscient, omnipresent, eternal, the creator, etc. (Veda Bharati, 1986; Grimes 1989). We will have much more to say about *Ishvara* later when we discuss *Ishvara pranidhana* in *pada* I of Patanjali's *Yoga-Sutra*. Relative to the Centre of Consciousness a related term is *antaryamin* which is the indweller, the dweller within, the inner guide or inner ruler pervading within all things and beings. It also refers to the immanent form of God, the cosmic form of the Self as associated with *maya*.

The third level in Yoga-Vedanta is *avatara*, an incarnation of the deity, the incarnate being manifest in history such as Krishna or Jesus.

In Christianity the analogous Trinity is God the Father, God the Holy Ghost/Spirit and God the Son. The Holy Ghost is the Teaching Spirit in the universe.

But the Comforter, which is the Holy Ghost, Whom the Father will send in my name,
He shall teach you all things, and bring all things to your remembrance.

John 14:26

In Buddhism *shunya*, the void, is the basic definition of ultimate reality. It exists on two levels as supreme, transcendental truth, and as a veiled, relative truth as seen in the universe (Veda Bharati, 1979a). The corresponding Buddhist triad consists of *dharmakaya* (transcendental, transpersonal being analogous to *brahman*), *sambhogakaya* (the universal spirit immanent in the universe) and *nirmanakaya* (the Buddhas who incarnate into history).

The idea of Centre can also be found in Kashmir Shaivism. Singh (1987, p 41) uses the term centre (*madhya*) in his translation of *sutra* 17 of the Pratyabhijnahridayam: "By the development of the centre [*madhya*] is acquisition of the bliss of the spirit [*cit*]." He then goes on to summarize the essence of the *sutra* in this way.

"By the development of the centre can the bliss of the spirit be obtained. *Samvit* [universal or supreme consciousness] or the power of consciousness is called the centre, because it is the support or ground of every thing in the world. [One is reminded of Paul Tillich's Ground of Being.] In the individual, it is symbolized by the central *nadi*, i.e., *sushumna*. When the central consciousness in man develops or when the *sushumna nadi* develops, then is there the bliss of the universal consciousness."

Thus the universal consciousness is the innermost reality and ground of every possible thing which emerges from it. At the stage of individual embodiment it exists principally as the *madhyama-nadi* (or central *nadi, sushumna nadi* or *brahma-nadi*) which has as its substrate Brahman in the form of *prana-shakti* (Singh, 1987, p 93). When that central consciousness develops one is liberated while alive.

As one thinks of the Centre of Consciousness using the word Presence, one is brought to the Vedantic term, *turiya* (also spelled *turya*). Singh (1987, p 137) notes that in Sanskrit (*Samskrita*) the word "*catur*" means "four." When the suffix *iyat* is added to "*catur*" both the "*ca*" and the "*t*" of *iyat* are dropped to give *tur+iya* or *turiya* which means "fourth." In the *Mandukya Upanishad* the sage Gaudapada in *sutra* 2 of the first chapter (*prakarana*) called the *Agama* (scripture) says: "All this is verily Brahman. This *Atman* is Brahman. This *Atman* has four quarters." (Nikhilananda, 1987b, p 11).

The *Upanishad* discusses the problem of Ultimate Reality, and states that knowledge of *Brahman* or *Atman* is the goal of existence. *Atman* is associated with the three states (*avastha*) of experience or consciousness of waking, dreaming and deep sleep, and these states merge in *turiya*, the Ultimate Reality. The non-dual *Atman* is identical with the three states and therefore all that exists is *Brahman*.

This *Atman*, signified by the *pranava, Aum*, which is both the higher and lower *Brahman*, has four quarters (*padas*). They are *vishva* or *vaishvanara* (the waking state or *jagrat*), *taijasa* (the dream state or *svapna*), *prajna* (the state of dreamless sleep or *sushupti*), and *turiya* which is the same as *Brahman* or *Atman*. The first three are parts and the fourth is the whole. *Turyatita* is beyond *turiya*. The states of waking, dreaming and deep sleep are exclusive. While you are in one of these states you have no experience of the other two. The first three quarters correspond in order to the three *matras* (letters) A, U and M of *Aum* (Om), while the fourth known as *amatra* (without a letter or corresponding sound) represents the Silence or *Atman* the Self corresponding to *turiya*. The sound (manifestation of the three states) proceeds from the Silence. Om is the sound-symbol for the Ultimate Reality. This is the *chatushpad* (four foot or part) doctrine which has roots in the early *Upanishads* and was later developed at length in the Advaita Vedanta school by Gaudapada and Shankara.

Turiya, then, is the fourth, the transcendental Self, the Supreme Reality, the real Self beyond changing existence. It is the ultimate non-dual awareness and reality, *Brahman* or *Atman*. In Advaita Vedanta it is the fourth state of consciousness. But it is not really a state, rather it is the underlying undifferentiated substrate of and beyond the three conditioned states of consciousness – waking, dreaming and deep sleep, which are different aspects of it, conditioning superimposed on it. It is the witness of the other three states. But *turiya* is a relative term; it is called *turiya* or fourth in relation to the other three states. It is an ever present witnessing consciousness of the other three states. It is pure consciousness (*cit*), unqualified, self-luminous, pervasive and unchanging. It is integral awareness. It is "indivisible, ungraspable, unthinkable, and unnameable. . . . It is *amatra* or modeless." (Grimes, 1989, p 369). While the other three states are named, the Absolute is referred to only as the fourth. The term is also used for the highest meditative stage. In Advaita "consciousness designates the unconditioned basis of awareness or mental activity (sensing, feeling, thinking, etc.). It is the animating substratum or source of the contents of an individual mind. This substratum/source of unity and continuity among the changing states is what Advaitas call *turiya*." (Fort, 1990, p 9).

The ego which is limited by the body, *prana* and the mind (*manas*) has no experience of *turiya* even though it is always present in the background of the other three states. But when primal ignorance (*avidya*) is removed, only then can one experience *turiya* consciousness. It is an experience of the essence of one's consciousness when present limitations are transcended. In the microcosm it is a fourth state of consciousness that holds together the experiences of waking, dreaming and deep sleep, running through them all like the string through the flowers of a garland, and from which they emanate and withdraw. But it is other than the three states and hence is called the fourth. In the macrocosm it is a fourth state that holds together the three divine actions (*krityas*) of creation (*srishti*), maintenance (*sthiti*) and withdrawal (*samhara*).

3

Experiencing the Centre of Consciousness

The Locus of the Centre: The Personality in Vedanta

To understand the locus of the Centre of Consciousness one needs to ask what is meant by the personality in the perennial wisdom. Figure 3.1 shows the personality according to Vedanta (Rama et al, 1976). The core is the Centre of Consciousness called the Self. It is enrobed in five sheaths (called *koshas*): three for mind, one for the subtle energy body and the outermost one for the physical body. Now clearly people are not onions in cross-section! Rather, this diagram is symbolic of interpenetrating energy fields of higher and higher vibrational frequency which are suffused with consciousness emanating from that core (Venkatesananda, 1993).

Swami Rama referred to this model as body, breath, mind and soul or spirit. It is the central core that we refer to as the Centre of Consciousness.

We have presented this as a two-dimensional model, a cross section that resembles a target. It would be a little more accurate to conceptualize it as a sphere of manifestation composed of a set of five concentric shells of progressively higher energy levels emanating out into manifestation from a *bindu* (an infinite point) as the Centre of Consciousness. By analogy with the "big bang" theory of the creation of the universe one might imagine it as a miniuniverse, an individual universe that manifests from that central point and then evolves through the stages of the human life span. Meditation is the journey in reverse which eventually bursts through the *bindu* and explodes into the infinite space of Consciousness. From this infinite point the metaphoric "light" of consciousness radiates outwards in all directions to "illumine" the sheaths or shells with consciousness. Although often presented as distinct shells, their boundaries form more of a continuum of vibratory energy ranging from gross to subtle, like regions in a vibratory spectrum analogous to those of the physical electromagnetic spectrum. In the physical body the energy frequencies are slow enough to "condense" as matter which can be conceptualized as standing waves. But rather than layers, these shells occupy, pervade and interpenetrate the space of the personality simultaneously just like all television channels or radio stations are everywhere present simultaneously in a room at different interpenetrating vibrational levels.

Thus the personality or microcosm (the individual person; and the macrocosm or cosmic person as well) in the Tantric view consists of energy (the *shakti* principle) and consciousness (the *shiva* principle). The microcosm within the macrocosm is a holographic concept. Master the forces of the individual, say the sages, and you also gain mastery of the corresponding cosmic forces. Manifested reality (the universe) is consciousness (*shiva, purusha*) enrobed in layers of energy (*shakti, maya, prakriti*), with the layers in a vibrational spectrum from mind to matter (body). The experience of physical matter is a construction of the five senses. In modern physics it is likened to "frozen energy" or standing waves. These five *koshas* or sheaths constitute the personality, a broader definition than is used in Western psychology.

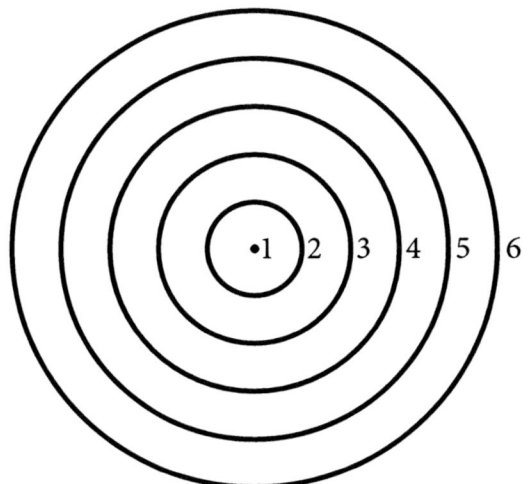

1. SELF
2. *anandamayakosha*
   (Blissful Sheath)
3. *vijnanamayakosha*
   (Intellectual or Intuitive Sheath; Buddhi)
4. *manomayakosha*
   (Mental Sheath)
5. *pranamayakosha*
   (Subtle Energy Sheath)
6. *annamayakosha*
   (Food Sheath; Physical Body)

Figure 3.1 The personality according to Vedanta. (Adapted from Rama et al, 1976)

Consciousness is primary. The Self at the core or centre of this personality is pure Consciousness. Spirit and Consciousness are the same. Ultimate Reality is Consciousness. It is for this reason that the ancient wisdom considers that the proper study of spirituality addresses this Centre of Consciousness or central core. Consciousness pervades the personality like space pervades a room, holding its contents as manifestations within it. One might imagine Consciousness to be like a space of awareness (*shiva*) within which energy in its potential form (*shakti*) manifests or precipitates like clouds from the invisible water vapor in the sky. To continue the metaphor, one's true nature is the aware space of the infinite sky, not the cloud. But Consciousness in Its omnipotence can identify Itself with the cloud and experience being the cloud. Then the individual ego is born with all of its boundaries. An even better conception of this diagram is to imagine it turned inside out. Imagine consciousness as the white of the page supporting and pervading all and holding the personality like a cloud in the sky which condenses down to the physical body in the centre with the layers in reverse order.

Singh (1987, p 118) points out that the word *Shiva* comes from two Sanskrit roots: √*shi* (to lie) and √*shvi* (to cut asunder). *Shiva* incorporates both meanings. He is the One in whom all objects and subjects lie and also the One who cuts asunder all sins. As the fundamental ground of all reality He is the Supreme, the Absolute, the Highest Reality. Also He is the supreme Benevolence and Highest Good Whose grace saves all. *Shakti* is the energy of *Shiva* which is not different from Him. They are like the two sides of one coin. Through *Shakti* He brings about cosmic manifestation and processes. The higher initiation of *shaktipata* is the descent of *Shakti*, the imparting of grace (*anugraha*) to an individual to bring about liberation. Thus in His creative function *Shiva* does not create the universe out of something else, some other "stuff" as a sculptor would make a pot out of clay as an object separate from himself. Rather the universe lies within *Shiva* as a potential which emanates from Him and yet lies within Him. The universe and *Shiva* are in essence one. Our everyday experience of the universe as separate is *maya*.

The Self or spirit is pure Consciousness.
• Ultimate Reality is Consciousness.
• The study of spirituality means the study of Consciousness.

The spiritual genius Shankara in the ninth century C.E. wrote:

> There is a self-existent reality which is . . . the witness of the three states of consciousness (waking, dreaming and deep sleep), and is distinct from the five bodily coverings (sheaths or subtle planes) . . . It is aware of the presence or absence of the mind and its functions. It is the Atman.
>
> That reality sees everything in its own light. No one sees it. It gives intelligence to the mind and the intellect, but no one gives it light.
>
> That Reality pervades the universe, but no one penetrates it. It alone shines. The universe shines with its reflected light.

> Purusha is the shining,
> yet formless cosmic spirit,
> the Self of the Universe.
> He is within everything,
> and without everything,
> unborn,
> untainted by either breath or mind.
> He is beyond even the tendency to take form.
>
> *Mundaka Upanishad*

For most of us there is little or no awareness of these *koshas* or energy shells that make up the personality. Our consciousness is identified at the extreme of manifestation, on the external surface of this sphere which is the physical body and waking consciousness. This *annamayakosha* occupies about 75 percent of our consciousness in daily life at our present stage of evolution (Niranjanananda, 1993a). The body is the focal point of our attention, experience and identity. It is like a kind of two-dimensional existence on the surface of a sphere. Sri Aurobindo called it "frontal man."

Later we will distinguish between awareness and consciousness. As awareness awakens and expands with spiritual practices, one begins to sense a kind of third dimension, a sense of depth in towards the centre of that set of spheres. For most of us the *manomaya* (mental sheath) experience occupies about 20 percent of our consciousness, and of the remaining five percent, perhaps two percent is a dim awareness of the *pranamayakosha* with its subtle energies.

It should be clearly understood that from the perspective of the perennial wisdom the new disciplines of energy psychology and energy medicine, which we will introduce later, operate at the *pranamayakosha* (which includes emotional) and *manomayakosha* (mental) levels of the personality. With regard to the latter, in Yoga the mind is also considered to be a very subtle energy field, so subtle, that at its highest and most refined levels (called the *buddhi*) it can reflect the subtleties of Spirit directly.

The contents of that mental field are called *vrittis* (operations, activities, fluctuations, modifications, thoughts). Yoga is the control of these modifications of the mind field (*Yoga-Sutra* I.2 (Aranya, 1981)). When this is accomplished then the seer (the spiritual self) rests in its own true nature (*Yoga-Sutra* I.3 (Aranya, 1981)). Thus because of the fundamental importance of their control the *vrittis* are discussed in some detail in *sutras* 5 through 12 of the first chapter of the *Yoga-Sutra*. Their conception is much greater than just thoughts and emotions and include the full range of modifications of the mental field including memory, dreams and even sleep (the thought of no-thing). A negative thought or emotion is conceived to be like a turbulence in the mind field, a small whirlpool of turbulent flow in contrast to the streamlined flow of a balanced and harmonious field. Thus the concept in modern energy psychology and energy medicine of a negative thought or emotion as a perturbation of the body's subtle energy fields is quite consistent with the ancient wisdom.

Awakening is the gradual extension and expansion of awareness deeper and deeper, layer by layer through these energy shells of the personality towards the Centre of Consciousness until all of it becomes aware. Then the waking, dream and deep sleep states are experienced equally from *turiya*, the fourth state which lies beyond manifestation. In this model the *annamayakosha* is the physical body (the conscious) and the *anandamayakosha* the causal body (the unconscious). The intervening three layers make up the subtle body and the realm of the subconscious. As the awareness extends deep into the subtle personality and its layers, mind-body control awakens with mastery of the autonomic functions and related processes in the psychoneuroimmune system. The progression from *bindu* to the surface of the personality is the journey of consciousness identifying outwards into manifestation (involution) as a separate self. The reverse movement from surface back to *bindu* is consciousness detaching and withdrawing itself from manifestation (evolution) back to the universal Self – all in an endless cycle of creation and dissolution. The same applies to the macrocosm. This manifestation process is described in great detail in the ancient texts of Samkhya and Tantra as a series of progressively unfolding evolutes.

An Experiential Definition of the Centre of Consciousness

In the highest state of yogic accomplishment, you are fully at peace. You are perfectly established in supreme consciousness. The experience of equanimity you gain at this stage cannot be compared with anything. It is indescribable. The experience of bliss is not outside you; it is inside you and it is you. There is no sense of duality in this state. You are in the world and the world is in you. You are in God and God is in you. You have transcended your mind and the realm of consciousness that is limited by time, space, and causation. There is no distinction between the past, present, and future. The world known by the senses and the world beyond the reach of the senses are fully integrated in this spiritually illumined consciousness. Upon reaching this state, you have not only known the meaning of life, but you also have found it. All your desires and cravings have been fulfilled, for you have found your eternal friend, your inner soul, and thus you are no longer lonely. Freedom from loneliness allows the descent of such a powerful peace and joy that you long for nothing anymore. This is called attaining perfection and attaining immortality. Upon experiencing this level of joy, you begin to see the whole world filled with indescribable beauty and joy. Regardless of whether you are young or old, man or woman, you find yourself beautiful. This experience of being a beautiful person is so real and fulfilling that you do not need others to admire your beauty. Rather, you find yourself brimming with the joy that your inner beauty is beyond all admiration.

Rama, 2005, p 26–27

The metaphor of a journey is used to describe the spiritual path. For any successful journey one needs a map and a method for taking the journey: in this case, *theoria* and *praxis* – theory and practice. We spend a great deal of time worrying about whether a map is real. The issue is not whether a map is real, but rather whether it is useful. For many years in physics, we envisaged the Bohr model of the atom as a small solar system, with electrons circulating around a central nucleus like planets whirling around a central sun. The issue was not whether this was truth or reality, but whether this was a model that allowed one to do useful calculations and predictions. Its value was in its utility, rather than its truth. For all theories are at best increasingly refined and approximate representations or maps of our understanding of reality. Korzybski (1980) in his General Semantics theory pointed out that the map is not the territory. Its value lies in its isomorphism, its one-to-one correspondence to the territory that it represents. A paper map is obviously not the reality of the city of Vancouver. However, it has a one-to-one correspondence to the city itself that allows one to recognize that one is in Vancouver and to be able to navigate around the city accurately.

The spiritual journey is no different. One needs methods and practices to undertake the journey. However, one also needs maps that allow one to recognize the signposts on the way and not get lost. There are various maps of the spiritual journey and of higher states of Consciousness. In our experience, theologians and philosophers have formulated most of these. They are very useful in the academic world, but they are often not very helpful to the practitioner who is undertaking the journey. For this, one needs experiential maps rather than theoretical or philosophical formulations. Experiential maps can only come from the teachings of realized sages who themselves have made the journey.

For any tradition, what are the signposts on the way? By what experiences would the practitioner recognize them? The core question is, if you had an experience of Spirit or God, would you recognize it? There are many stories of aspirants who have had these experiences and have not recognized their significance (Tweedie, 1986). Alternatively, they have had doubts about what these experiences actually represent, for in the beginning, they can be very subtle. This is one situation where the availability of a *sadguru*, a true master, is indispensable. Certainly, in our case H.H. Sri Swami Rama was able to clarify and verify the authenticity of our own inner experiences with him. It should also be noted that if one has the wrong map, one can miss or misunderstand the experience when one meets it. A faulty map can prevent one from recognizing what one is looking for. Therefore, as we study the writings of the enlightened sages in the context of our own experiences we are constantly building and refining an experiential map of the journey.

A master decided to test his five disciples. He gave each a small object and told them to hide it in secret so it could not be found. Some hours later one disciple returned full of confidence and related to the master how he had gone into the forest and found a hiding place that no one would ever find. "You have done what was asked," said the master. The next disciple arrived back extolling the virtues of her hiding place in the desert where no one would even think to look. "You have done what was asked," observed the master. And so it was with the next two disciples when they also returned. But after many hours the fifth disciple did not return and the group started to worry. As darkness began to fall the group organized themselves to begin a search. But just then the fifth disciple appeared, shuffling through the door, eyes downcast, and the picture of dejection. He slowly approached the master, fell to his knees and gave his object back. "What!" exclaimed the Master, "Have you disobeyed me?" "Sir," replied the dejected disciple, "I searched everywhere but I could not find a hiding place that was secret where I was not observed. I tried the forest, I tried the desert, by the river, in the pasture, on the hill, but wherever I went I felt I was being watched. Sir, I have failed." "Not at all," replied the Master gently with a smile. "You are the only one who has passed the test!"

A Story from the Yoga Tradition

Philosophical discussions of the Centre of Consciousness are of less interest to us than direct experiential descriptions. In our *Sutras of the Inner Teacher* (Jerry & Jerry, 2001) we have presented our own concise experiential description of the Presence in *sutra* 36.

"36. The Centre of Consciousness is a still, but effulgent, Conscious Presence, Silence or 'Thatness.' It is a Void or Emptiness that paradoxically is also a Plenum or Fullness. It pervades all of inner space and holds all manifestation, all inner mental content within Itself like space pervades and holds the contents of a room, and yet is unaffected by them."

The description of a conscious space is commonly used as one way to describe the Witnessing Presence.

"37. Space is Self and Self is Space. In inner space the wise find the Intelligence of pure Consciousness, and ultimate Truth in the effulgent Void."

Jerry & Jerry, 2001, p 84

"Is there a difference between pure consciousness and utter void? . . . I am the pure space of Consciousness. . . . It is as if void is the ultimate truth!"

Yoga Vasishtha VI.2:29 (Venkatesananda, 1993)

"Absolute Consciousness and space resemble each other in being perfect, infinite, subtle, pure, unbounded, formless, imminent in all, yet undefiled within and without. . . . In fact, the conscious Self is space. . . . Space is Self; and Self is space. . . . The wise . . . find in space the Self, the Abstract Intelligence."

Tripura Rahasya, XVIII:72–79 (Sri Ramanananda Saraswathi, 1980)

Paramahansa Yogananda (2004, Vol. 2, p 970) spoke of the Eternal Presence as the Eternal Now. "In Spirit there is no past or future, only the everlasting Present. It is in the relativistic consciousness of persons under the influence of *maya* that Eternity appears separated into past, present, and future. God always is, and His immortal omniscience is not compartmentalized by the dimensional delusions of time and space; He beholds everything as happening in the infinitude of His Being *now*."

If one could imagine an infinite volume of Conscious space representing *Brahman* as God transcendent, and then a galaxy "precipitating" or condensing in place like a cloud floating in the space of the sky, then that part of the space permeating that galaxy would be called *Ishvara*. It is one with the whole space and yet is the foundation and source of the galaxy. It is and is not, its "existence" a linguistic distinction. From the viewpoint of the galaxy there is a God immanent. From the viewpoint of the whole there is just the Unity with the galaxy floating within it. If a second galaxy were to appear in the whole space, that pervading part of the space of the One Consciousness would also be called an *Ishvara*. Thus some formulations of Vedanta allow for the possibility of an infinite number of *Ishvaras*, one for each of an infinite number of galaxies.

In Vedic language one speaks of a *Brahmanda* (Cosmic Egg or Egg of *Brahma*), and in the texts these variously denote solar systems or perhaps larger astronomical bodies like a galaxy (Nikhilananda, 1977a, b, p 71). The name derives from its oval, elliptical shape like an egg. The *rishis* (Seers) say there are innumerable *Brahmandas* continually appearing and disappearing, and each has its own Lord, its Governor or Controller who is a manifestation in *maya* of the Absolute, *Brahman*.

Each Lord or *Ishvara* has three functions described by the aspects of creator (*Brahma*), preserver (*Vishnu*) and destroyer (*Shiva*). And under these there are many subsidiary deities (i.e., conscious forces) to carry out the many other lesser functions and duties within the *Brahmanda*. Deities can be thought of as personified or conscious forces. But the Puranas say that the *Brahmandas* are uncountable and so too the *Ishvaras*, *Brahmas*, *Vishnus* and *Shivas* are without number. The Lord of all these countless deities is called *Maheshvara*, the Supreme lord, which is *Saguna Brahman*. While the deities are innumerable, *Maheshvara* is one without a second. Each *Ishvara* is the Lord of one *Brahmanda* alone, whatever one conceives that to be from solar system up to galaxy. But *Maheshvara* is the Lord of all *Ishvaras* and *Brahmandas*. The texts say that the Supreme *Brahman* accepts the limitation of *maya* and becomes *Maheshvara* who is the first person in the creation. *Ishvara*, *Hiranyagarbha* or *Brahma* is the ruler of a *Brahmanda* and is the Second Person. The

Godhead dwelling in every heart as the *Antaryamin* or Inner Teacher is the Third Person in the creation, and thus another formulation of the concept of the trinity (Nikhilananda, 1977a, b, p 75). The *Upanishads* do not teach many Gods or ultimate realities. In the *Upanishads*, *Brahman* is one without a second. Understanding this as a multiplicity of functions of a Unity along with the spatial metaphor offered here can make sense of this apparent paradox.

Take another similar metaphor more suitable for the *jiva* or individual soul. Immerse an empty bottle under the surface of the ocean and allow it to fill completely with the water. Is the water inside the bottle separate from the ocean? No, because the mouth of the bottle is open. Now screw on the lid. Is the water inside the bottle now separate from the ocean? Yes and no! It depends on your perspective. It could be called separate as a linguistic distinction. Again remove the lid from the bottle. The water inside is no longer separate. One could use the same metaphor for the air inside a clay pot with or without a lid. Hence the question: Are there many souls or just one Atman? Some formulations of the perennial wisdom support one interpretation and some support the other. Does the divine fire issue sparks or is there just one fire? Souls would not be the fire itself, but would share its essential fieriness. Again the spatial metaphor can help one to think about this issue and to resolve the apparent paradox.

There is a trap that the aspirant must be very wary of. One reviews the descriptions of the experience of the Centre and notes words like "space, peace, stillness, bliss," etc. Then one uses one's imagination to construct a similar internal experience in the mind. One practices with that constructed internal representation as the object and confuses it with the real experience. One is led far astray. The experience of the Centre is qualitatively unique. It can not be imagined even though paradoxically these words are exact descriptions of the experience. It reveals Itself as a Presence behind the mind from which It is clearly distinguishable. If It is concealed, that experience cannot be recreated from memory or with the imagination with anything like the vividness or qualities of the actual experience. Either It is present and perceptable or It is not. Patanjali's *Yoga-Sutra* repeatedly emphasizes the importance of developing *viveka*, the ability to discriminate between *pursuha* and manifestations of *prakriti*, especially the *sattva guna* (pure and luminous quality) of the mind field. An imagined construct is part of the mind; the Centre transcends the mind.

Another useful metaphor that one sees frequently is that of a still centre or stillpoint in the midst of the storm of everyday life. Most frequently it is in terms of the eye of a storm. Swami Rama used the still centre of a wheel versus the movement of the rim as a similar metaphor. Paul Brunton (1935, p 109) refers to the centre of a whirlwind.

> Strangely enough, you find that, in the very centre of the whirlwind, there is a place perfectly calm and untouched. So, too, the man who knows himself attains mental equilibrium and remains unmoved amid the feverish activity of the world. His inmost being is in peaceful undisturbed repose, whatever whirlwind of life swirls around him, whatever work he is doing and whatever thoughts engage his intellect.

He also uses the model of the atom. "The electron theory of modern science provides us with an apt analogy for the Overself. . . . The point of Absolute Rest round which the electrons revolve may be likened to the true self, and the electrons to its appurtenances, intellect, emotions, body." (Brunton, 1935, p 88).

One easily accepts these images as apt metaphors and moves on. Yet surprisingly this metaphor of the Centre can be an exact description of the early experience of the Centre of Consciousness in its expression as Being. Its manifestation may be sensed in no-time and no-space in the centre of the torso or the region of the heart *chakra* as an energetic focus or stillpoint at the core of one's personality, and from which that personality is energized.

We join spokes together in a wheel, but it is the center hole that makes the wagon move.
We shape clay into a pot, but it is the emptiness inside that holds whatever we want.
We hammer wood for a house, but it is the inner space that makes it liveable.
We work with being, but non-being is what we use.

Throw away holiness and wisdom, and people will be a hundred times happier.
Throw away morality and justice, and people will do the right thing.
Throw away industry and profit, and there won't be any thieves.
If these three aren't enough, just stay at the center of the circle and let all things take
      their course.

Tao Te Ching
(Mitchell, 1988, chapters 11 and 19)

4

Contemporary Maps of Awakening

In the perennial wisdom the traditional map of transcendent states of consciousness (*samadhi*) comes from the first chapter (*samadhi pada*) of Patanjali's *Yoga-Sutra*. It is a complex and subtle typology which is discussed in detail elsewhere to which we refer the reader (Veda Bharati, 1986; Whicher, 1998). Its major thrust is that enlightenment or Self-Realization is not a simple awakening, a grand "Aha!" This is a frequent misunderstanding in the West with our penchant for instant results for everything. A student may be given a *mantra* and taught to use it for meditation, only to return to the teacher six months later asking, "What's wrong with it, because I haven't gotten my enlightenment yet!"

The maps for the absorption of *samadhi* in the *Yoga-Sutra* show a gradual state-by-state unfoldment of Self-Realization that passes through several levels of transcendent subject-object consciousness (consciousness-with-an-object) – to use Merrell-Wolff's terminology – called *sabija* (*samadhi* with seed) or *samprajnata samadhi*. It ends with the appreciation of pure Consciousness as consciousness-without-an-object, called *nirbija* (*samadhi* without seed) or *asamprajnata samadhi*.

An example of the contemporary typology of higher states of consciousness is the one put forward in the writings of Ken Wilbur (1996) based on the Great Chain of Being (Lovejoy, 1936). It is an intellectual tour de force of synthesis of the ancient and the modern. As a paradigm, it has utility for research, but does not describe direct mystical experience. One could quote many examples of maps like this based on hierarchies of states of consciousness. David Hawkins (1995, 2001, 2003, 2005, 2006) presents one, for example, that constructs a scale mainly from the spectrum of negative and positive emotional states. Lester Levenson (Dwoskin, 1991) has an emotional scale that is strikingly parallel, and the writings of Abraham (Hicks, 2004, p 114; 2006) are similar.

In the Pratyabhijnahridayam, a text of Kashmir Shaivism, *sutra* 8 says: "The positions of the various systems of philosophy are only various roles of that (consciousness or Self)." (Singh, 1987, p 37 and 65). The commentary to the verse goes on to enumerate the positions of thirteen different philosophies as to what the highest reality is ranging from materialist through dualist to various non-dualistic and monistic postions. The commentator then writes that in effect they are all right! The positions of the various systems of philosophies are simply roles assumed by the one Self. In other words, your philosophic position (and model of the world) reflects your level of consciousness. Expand your consciousness and how you experience and interpret the world (summarized in your model of the world) and hence your philosophy will change. There is no absolute interpretation of correctness; interpretations are all relative to the degree of expression of higher consciousness just as an adult's world is very expanded compared to that of a child.

To interpret the significance of the awakening of the Centre of Consciousness or Inner Teacher in terms of a map of awakening to make sense of one's inner experiences, one needs a map based on the personal mystical experience of an awakened sage. The map in Patanjali's *Yoga-Sutra* is considered to be the benchmark in Yoga, but it needs an awakened preceptor to interpret it. Unfortunately most of the many commentaries available for the *Yoga-Sutra* are academic rather than experiential. We provide a reading list at the end of this chapter of a few books that for us have been the most helpful in understanding the spiritual nature of Consciousness in the perennial wisdom and we would highlight especially the writings of Franklin Merrell-Wolff (1994), as well as the Yoga Vasishtha and Tripura Rahasya.

Of the many possibilities we choose and present here one example, a brief account of a recently published map of awakening from a contemporary sage (Kristof, 1999, 2000; Kristof & Emami, 1999), which has been most helpful to us. Our purpose in presenting it is to help the aspirant to understand where the experience of the Centre of Consciousness fits on the overall map of the spiritual journey. Since transcendent states of consciousness are not part of ordinary experience we have no language to describe them in common speech. Nevertheless, Kristof (1999) tries to formulate his model using everyday English. This helps at the same time as it obscures, since the words are not used with their everyday connotation. Our own preceptor stressed over and over that Spirit can only be known through direct experience from practicing a spiritual discipline like Yoga. Transcendent states cannot be captured in language by the intellect. Transcendent states are secrets which when revealed by the intellect remain secrets. One can only know by direct Realization. The only maps of real value are those from a realized sage.

Having introduced the Presence, the Centre of Consciousness, we now consider where it fits a within a broader cartography of transcendent states of consciousness using the model of Aziz Kristof (1999, 2000). The map is outlined in figure 4.1, which represents our own interpretation of his model from the perspective of Advaita Vedanta. (Kristof himself denies any connection between his teaching and traditional perennial wisdom. Rather he sees his teaching as a new dispensation for a modern age.) It is an evolutionary model of consciousness in which enlightenment does not occur immediately and is not a static goal or destination. Rather there are a series of levels of enlightenment that represent the progressive depth of experience of the integration of awareness with Spirit. The two horizontal lines mark the beginning and end of the process. At the level of the lower line, the early stages of enlightenment begin. At the upper line, the process is complete and represents the end of evolution of human intelligence. But beyond that, a new process takes over and there is expansion without end.

The first three states of consciousness lie in the realm of what Aziz calls ignorance. These include the states of waking, dreaming and deep sleep which are elaborated in the *Mandukya Upanishad* in the context of Vedanta (Nikhilananda, 1987b). The word "ignorance" is used because these states of consciousness are disconnected from the I AM, his word for the Divine. Because of this disconnection there is no centre of identity in the mind. He also uses the word "forgetfulness" and describes this state as the Subconscious because of the disconnection – an unfortunate term since we use the word subconscious in a very different way in psychology. He says that the dream state

A MAP OF AWAKENING

Expansion without End

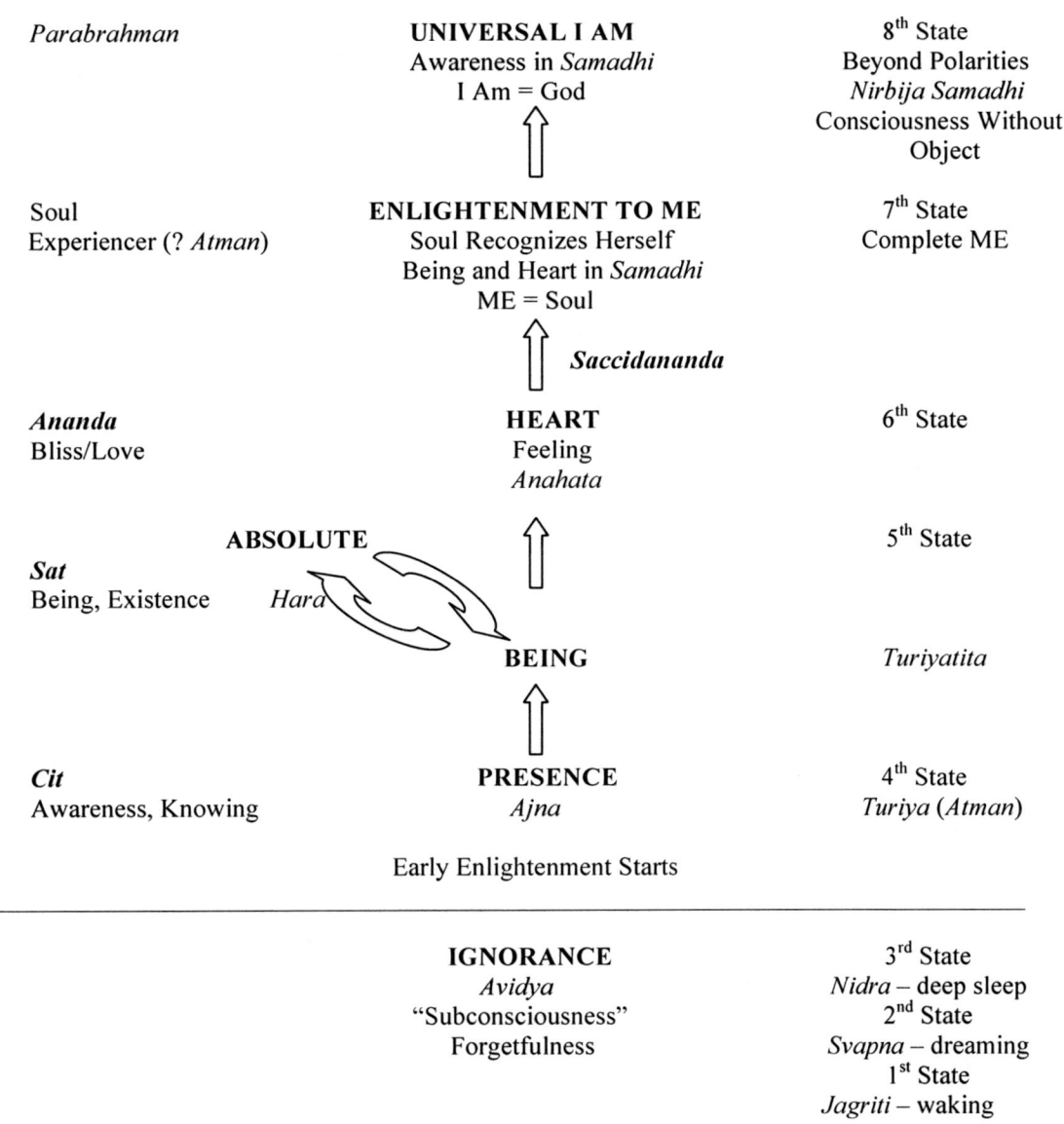

Figure 4.1 A Contemporary Map of the Spiritual Path
(Our Adaptation from Kristof, 1999)

perhaps best represents this stage of consciousness in which the awareness is fully associated into sensory experience. This level includes the ego and the intuitive intelligence. It also includes the realm of everyday ordinary awareness and is the field of cognitive neuroscience and modern psychology, as well as the *koshas* of the Vedantic model of the personality. The essential feature of this stage of ignorance is the lack of conscious awareness of Spirit.

The first awareness of Spirit comes with the opening of the Centre of Consciousness, which he describes as Presence or Awareness. *Brahman* is described in Vedanta as pure Consciousness, a combination of *sat, cit* and *ananda* (*saccidananda*). We interpret this Presence described by Aziz as the *cit* aspect of Consciousness, the Knowing quality of the I AM. It is the centre of ME (his word for the Soul) expressing in the mind as a pure Awareness without content that is experienced in the head and involves the *ajna chakra*. He identifies it with the Vedantic *turiya* or fourth state and calls it the *Atman*, although others would assign that term to the Soul. Concentration and meditation are used to activate attention. (This is reminiscent of mindfulness meditation.) Continuity of attention lets Awareness (Knowing) shift to a higher state where its Centre, the Presence or what we call the Centre of Consciousness, is recognized. Once this sense of ME is recognized in the mind behind thoughts, one holds It as one's own Centre and then relaxes to let It expand and become natural (*sahaja*) and effortless.

The four methods used for Awakening the Presence involve 1) observation of the mind with the dissociation achieved through meditative techniques, and then one observes the Observer. Who is the One that is aware? Thereby the attention is turned back on itself to produce a state of self-attention. The Observer is the ME, the soul, the *Atman* reflected in the mind. This is reminiscent of Ramana Maharshi's method of self-inquiry, "Who am I?" (Ramana Maharshi, 1988). 2) A second process for awakening the Presence is the *mantra* or the repetition of a thought. Again the question is, who is the Observer? This leads to a recognition of the sense of ME in the mind, the pure I, Awareness Itself independent of the thinking process. 3) The third method is contemplation, conscious think-ing when fully present and focused on any subject. Who is the I that lies behind and is the mover of the thinking process? Distinguish the Thinker from the thinking and step back in the mind to the sense of ME. 4) Finally the Presence can be directly recognized as an instantaneous recognition of the Centre in the mind.

It is the first awareness of the inner space in the mind where one observes thoughts come and go. One stays with that Presence in Silence to distinguish the bare attention of Awareness, of the sense of I. Integration and stabilization of the Presence involve holding to crystalize the Centre in the mind and then letting go to allow It to expand as the experience comes and goes, until it is spontaneous in all things and can be accessed at will. Success in working with the Presence means completion, to be fully established in the State of Presence with no moments of forgetfulness. Absolute stabilization is not necessary. One needs only the ability to be in that State at one's wish, and to be in the State most of the time.

Next come the related states of Being and the Absolute. They are experienced in the *hara* centre (the vital energy centre of the body four cm. below the navel). We interpret them to represent the *sat*, Existence or Being quality of the I AM. This is the fifth state and represents a realization within Being. It integrates the experiences of Awareness with Being. This level of Being Aziz identifies with the Vedantic term *turiyatita* – beyond the fourth – in which Presence (Awareness) surrenders and dissolves into Being/Rest, which is a primordial state of Rest (others might use the word "Silence"). A vertical dimension is added to the state of Presence, with an experience of dropping down to the *hara* along with expansion until the meditator rests with the body immersed in this State of Being.

In ordinary consciousness we are identified with the mind. To disidentify, one first activates and stabilizes Attention and the Presence as a stable centre of awareness behind the mind. One then relaxes and lets go into Being. Attention dissolves into the open space of pure abiding or "isness" rooted in the unmanifested which is called Being, and yet Awareness remains. Be in the Presence, the Centre of Attention, the Now, and then surrender into Being.

To awaken the Presence one uses traditional spiritual methods such as concentration, meditation and contemplation. But the subsequent stages are reached through surrender and Grace. Doing becomes being. This is difficult for the western mind which is used to achieving its goals through doing, to comprehend this process. One always raises the question, "But how?" One is looking for a recipe, a method, a process, an algorithm. But with being, no such thing applies. And so the process now becomes very subtle indeed. There is no "method" for surrender.

Like the State of Presence, the State of Being is awakened. The process is like a coin with two simultaneous sides. The first has to do with the maturation of the student's consciousness-energy system, the *koshas* or energy sheaths that make up the Vedantic model of the personality. This process of maturation is based on whether the student's *prana* is polarized towards individuality (i.e., the physical body at the periphery of the sheaths) or more on the side of the Beyond, towards the centre of the personality transcending the borders of the separate self. We interpret this as a raising of the vibrational set point of the energy sheaths of the personality, a kind of divinization of the whole personality as the Centre of Consciousness expresses more fully through the personality, of which we will have more to say later. There are specific practices in Tantra, such as *Bhuta Shuddhi* or purification of the elements (Rama, 2002c), which directly address this process.

The other side of the coin is conscious surrender. One first crystalizes the attention in the mind into the Presence or Centre of Consciousness which allows the student to be fully present. Now the student surrenders Awareness into Being. It is a subtle act of a vertical letting go into a state of non-doing where one is deeply relaxed and passive, yet centered. The energy then drops to the *hara*, but is not experienced there. Rather the experience is in Being, beyond personality, as a state of calm non-abiding. The student feels nowhere and everywhere at the same time. The mind is utterly silent, still, at rest, and yet fully aware. One is immersed in It, identified with It. Completion of this state of the process means an integration of both Presence and Being. It adds a vertical or depth dimension to Consciousness. One is immersed and surrounded by Being, cocooned in It.

The Absolute is a related state which Aziz labels as the fifth state. The energy remains in the *hara*. The Absolute is realized within Being as a final expression of the process of surrender into

Being. There is a transcendence into motionlessness and inner silence. The absolute is placed off to one side in this scheme, since it is not a necessary step in the process and is the destiny of very few souls. Aziz likens it to the other side of a black hole beyond time to the unmanifested, to pure Rest with no movement or fluctuation of energy. It is an extreme state of Being.

Our interpretation is that at this point the student has integrated the *sat* and the *cit* aspects of *Brahman*. Now comes the sixth state which Aziz calls Heart that we interpret as representing the *ananda* (love/bliss) or final aspect of the triune *Brahman*. This adds the dimension of feeling in the broadest sense of that term and is located in the heart centre (*anahata*). The heart is a mix of feeling and being. Feeling is the dynamic part and being is the static part. Each depends on the other. The heart must be fully activated to fully experience Being, and one must have Being to be able to rest within to experience sensitivity and feeling. One adds the elements of bliss, love, fullness, beauty, and a sensitivity or warmth of divine flavor. The continuity of Awareness and Being achieved in the previous stages of Intelligence and Rest, allows the student to go fully into the heart to discover the Spiritual Sun within. The *jiva* or embodied soul rests within the heart centre. This is a subtle energy phenomenon and brings the sense of identity from the head into the heart.

Aziz describes the heart as awakening on two levels. The first is energy, which is the foundation and involves an energetic activation of the heart centre. The heart is the midpoint or mid-balance between the inner as the absolute and the outer as manifestation or creation. The second level is feeling or sensitivity, an awakening to the soul itself. The student feels the energy and also senses it as a feeling centre. The soul itself is awakened, touched and discovered through this profound sensitivity – this profound essence of ME in the heart. The completion of these three stages represents the unity of understanding and clarity of the I AM in this state of inner wholeness which we interpret as the *saccidananda*. The triune *Brahman* is now experienced as an integrated state of Consciousness.

Aziz's seventh state is enlightenment to ME. It is Being and the Heart absorbed in *samadhi*. It is the complete ME, the soul, the experiencer, what others might call the *Atman*. There are now three centers in the personality: ME in the mind is the Presence or pure Awareness, or what Aziz calls the *atman* centered in the *ajna* chakra in the head. ME absorbed in Being is the *hara* centre. The feeling Centre of ME in the heart is the *anahata* or heart centre and is the true centre of the soul.

This is a long journey because it is complex and multidimensional. At a certain point a clear intention to awaken the heart arises within and then the power of evolution and grace take one to the goal. We believe that the stages from four through seven represent the processes of *sabija* or *samprajnata samadhi* as described in Patanjali's *Yoga-Sutra* and take place within subject-object or dual consciousness in Merrell-Wolff's scheme (1994). Within these processes both the soul and the immanent triune *Brahman* are realized.

The final step is realization of the Universal I AM. The term I AM is used by Aziz for God. We believe this to be the *parabrahman* of Vedanta, God transcendent. Aziz uses many synonyms: Beloved,

Creator, Divine Mother, the One, Universal Light, the Light of Creation, the I AM, the Universal I AM, the Now, and the Supreme Presence of God. This eighth state is beyond polarities and to us represents *nirbija* or *asamprajnata samadhi* in the *Yoga-Sutra* or consciousness-without-an-object in Merrell-Wolff's terms (1994).

ME or the soul, is the child of the Beloved, the Experiencer, and she dwells in the depths of *anahata*. The soul is the experiencer of the I AM, and in that divine mirror awakens to her self identity. She has conscious unity with the Creator and yet paradoxically she knows herself. To know herself is to merge with the One. This awakening of the Beloved is the final step. The soul surrenders completely to the depth of the heart space and in letting go of herself merges with the divine Beloved which dwells in the depth of the heart and awaits the soul, her child, to return to unity with her. The soul recognizes the Beloved through Intelligence (Awareness), surrender and utmost sensitivity. The goal of life is this spiritual journey of awakening or enlightenment and is an urgent necessity for humanity.

This is a remarkable experiential map of the inner higher states of consciousness based on the teachings of a modern realized sage. Our point in presenting it here is to fix the position of the Centre of Consciousness and Its awakening within the process of this evolutionary model of consciousness. The Presence would appear to us to be the first manifestation of the *saguna Brahman* (God immanent). The sequence of Presence, Being and Heart seem to describe the integrated awakening of the *saccidananda*. Only these higher states deal directly with spirituality and show that the study of spirituality is actually the study of Consciousness. The scheme also shows that enlightenment is not a sudden thing. The process is long, complex and occurs in gradual steps. There are variations in descriptions of the enlightened state among various masters. Yet the teachings imply that once the mountain is climbed by whatever route, the view is the same from the top. Does this variation then mean that the principle of unitary view is wrong? Are there different enlightenments? The scheme suggests that this puzzle is resolved by recognizing that different masters reach different levels of attainment in the scheme, accounting for this variation.

Aziz asks one to imagine a room. The space of the room creates and holds it. This is Being. The contents of the room which are held within Being represent creation. The light in the room that allows you to see and to know its contents represents Awareness, the Presence. There is a table in the centre of the room. A vase containing a rose sits on the table and its perfume fills the room. This is the Heart aspect that provides the qualities of feeling, sensitivity and love. Yet the space, the light and the perfume in and of themselves are invisible.

In the beginning of the Now, a rainbow was created from the Original White Light. It was made of three colours: Awareness, Being and Heart. Awareness is the light of knowing, the pure presence of thought-free consciousness. Being, the condition of Pure Rest is the sacred vessel containing the whole of Creation and its living beings. The Heart is the presence of divinity, infinite sensitivity, beauty and love – she is the very meaning of Creation. When this inner rainbow is fully realised through the existence of the Soul, the space of I Am is born, the manifestation of wholeness. When it is done,

I Am merges back to the Original White Light realising her innate transparency. Here, the rainbow dissolves into the very space from which it originally emerged.

To enter the cave of a Lion, you must be a Lion yourself. To enter the Dimension of I AM, you must become the I am!

Aziz Kristof, *The Human Buddha*, 2000, p 162

Suggested Readings on Consciousness in the Perennial Wisdom

Aziz Kristof. *The Human Buddha*. Motilal Banarsidass, Delhi, 2000.

Aziz Kristof. *Transmission of Awakening*. Motilal Banarsidass, Delhi, 1999.

Aziz Kristof & Houman, Emami. *Enlightenment Beyond Traditions*. Motilal Banarsidass, Delhi, 1999.

Bucke, RM. *Cosmic Consciousness*. E. P. Dutton, New York, 1923.

Eckhart Tolle. *The Power of Now: A Guide to Spiritual Enlightenment*. Namaste Publishing, Vancouver, BC. 1997.

Eckhart Tolle. *Stillness Speaks*. New World Library, Novato, CA. 2003.

Eckhart Tolle. *A New Earth: Awakening to Your Life's Purpose*. Dutton, New York. 2005.

Fort, AO. *The Self and Its States: A States of Consciousness Doctrine in Advaita Vedanta*. Motilal Banarsidass, Delhi, 1990.

Franklin Merrell-Wolff. *Experience and Philosophy*. State University of New York, Albany, 1994.

Franklin Merrell-Wolff. *Transformations in Consciousness*. State University of New York, Albany, 1995.

Martin and Marian Jerry. *Sutras of the Inner Teacher: The Yoga of the Centre of Consciousness*. Unlimited Publishing, Bloomington, Indiana, 2001.

Swami Sri Ramanananda. *Tripura Rahasya: The Mystery Beyond the Trinity*. Sri Ramanasramam, Tiruvannamalai, India, 1980.

Swami Venkatesananda. *Vasishtha's Yoga*. State University of New York, Albany, 1993.

William M Indich. *Consciousness in Advaita Vedanta*. Motilal Banarsidass, Delhi, 1995.

5

Awareness

A Paradox?

By now the reader may be puzzled by the apparent variability of experiences described by enlightened sages, both ancient and modern, albeit on an underlying foundation of unity. Which of these many experiences is correct? If the realized sage participates in divine omniscience surely s/he ought to know which is correct. Does this point to their lack of real attainment? Have not the sages themselves said that the view from the top of the mountain is the same no matter the path taken?

May we suggest the possibility that all viewpoints are correct! When one examines the coloured lights formed when a prism refracts white light, which colour is the true light? They are all aspects of the original white light, and together combine to give it. They are all correct. The Tradition has an oft quoted story of blind men examining an elephant, each giving a disparate view of the nature of the beast depending upon what aspect is examined: the leg, the ear, the tail, the trunk or the side. Yet all are correct interpretations of an aspect of the whole beast. The challenge is to put together all of these aspects to yield the whole beast. Some of the variability in reported experience represents different levels of attainment within the broad continuum of enlightened states. Some is due to the linguistic confusion of attempts to describe felt experiences for students and disciples as filtered through many models of the world in disparate cultural contexts. The experience of higher states of consciousness is ineffable. Rather than confronting the apparent discrepancies in these descriptions, it is more useful to "hear" them with the heart, with the intuition, and to search out their underlying unity. The more varied these descriptions that one can absorb and integrate, the more complete becomes one's understanding of the map of the One in all of Its infinite manifestations. Rather than be put off, one should revel in the richness of that diversity.

Awareness

At this point it is important to distinguish awareness from consciousness. In Yoga, *chetana* is consciousness – a continuous, changeless state of Being and Knowing in endless continuity. Within the personality consciousness is divided into the three states of waking, dreaming and deep sleep. But awareness is not part of this scheme! For most people, there is no or only limited awareness as such in these states. Even in wakefulness we often are aware of not much more than basic sensory percepts and their superficial, flat significance expressed in language. In dreaming sleep awareness is limited to just perception, and dreams may be difficult even to remember (excluding here a discussion of lucid dreaming). To be aware in one of these states is both to experience and to know that I am experiencing.

> The unfortunate thing about the emotional content of our mind is that we are most often not aware of it. People who deny a certain emotional state are not dishonest, nor are they liars. People who deny being angry, people who deny being ill, people who deny being depressed, people who deny being in a mental state called selfishness, they are not liars, they are not deceivers; they simply are not aware. They simply are not aware that they have this mental content. And awareness is our first step. We are not aware that the presence of mental situations is affecting indirectly our other situations and is reducing our effectiveness in life.
>
> Swami Veda Bharati

One of the presuppositions of Neuro-Linguistic Programming™ (NLP) expresses this idea in another way. Present behaviour always represents the very best choice for the person. We always do the very best we know how in any given situation. If that behaviour is inadequate, inappropriate or insensitive, then it means that our model of the world lacks information, the benefit of experience, appropriate skills or the requisite depth of awareness to handle the situation better.

Real awareness begins to add depth of knowing to ordinary perception, and really begins to awaken when the higher intellect (or *buddhi*) begins to function. Sri Aurobindo talks about "frontal man." By this he refers to the superficial nature of ordinary waking consciousness, as though metaphorically it were spread over the surface of a sphere in two dimensions. That surface area may be small or extended in proportion to intelligence, but it lacks depth. The awakening of the kind of awareness to which we refer here is like adding depth to that area, a third dimension, like beginning to travel along a radius of that metaphoric sphere in towards its centre. It is in this sense that we say awareness adds depth of knowing to ordinary perception. Much of this expanded awareness comes from the opening of intuition.

Here is this metaphor of the wheel again.

> Life is like a wheel. In the Centre of the wheel there is a hub that does not move, but wherever you go that center is with you. The center itself never moves, but it moves when the wheel rotates. It goes with the wheel. How will you classify and define that center which moves, yet does not move? It is the cause of all movements but it does not move itself. You cannot study that thing which moves. That which moves is not everlasting, is not Truth. Body, senses, and mind move. They are not the everlasting part of the Self. That which does not move is immortal. Deep within us, that which is the center of consciousness, does not move. It is not subject to change or decay; it does not go to destruction. Your essential nature is the center of consciousness within. You have consciousness now, but that consciousness is so low that you are not aware of your true nature. You are only aware of the body. You cannot say that you have no awareness. You all have awareness of your individuality. That is why you project yourself. That is why

you say, *this is me, this is not me*. You are aware. Just by saying that you are aware you do not receive anything. How much are you aware? Are you aware of all the levels of your being? Are you aware of that center from which consciousness flows in various degrees and grades? That is perfect awareness. Until you have realized that center, you are not spiritually aware. You are not enlightened. You have to know yourself on all levels in this lifetime and get enlightened here and now. You should have that determination.

Swami Rama (2002d), p 162.

Modern cognitive neuroscience studies aspects of attention and selective perception (Gazzaniga et al, 1998). These studies have three principal goals: (1) to understand how attention leads to detection, perception and encoding of stimuli; (2) to work out the underlying neural computational algorithms; and (3) to find out how these algorithms are used in the brain's neural circuits. The studies thus far have looked at selective aspects of perception that result from attention, examining executive systems responsible for selection within sensory pathways. Distributed brain systems participate in the control of attention. These systems require the parietal lobe along with subcortical structures. Regional cerebral blood flow (rCBF) obtained from PET (positron emission tomography) studies in humans indicates that a network which includes the pulvinar nucleus of the thalamus, the posterior parietal cortex, and the dorsolateral prefrontal cortex may mediate cortical excitability in the extrastriate cortex as a function of selective attention to color, form or motion. Attentional phenomena are diverse and involve many brain computations and mechanisms. All of this refers to attention experienced at the sensory level as a kind of "spotlight" with a fuzzy periphery that plays over the fields of accessible consciousness at the level of perception. But with awareness, we mean something quite different.

Real awareness is more a depth and sensitivity of knowingness which begins to add depth of knowing to ordinary perception. It really begins to awaken when the higher intellect (the *buddhi*) begins to function. Awareness in this sense is an attribute or expression of the intellect (Niranjanananda, 1993a). The word "intellect" is used here in a very broad sense of intelligence or knowing, and not in the limited sense it is usually used in ordinary language. Broadening the awareness means expanding the receptivity and analytical function of *buddhi*, expanding the ability to "know" ever larger aspects of the fields of consciousness, until from the perspective of *turiya*, the fourth state, the Centre of Consciousness, one can be aware as one chooses any part of the three fields of consciousness. Ordinary wakefulness expands, and then moves into lucid dreaming and then into *yoga nidra* or conscious deep sleep. As one's consciousness expands to take in all of the *jagriti* (waking) and then the *svapna* (dreaming) followed by the *nidra* (deep sleep) levels, there is an expansion of the field of awareness to encompass all three states of *jagriti*, *svapna* and *nidra* – a broad awareness known as *turiya* (the fourth). This is not the supermind but a simultaneous awareness of all three states which takes us closer to enlightenment.

Awareness adds depth to knowing. One person sees another and realizes only a waitress in a uniform with little of any personal interaction. Another person greets the same waitress and within a moment's interaction senses layer after layer after layer of the personal depth of that other human being. The difference is the degree of awareness.

Although translated as "intellect," the word *buddhi* comes from the Sanskrit root *"bodh,"* meaning "to be aware of," "to know," "to have the experience of." It has more the sense of "being aware of" reflecting recognized experience. *Buddhi* is the faculty of being aware and is different from the intellect as we commonly know it as a faculty of mind. *Buddhi* is more a quality of consciousness. The differences among the overlapping concepts of mind, consciousness and awareness are difficult to explain in language. But they can be experienced. The state of superconsciousness, of *samadhi*, of *turiya*, is a kind of combination of these three areas of conscious, subconscious and unconscious with equal intensity of awareness all the way through – all as one homogeneous experience, one state of perception. This final state is experienced with the awakening of the *bodhi* aspect of the Self in Yoga known as *drashta*, "the seer," the Witness, the Centre of Consciousness behind the action of life and living. This kind of awareness leads to the awakening of the intuition, also a function of the higher *buddhi*.

Thus consciousness does not change. But the quality of its expression as awareness becomes expanded to realize higher potentials of that consciousness. It is said that consciousness sleeps in stones, dreams in plants, begins to awaken in animals and can be fully realized in human beings. Only human beings can know that they are awake. In Yoga, awareness is the ability to witness, to stand back and observe one's mental, emotional and physical actions. Its implications are profound. It means your nature transcends body and mind which can be observed by something in the background that witnesses their actions. This background witnessing principle is called awareness in Yoga. Few experience it for most of us lose ourselves and are totally absorbed in the experiences of body and mind. It transcends the concepts of perceptual positions like "meta" in Neuro-Linguistic Programming.

Yoga tries to increase the awareness that our nature is something that transcends body and mind, which are then seen as only our grosser vehicles. Clearly it is an issue of identification or dis-identification of consciousness, of the observer with the observed and the process of observing. Identification with the mind and body imprisons us in the limited realm of manifest existence. Cultivation of awareness lets us transcend the mind to realize and to know things that are completely beyond present comprehension. We do not expand consciousness which is infinite and all-pervasive. What we actually do is to expand awareness, to tune in with and to identify with more and more of the field of consciousness. This assumes that consciousness is independent of the function of the brain. From the perspective of the perennial wisdom consciousness uses the brain and senses as intermediary instruments between itself and the outside world.

> For Western philosophy the mind is the hub of man; for Yoga it is consciousness that is the central and most basic aspect. . . . Our deepest nature is infinite, for it is consciousness. It is not mind. The mind is merely the instrument of consciousness and the storehouse of our finite personality.
>
> Satyananda Saraswati, 1981, p 73

All the practices of Yoga involve an increase in awareness. To be a witness is to be aware. To be totally lost, involved and identified with an action is to be unaware. Spiritual *sadhana* without awareness loses 90 percent of its benefits. Initially the experience will be like third position in Neuro-Linguistic Progamming perceptual filters – dis-association into an observer or meta-position. But awareness is self-reflexive and eventually transcends even this perceptual position. We will have more to say later about how this process of expanding awareness eventually awakens the Presence or the Centre of Consciousness.

> [Understand] . . . the relationship of the active peripheral consciousness with the inner consciousness. . . . consciousness is seen in the form of a vortex. At the outside of the vortex is the whirlwind that lifts up all the dust . . . This whirlwind carries with it a force which represents the dynamic, active nature or principle of consciousness. But behind and beyond this active principle of consciousness, within the self there is absolute stillness at the centre of the vortex. Our [everyday] experience is just the surrounding periphery. The force of movement of the mind, which lifts up dust, paper and other objects in its path, is the *vritti* aspect. As long as that has a form, a shape and a movement, it is known as the individual identity or the individual self. When this movement is stopped and one enters the zone of silence, stillness and passiveness, that is known as the awareness or knowledge of the superconscious mind.
>
> Niranjanananda, 1993a

In the *Yoga-Sutra* (Aranya, 1981) the afflictions (*kleshas*) or causes of suffering are presented as fivefold: *avidya* (ignorance), *asmita* (ego; the sense of I as the doer), *raga* (attraction), *dvesha* (aversion; looking for something new) and *abhinivesha* (survival, fear of death; "May I not cease to be"). *Avidya* is considered to be the chief of these. These five qualities ground the consciousness into the physical plane. Emotional reactivity is based in *raga* and *dvesha*.

A similar concept is found in Tibetan Buddhism:

> According to the Buddha and Abhidharma, what obscures or prevents the perfection of the human mind are the *klesha* (Tibetan: *nyon-mongs*). In English they are called afflictive emotions, defilements, mental distortions, negative emotions or even disturbing concepts. In the *Abhidharmasamuccaya* a *klesha* is defined as a "mental factor that, upon occurring in the mind, has the function of producing turmoil in and lack of control over the psyche." These mental-emotional obscurations are reflexive modes of consciousness, habitual reactive and emotive complexes; they are the psychic roots of illness. . . . [They] can be condensed into the so-called "three poisons" – confusion, attachment and aversion, which all arise from fundamental ignorance or unawareness.
>
> Clifford, 1994

Avidya is usually translated as "ignorance." But this is not ignorance in the sense of lack of knowledge or even information, nor is it a polite word for stupidity, as one would usually mean in English. What it really means is absence of conscious awareness (Niranjanananda, 1993a). The consciousness is overidentified or bound to the senses and cannot see beyond. Thus lack of awareness or limited awareness in the sense that we have defined awareness above is the central cause of suffering. This makes the concept of models of the world even more subtle. Despite the coding of at least some beliefs in submodalities in Neuro-Linguistic Programming, beliefs are not always just objects on a shelf that can be changed or moved about at convenience. As awareness deepens one's world view and its component beliefs will change. Some aspects of pictures of reality will only be possible with deepening awareness. This is another way to think of states of consciousness and the *chakras* as described by Ajaya (1983).

The Significance of the Awakening of the Centre of Consciousness

We have described the Centre of Consciousness, and Its manifestation as the Inner Teacher in the Yoga tradition, as well as Its placement in the hierarchy of higher states of consciousness. To address this Presence which is the Centre of Consciousness is to talk about spirituality directly. What then is the significance of this inner awakening for the traveler on the spiritual path?

There is considerable confusion in spiritual traditions about the nature and role of the spiritual preceptor, the *guru*, in the master-disciple relationship. The *guru* is seen as a separate physical person. But what must be understood is that the *guru* is a physical embodiment of the same Inner Teacher that has just awakened within the disciple. The Outer Teacher, the *guru*, is but an expression of the Inner Teacher. In Consciousness they are one and the same. Communication to the Inner Teacher is communication to the outer master. Teaching from the Inner Teacher is teaching from the outer master and vice versa. Our preceptor, Swami Rama, would sometimes say to particular students, "You I will teach in silence!" Such advanced students would then be given a major task to perform and kept at a physical distance. The preceptor would refuse to discuss the project with the student and thereby force the student to learn effective communication with the Inner Teacher. The student soon learned to turn inward with questions and to receive a continuous flow of loving, intuitive guidance. Direct verbal instruction from the master would seldom be necessary, and only when the student had done his or her best to understand the inner guidance.

Just as there is an outer ashram where students and disciples are taught by the master, so the student learns that there is also a corresponding Inner Ashram. That Inner Ashram has now opened by virtue of the student's qualifying state of higher consciousness. The student has been tested (and how they do test!), and is now accepted as a disciple and the master will make clear that the relationship is eternal. Through spiritual yearning and long preparation, the student has asked; the Inner Teacher has responded with the grace of a master.

> "Ask, and it shall be given you; seek, and ye shall find; knock, and it shall be opened unto you."
>
> Matthew 7:7

> "When the student is ready the master will appear."
>
> The Yoga Tradition

This is not enlightenment. To use a modern metaphor, it is the light at the end of the tunnel and that is not a train coming down the track! But you are still in the tunnel. The metaphor of a sunrise may be helpful here. During the long cold hours of the night (perhaps representing many lifetimes of ignorance) one has awaited the dawn. When the time is at hand one goes to the hilltop (prepares) to witness the sunrise. The glow begins to appear, lighting up the eastern sky. Soon there is a flash of brilliant light on the horizon as the disk of the sun first appears. This represents the opening of the Centre of Consciousness. It is yet many hours before the sun stands directly overhead in all of its brilliance.

The entry to the path has at last been found. Now the Centre of Consciousness calls the student to discipleship. To answer, to cross over the threshold and begin to tread the path in earnest, the student must die to the world – be strong enough to leave behind the distraction of worldly attractions and attachments. But if he or she is not strong enough, not yet ready, the portal will close. But only for awhile, while the student gains detachment through further worldly experience. For once opened, the relationship is eternal.

> Once having passed through the storm and attained the peace, it is then always possible to learn, even though the disciple waver, hesitate and turn aside. The voice of the Silence remains within him, and though he leave the path utterly, yet one day it will resound and rend him asunder, and separate his passions from his divine possibilities. Then with pain and desperate cries from the deserted lower self he will return.
>
> Collins, 1976

The new disciple now enters a period of advanced training. We have described some of the curriculum in detail elsewhere (Jerry & Jerry, 2001). The *Bhagavad Gita* is an essential text on the Centre of Consciousness. Krishna plays the role of the Inner Teacher and Arjuna is the qualified disciple on the battlefield of life. We quote here a powerful excerpt from *Light on the Path* that describes the Centre as the Warrior Within. Read between the lines with intuition. Although it is metaphorical, it describes exactly how to work with the Centre in real life.

THE WARRIOR WITHIN

> Stand aside in the coming battle, and though thou fightest be not thou the warrior. Look for the warrior and let him fight in thee. Take his orders for battle and obey them. Obey him not as though he were a general, but as though he were thyself, and his spoken words were the utterance of thy secret desires; for he is thyself, yet infinitely wiser and stronger than thyself. Look for him, lest in the fever and hurry of the fight thou mayest pass him; and he will not know thee unless thou knowest him. If thy cry reach his listening ear then will he fight in thee and fill the dull void within. And if this is so, then canst thou go through the fight cool and unwearied, standing aside and letting him battle for thee. Then it will be impossible for thee to strike one blow amiss. But if thou look not for him, if thou pass him by, then there is no safeguard for thee. Thy

brain will reel, thy heart grow uncertain, and in the dust of the battle-field thy sight and senses will fail, and thou wilt not know thy friends from thy enemies.

. . . He is thyself, yet thou art but finite and liable to error. He is eternal and is sure. He is eternal truth. When once he has entered thee and become thy warrior, he will never utterly desert thee, and at the day of the great peace he will become one with thee.

Collins, 1976.

To answer the call, total surrender, total commitment is required. For the Inner Teacher ultimately is one's own Self.

Now begins the curriculum for the new disciple which we have elaborated in detail elsewhere (Jerry & Jerry, 2001). Light on the Path (Collins, 1976) puts it this way:

Out of the silence that is peace a resonant voice shall arise. And this voice will say. It is not well; thou hast reaped, now thou must sow. And knowing this voice to be the silence itself thou wilt obey.

Thou art now a disciple, able to stand, able to hear, able to see, able to speak, who hast conquered desire and attained to self-knowledge, who hast seen thy soul in its bloom and recognized it, and heard the voice of the silence, Go thou to the Hall of Learning and read what is written there for thee.

The commentary provided with Light on the Path amplifies the meaning of these pithy statements further:

To be able to stand is to have confidence; to be able to hear is to have opened the doors of the soul; to be able to see is to have attained perception; to be able to speak is to have attained the power of helping others; to have conquered desire is to have learned how to use and control the self; to have attained to self-knowledge is to have retreated to the inner fortress from whence the personal man can be viewed with impartiality; to have seen thy soul in its bloom is to have attained a momentary glimpse in thyself of the transfiguration which shall eventually make thee more than man; to recognize is to achieve the great task of gazing upon the blazing light without dropping the eyes and not falling back in terror, as though before some ghastly phantom. This happens to some, and so when the victory is all but won it is lost; to hear the voice of the silence is to understand that from within the Hall of Learning is to enter the state in which learning becomes possible. Then will many words be written there for thee, and written in fiery letters for thee easily to read. For when the disciple is ready the Master is ready also.

Part Two
The Chariot of SADHANA

6

The Chariot of Sadhana: An Organizing Principle

In the first chapter (*pada*) of Patanjali's *Yoga-Sutra* an organizing principle is put forward for advanced spiritual practice. Swami Rama referred to it as the chariot of *sadhana*. It consists of two simultaneous processes. One is *vairagya* (non-attachment), and the other is *abhyasa* (practice). Each constitutes a wheel of the chariot. For a chariot to move forward, both wheels must turn together. The concept lies at the foundation of what we refer to as the Yoga of the Center of Consciousness for which we have coined the term *samahita* Yoga. This notion is basic to the structure of our *Sutras of the Inner Teacher* (Jerry & Jerry, 2001). It is also foundational to the practice of Yoga as described in *pada* I of Patanjali's *Yoga-Sutra*. Our objective in this present book is to explore this concept in depth and in practical detail.

The very first words that our spiritual master, Swami Rama, said to us were, "I will answer all your questions." Only very much later did we realize this to be our first introduction to the Inner Teacher and to the ultimate promise of *samadhi*. Thus we chose to coin the term *Samahita* Yoga to honor this profound impact of our first personal experience of our *guru*, and the essence of his teaching to us in this lifetime.

Our preceptor, Swami Rama, defined the ultimate goal of spiritual practice, *samadhi*, as the state in which all questions are answered and no questions arise.

> "The word *samadhi* means *samahitam* – no question remains unanswered, no mystery remains unsolved."
>
> Swami Rama, 1999a

Swami Veda Bharati (1986) expands further on the meaning of this word, *samahita*.

> The word *samahita* means "harmonized"; that in which conditions of conflict have been resolved, as though previously broken pieces have been set and fused together (from *sam + a + dha* "to set together, join together" [as of broken bones]; and "that which is in *samadhi*." The two, again, are actually one condition. From *sam + dha*, "*samadhi*" is the abstract noun and *samahita* is the perfect participle expressing the fact that this harmonizing, resolving of the conditions of conflict has been accomplished by reaching *samadhi*.

Thus *samahita* yoga is the harmonizing yoga or the yoga of harmony, the yoga of aequanimitas, the union with that State in which all questions are answered and no questions arise.

This Yoga of the Centre of Consciousness is based on the foundation of an integrated practice of Raja Yoga. The royal or eightfold path is described in the second and third chapters of the *Yoga-Sutra*. In its various aspects, it is the basis of all spiritual practices and meditation is its core methodology. The beginning student starts with this eightfold path. When the Centre of Consciousness opens one's practice moves to the first chapter with its basis in the chariot of *sadhana* (*Yoga-Sutra* I.12–16).

The Essence of Patanjali's *Yoga-Sutra*

We begin our discussion by locating the idea of the chariot in the overall presentation of *pada* I of Patanjali's *Yoga-Sutra*. The essence of the book and of Patanjali's philosophy is presented in the first four *sutras*. A grasp of these four *sutras* lets the aspirant understand the entire book in principle, but to practice s/he will have to learn much more.

> I.1 *atha yoganushasanam*
> Now then Yoga is being explained.

> I.2 *yogash chitta-vritti-nirodhah*
> Yoga is the control of the modifications of the mind.

> I.3 *tada drashtuh sva-rupe-vasthanam*
> Then the Seer abides in Itself.

> I.4 *vritti-sarupyam itaratra*
> Otherwise It appears to assume the form of the modifications of the mind

The essence of these first few *sutras* is actually quite straightforward. The first *sutra* implies qualification on the part of the student. It means that the student is prepared to receive the teachings. That preparation means that the teachings will sink deeply into the student's personality and by effecting the appropriate changes will come to fruition. The student must be able to absorb the teachings on a level that is much deeper than pure intellectual understanding. An intellectual grasp of the teachings is not sufficient for their fruition. We have seen students who have applied themselves diligently to Yoga and its teachings for much of their adult lives, and who have acquired a sophisticated intellectual understanding of its philosophy and practices. Yet in later life all of this experience appears not to have touched their basic personality and way of life. It is as though the teachings have had no more impact than water washing of the back of a duck. These students were not qualified, not prepared in the sense meant here. The teachings could not take deep root and grow from within.

Think of the metaphor of a gardener. The gardener may plant seeds, but these seeds will not grow unless the ground is first prepared. The ground must be tilled, watered, made free of weeds and fertilized. The seeds must then be planted properly. And then the gardener must nurture their growth by removing the weeds, and providing light, water and fertilizer. The seed must be planted in order to obtain the fruit of knowledge. But for the seed to grow to fruition the ground must also be prepared, qualified, and maintained in that receptive state. Jesus' parable of the sower and the seed is applicable here (Matthew 13:18–23; Mark 4:10, 13–20). Yogananda (2004: Vol. I, pp 697–700) provides a Yogic commentary on this parable.

The next three *sutras* contain the essence of Patanjali's text, the seeds of knowledge that will be planted in the prepared student. One's essential nature is peace, happiness and bliss, but one is not aware of that essential nature. A *jnani*, one who knows, is aware of the Reality and has become a *drashta*, a seer. One is not aware of this Reality because one identifies oneself with the objects of the mind and the world, forgetting one's true nature. This lack of awareness and knowledge is called ignorance (*avidya*). It is self-delusion and a self-created cause of suffering.

By not identifying with objects of the mind one can establish oneself in the Reality, one's own true nature. One does this by gaining control over modifications of the mind (*vrittis*), thereby attaining a state of *samadhi* and establishing oneself in the Reality. As we indicated above based on the etymology of the word *samadhi*, this is a harmonious state, one free from conflicts and problems. If one is not in *samadhi* then one continuously identifies with the physical world and its objects which are impermanent and subject to continuous change. They arise, change, decay, and die, and in this sense they are unreal. Identification with things that are changing can only bring unhappiness because of the loss of awareness of that which is eternal, unchanging, and everlasting, and, therefore, real. Through this identification one becomes attached and becomes a victim. Learning to establish oneself in one's essential nature brings freedom from misery. "Identify with your true nature that is Truth, and that is not subject to change or death. In actuality you are *Atman*, a child of eternity. To remember, to be aware of the center, is the only way of freedom. When awareness is turned inward, that is called freedom." (Rama, 2002d, p 177).

The Chariot of *Sadhana* and the *Yoga-Sutra*

Now where does the Chariot of *Sadhana* fit in? Let us look at the flow of the argument through the first few *sutras* of the *Yoga-Sutra*.

First the essence of the text is provided as explained above:
  I.1 Now then Yoga is being explained.
  I.2 Yoga is the control of the modifications of the mind.
  I.3 Then the Seer abides in Itself.
  I.4 Otherwise It appears to assume the form of the modifications of the mind.

Now comes a relevant digression in YS I.5 – 11 to discuss the five major categories of these modifications of the mind (*vrittis*): valid proof, perversive cognition, imagination, memory and sleep.

Then the concept of the Chariot of *Sadhana* is introduced:
  I.12 By practice and detachment these can be stopped.

By "these," of course, is meant the modifications of the mind which must be controlled so that they do not obscure the inner Reality beyond.

The text next asks what practice (*abhyasa*) is.
>   I.13 Exertion to acquire mental tranquility devoid of fluctuations is called practice.
>   I.14 That practice when continued for a long time without break and with devotion becomes firm in foundation.

Then the text asks what detachment (*vairagya*) is.
>   I.15 When mind loses all desire for objects seen or described in the scriptures it acquires a state of utter desirelessness called detachment.
>   I.16 Indifference to the constituent principles (of nature, the *gunas*) achieved through knowledge of the nature of *Purusha* (the inner Reality) is called supreme detachment (*paravairagya*).

Now the text goes on to discuss the nature of *samadhi* and how it is obtained to complete the first chapter (*pada* I). In this way we have placed the Chariot of *Sadhana*, our subject of interest here, in its proper place in the flow of the argument of the first chapter so that the reader can understand this concept within its larger context in Patanjali's Yoga. When we discuss the Centre of Consciousness, we seek this Seer or inner Reality.

When the argument of the initial *sutras* is written this way one can see the flow of logic and exactly how the Chariot of *Sadhana* is placed within that flow. *Sutras* 2, 3 and 4 contain the essence of the whole text. One's essential nature is that Reality which is peace, happiness and bliss, but one is not aware of that Reality because of attachment to the world. One identifies with the objects of the mind, becomes a victim by letting them condition and control one's life, forgetting one's true nature. The cause of suffering is this lack of awareness and knowledge of the Reality within which is a self-created form of ignorance (*avidya*). By not identifying with the objects of the world (detachment) which are fleeting and subject to change, one can be established in one's true nature. Control the modifications of the mind to attain a state of tranquility and harmony, and to resolve duality and conflict. This is *samadhi*, to be established in one's essential nature. Be aware of the Reality within which is eternal and unchanging. That is *abhyasa* in this context. Turn the awareness inward and remember that Centre, be aware of that Centre constantly in all things. As Sri Swami Rama put it, "These four *sutras* are the foundation of Patanjali's philosophy. If you understand these four *sutras*, you will understand the entire book in principle, but to practice, you will still have to learn more." (Rama, 2002d, p 177).

The commentary on *sutra* 12 on this twin practice of the Chariot, practice and dispassion, points out that the mind can flow out to the world or inwards toward liberation (Veda Bharati, 1986). The mind is compared to a river that can flow two ways It can flow outwards towards the world (*samsara*). Through worldly involvement one gathers *karma* and becomes entangled in the endless cycles of creation and dissolution with its transmigration through rebirth. This is the mind stream flowing as indiscrimination (*aviveka*). Alternatively the mind can flow inward towards liberation (*kaivalya, nirvana, moksha*). It leads to all that is beautiful (*kalyana*). It is the way of the beatitude, of liberation. This is the flow of the mind stream as discrimination (*viveka*).

The practice of dispassion stops the normal outward flow of the mind towards the world (*samsara*). It reduces or blocks the stream of worldly attractions so that the mind is turned off when it perceives the distraction of worldly interests and activities. *Abhyasa* (practice) then turns the flow of the mind stream inwards towards *nirodha* (control) by cultivating and opening up the flow of discriminative wisdom (*viveka*). This wisdom is the philosophy and experience of discernment of the distinction between *Purusha* and the *sattvic* nature of the mind field. Mental turbulence is calmed. The mind flows pacifically into peacefulness and tranquility, yet with the qualities of firmness and strength in both practice and dispassion. Both are needed to attain the state of *nirodha*. Dispassion stops the normal mental flow outward towards *samsara*. *Abhyasa* then turns the mind's flow inwards and upwards towards *nirodha* (control).

If *vairagya* (disinterest in the world) is practiced alone without the benefit of discernment and meditation, mental agitation is pacified, but the mind enters into sleep and *samadhi* will not occur. Unprepared students who have not practiced easily fall asleep during mental exercises done in meditation or in the corpse posture (*shavasana*). They may also fall asleep in the presence of the intense field of a master's mental and *pranic* energy. The student must carry out gradual practice to absorb and assimilate the rising energies of *prana*, *kundalini* and consciousness so that the meditation practice can go higher (Veda Bharati, 1986).

When the outward flow of mental modifications (*vrittis*) ceases, they turn inwards to dwell in their origin as potentials (*shakti* – potentia, power, potential energy), their originating cause, in the mind field. Then the mind flow gradually merges into *nirodha* (control), which is *kaivalya* (isolation) or liberation. One is reminded of David Bohm's theory (1983) of implicate and explicate realities, with the manifest explicate order subsiding into the unmanifest implicate order at the level of the mind field. The movement between kinetic and potential energies in a system is another physical metaphor.

No doubt, O mighty-armed Arjuna, the mind is fickle and difficult to restrain, but, O Son of Kunti, it is brought under control through practice (*abhyasa*) and through dispassion (*vairagya*).

Bhagavad Gita VI.35

7

The Yoga of the Centre of Consciousness

Samahita Yoga

The Yoga of the Centre of Consciousness has as its foundation an integrated practice of Raja Yoga, the *Ashtanga* Yoga described in Patanjali's *Yoga-Sutra*. Although we will not elaborate on this further, this foundation is a fundamental assumption that underlies all that is written here in terms of practice. If Raja Yoga is its foundation, then its essence is the Chariot of *Sadhana* composed of the twin wheels of detachment (*vairagya*) and constant practice (*abhyasa*). Meditation is the core method to explore inner space, so meditation bridges the wheels of the Chariot of *Sadhana*. Although we will treat detachment and practice separately, in fact the separation and distinction between them is artificial. Just as the wheels of a chariot must turn together simultaneously so that it can move forward, detachment and practice in this Yoga are really two sides of one coin. The following table highlights the key aspects of detachment and practice in the context of the Chariot of *Sadhana*.

Samahita Yoga
The Yoga of the Centre of Consciousness
Chariot of *Sadhana*

Vairagya Detachment	*Abhyasa* Practice
Emotional and mental purification	Unceasing awareness and remembrance to invoke the Centre of Consciousness as Presence, Wisdom and Bliss
Dis-identification leading to the identity shift	Practicing the Presence of God. (*Ishvara pranidhana*)
Releasing, letting go	Absorption, surrender

In the next chapters we will examine in more depth these multiple dimensions and aspects of both detachment and practice, as well as some of the variety of methods that are used in Yoga to bring them about.

The Meaning of Control (*nirodhah*)

In *Yoga-Sutra* I.2 Patanjali describes Yoga as the control of the modifications of the mind field. What is meant by the word, "control" (*niruddhah* or *nirodhah*)? Does it have the sense of annihilation or negation of the mind, or does it mean transformation of the mind?

The word *nirodhah*, meaning cessation, comes from *ni* (down, into) + *rudh* (to obstruct, arrest, stop, restrain, prevent). It has been frequently mistranslated by words such as, "suppression," "inhibition," "restriction," "cessation," "restraint," or "control," all taken in the sense of dissolution or stopping of the mind and its functioning. It has been taken as meaning annihilation or suppression of the mind and its modifications (*vrittis*) to gain spiritual liberation (Veda Bharati, 1986; Whicher, 1998). This is a misunderstanding of the word.

The proper translation of the word *nirodhah* as "cessation" or "control" is in the sense of undoing or dissolution of the confusion of identity between *Purusha* and the mental processes. It means the cessation of this misidentification and of the effects of the thought forms (*vrittis*) on consciousness, not the complete cessation of the *vrittis* themselves (Veda Bharati, 1986; Whicher, 1998).

Nirodhah means to cultivate, to coordinate all the aspects of the mind so that it attains a state of equilibrium and tranquility, and is prepared for *samadhi*. One can attain *samadhi* only after one achieves *nirodhah* (Rama, 2002d). The word does not mean suppression, repression or restraint of the mind with its feelings and thoughts. That would mean that the *manas* could not think and the *buddhi*, ego and *chitta* would not function. One does not want to suppress all the faculties of the mind so that one cannot think, act or function. Suppression and repression are dangerous for mental function; what is suppressed will reappear in dreams and conditioned behavior.

Rather the mind should be cultivated to a state of perfect equilibrium. This is what is meant here by control. To control something is to master it. To suppress or stop the mind means it will come up again and control you. Thus *nirodhah* means control in the sense of regulate and use properly with conscious command of the various powers within. "Mind should be controlled exactly as a rider controls the horse, not allowing the horse to run wild here and there." (Rama, 2002d, p 46).

Swami Rama likened the mind to a lake. The *vrittis*, modifications or thoughts, are like waves on the surface of the lake of the mind preventing you from seeing what is hidden beneath. One cannot know what is in the unconscious mind and beyond when the waking conscious mind is so disturbed. *Nirodhah* requires establishing coordination among *chitta*, *manas*, *buddhi* and *ahamkara* through determination (*sankalpa-shakti*) or will power.

We will have much more to say about this state of mental tranquility below. But for now, consider a metaphor. The energy that drives the activity of the mind field can be thought of as having both a potential and a kinetic form. The kinetic form is the continuous state of manifestation of the activity of thoughts, emotions and perceptions experienced in everyday wakefulness and in dreams. The potential form is the unconscious part of the mind in the sense that most of the mind lies dormant and out of ordinary awareness, and acts as the source of the kinetic experience of the stream of consciousness. Thoughts arise continually from that potential ground and then subside back into it, but at such a rate that it seems a continuous connected stream in the same way that the sequence of still frames on a movie film pass at just the right rate to give the impression of continuous movement. In other words, thought is quantized.

We revisit again the work of David Bohm (1983) who formulated a hidden variable theory of quantum mechanics that postulated an implicate and an explicate reality based on the same kind of idea. The explicate reality is manifested reality which arises from its unmanifest potential ground, the implicate reality. In other words nature (*prakriti* or *maya*) or energy (*shakti* – as opposed to consciousness or *shiva* in the Tantric formulation) has manifest (or kinetic) and unmanifest (or potential) forms with a process of "in-winking" and "out-winking" back and forth between them. When we talk about *nirodhah* we mean the subsiding of the kinetic activity of the mind field back into its potential ground, not the annihilation of the mind.

But one should be careful of these metaphors. Bohm's implicate/explicate realities have been widely applied in New Age thinking as though true without any evidence to support them. Indeed hidden variables theories in quantum mechanics have been ruled out. Here we most certainly do not wish in any way to imply that Bohm's implicate/explicate realities apply in any way to the mind field. There is no such evidence available to our knowledge. This is just a convenient metaphor to help understand a concept.

States of the Mind Field

The word *nirodhah* raises the issue of the five states of mind described in Vyasa's commentary to YS I.1: *kshipta* (disturbed), *mudha* (somnolent, stupified), *vikshipta* (distracted – away from meditation), *ekagra* (one-pointed), and *niruddha* (controlled – related to the word *nirodhah*).

Swami Veda Bharati puts it this way:

> We experience, ordinarily, only two states of mind: *kshiptum* and *mudham*. Both of them are simultaneous. *Kshiptum*: "totally distracted." This thought now, that sensation then, another emotion, another something, attraction, distraction, aversion, moment-to-moment goes on. These random movements of the mind do not let the mind be alert. So while a small part of the mind remains thus and agitated, the remaining vast area of the mind remains in a state of *mudham*: "stupor." Unaware, not awake, comatose – we're all in a coma! That's why we do not perceive; that's why we do not understand, do not understand from where the other party is speaking, do not understand what is the cause of that person's anger, do not understand what pain and anguish has caused someone to make a negative and unfair remark about you.

8

Kriya Yoga

The practice of the Chariot of *Sadhana* is based not only in the eight rungs of Patanjali's Raja Yoga, but also in Kriya Yoga, the Yoga of (transformative) action or of practices, as described in his *Yoga-Sutra* II.1. This is not to be confused with the different kriya yogas of the same name described by Paramahansa Yogananda, or Babaji's Kriya Yoga from the Tamil Yoga Siddha lineage (Govindan, 2000), or by the Bihar School of Yoga (Satyananda Saraswati, 1981). Patanjali's Kriya Yoga consists of the last three of the five *niyamas* (observances or restraints and disciplines) constituting the second rung of Ashtanga Yoga (the eightfold rungs of Raja Yoga): *tapas* (intense practice), *svadhyaya* (self-study) and *ishvara pranidhana* (surrender or devotion to the Lord). Feuerstein (1989, p 60) conceptualizes Kriya Yoga and the Chariot as follows:

Kriya Yoga

| **abhyasa** | **vairagya** |

| **tapas   svadhyaya   ishvara-pranidhana** | **apara-vairagya   para-vairagya** |

He proposes (Feuerstein, 1979) that the second book of Patanjali's *Yoga-Sutra* is a blend of two independent traditions. One is Patanjali's Kriya Yoga and the other is the eightfold path of Ashtanga Yoga which is more popularly associated with Patanjali. However, Kriya Yoga is not to be considered as a preliminary to the practice of the eightfold path, but is a full tradition of its own and Patanjali's teaching proper (Feuerstein, 1979). The various methods of transforming consciousness into pure Self-awareness are given in the first chapter (*pada*) of the *Yoga-Sutra*. The commentator Vachaspati Mishra observes that the means to Yoga given in the first chapter are practice and dispassion in the most general sense, but they are only possible for the advanced and prepared practitioner. Until so qualified, one needs the means taught in the second chapter or *sadhana pada* (*sadhana* here means path to realization) in order to purify the *sattva*, especially of the mind field. Beginners start in chapter two, not chapter one.

Vairagya is conceptualized in the *Yoga-Sutra* as occurring in two stages: a relative renunciation (*apara*) in the manifest world progressing to an absolute renunciation (*para*) experienced in higher *samadhi*. We agree with Feuerstein (1989, p 60) that the three means of Kriya Yoga come under the category of practice (*abhyasa*), and that *tapas* does not refer to a specific practice. Rather, *tapas*, like *abhyasa* and *vairagya*, should be considered as a general or formal category which contains all the exercises other than those under *svadhyaya* or *ishvara-pranidhana*. We also consider the components (which are not stages as is so often thought) of the eightfold path as subcategories under *abhyasa*.

Let us review briefly these components of Kriya Yoga, Patanjali's original yoga, as pictured in the diagram above. The spiritual path is sometimes conceptualized as a journey. Yet paradoxically it is a journey without a destination, in the sense that we are not trying to acquire something we lack, but rather trying to uncover something we already are. To make a journey one needs a map and a method. *Tapas* is the method or praxis. It describes the way to practice in general, and does not refer to any specific practice. It tells not what to practice, but how. *Tapas* is intense practice, practice with an intensity that leads one beyond one's limitations. What is practiced here is the eightfold path of Raja Yoga. *Tapas* has the connotation of asceticism and the meaning of straightening by fire.

Ballentine (1999) refers to its special meaning as a Tantric key to transmuting energy, where it is used to transform habitual impulses that are relevant to the practice of the *yamas* and the *niyamas*. One may consciously choose not to express an urge to act out an old habit, regardless of the discomfort of its urgency. This is not about avoiding experiencing the urge by suppressing or denying it. One intentionally observes, witnesses, allows, accepts and contains the building discomfort, refusing to be moved by it. One remains a witness. Although one may feel that one will "explode" with the growing urgency of the energy, with persistence there comes a point when that energy and urgency burst into another channel. The use of the spinal breath in meditation helps prepare a basis for that energy to explode upward into a higher *chakra* to produce exhilaration and a sense of empowerment.

This is reminiscent of a Buddhist method. When a problem arises – e.g., a sexual urge, greed or anger – note its presence with fullest awareness three times – e.g., say inwardly, "anger, anger, anger." Then go on with what you are doing. Do nothing with the anger; simply note it three times and with this awareness it will subside. It can only grip you if you are unconscious, if it is a conditioned response that carries you away. Full awareness objectifies the anger and separates you from it. Our current culture teaches us to repress problems. We become unconscious of them, forget them, and think they do not exist. But they re-express as conditioned responses with the right trigger and context. Instead make them absolutely conscious and focus on them and they melt. The Buddha's disciples were taught to do this with everything. It is another aspect of living in the Presence, in the moment. Another related approach in deep meditation is following a thought back to its origin and dissolving it into the mind field.

Svadhyaya or self-study creates the map or theoria for the journey. This process uses the *buddhi* faculty to know the Self. It asks the question, Who am I? This is done by learning to discriminate between what is Self and what is non-Self. You objectify all levels of the personality to distinguish what is Self or pure Subjectivity. What you can perceive in the mind as an object is not your essential Self. Pure Subjectivity cannot be made an object by definition. This is the *via negativa* or process of *neti neti* (not this, not that) of Jnana Yoga and Vedanta. Ramana Maharshi's (1988) process of "Who am I?" inquiry is relevant here. *Svadhyaya* involves three processes: study of revealed scriptures, repetition of one's *mantra*, and witnessing or observing one's mental psychodynamics. All three of these processes help the aspirant to discriminate between the Self (i.e., the Centre of Consciousness) and what is non-Self.

Ishvara pranidhana means devotion or surrender to the Lord or Supreme Being. It is what is called practicing the presence of God in the Christian tradition. It is unconditional love and the realm of devotional or Bhakti Yoga which comes to see the Lord everywhere. Here it means surrendering all fruits of one's actions to the Lord. It also embodies the idea of letting go of ego and mental concerns, as enshrined in the phrase, "Let go and let God." The form of the Lord that is chosen in this act of worship is a personal choice. That form becomes a symbol for what is beyond form and cannot be grasped by the mind.

Vairagya comes in two stages. Preliminary detachment (*apara-vairagya*) is toward objects seen in the external world. Superior detachment (*para-vairagya*) is to things in the heavens and the subtle worlds (for example, the *devas*). The ultimate aim of detachment is total transcendence of desire, craving or attachment to any manifestation, subtle or gross, so that one can live fully conscious of the Higher Reality. The ultimate *vairagya* is *kaivalya* (aloneness or enlightenment) as total transcendence of manifestation. This is the identity shift from the small self or ego to the transcendent Self. Swami Hariharananda Bharati has said not to let go of desire, but rather of the objects of desire. He describes love as desireless desire. Devotion is desire without an object.

9

Kriya Yoga in the YOGA-SUTRA *1*

Let us look now a little more closely at these *sutras* in Patanjali's *Yoga-Sutra* which directly describe Kriya Yoga. These are *sutras* 1, 2, 32 and 43–45 of chapter (*pada*) II. Here we use the translation and commentary by Swami Veda Bharati (2001) which is the most comprehensive and which reflects the Himalayan Tradition.

> II.1 *tapah-svadhyayeshvara-pranidhanani kriya-yogah.*
> "Ascetic observance, silent recitation, self-study of scriptures and *japa*, and surrender of all practices and acts to God constitute the yoga of practices (*kriya-yoga*)."
>
> II.2 *samadhi-bhavanarthah klesha-tanu-karanarthash cha.*
> "[*kriya-yoga* is practiced] for the purpose of developing and nurturing *samadhi* and for attenuation [and elimination] of afflictions."

The Yoga in chapter one of the *Yoga-Sutra* is for those who have tasted *samadhi* and in whom both practice (*abhyasa*) and detachment (*vairagya*) can arise and be worked with in the mind. In other words it is for appropriately qualified (*adhikara*) aspirants who have prepared the ground by prior practice. But others begin here with Kriya Yoga, a practical Yoga for a mind which is still involved in the external world. This is Kriya Yoga, the Yoga of practices. We have learned above that it consists of three components. The first is *tapas*, which traditionally refers to ascetic observances and efforts toward self-purification. The actions (*karma*), afflictions (*kleshas*), as well as residues (*samskaras*) and propensities (*vasanas*) that lie deep in the unconscious mind constitute a beginning-less chain so that these impurities are complex. Moreover, objects of attraction are always present in the world to stimulate, evoke and excite their expression further. These ascetic observances are practiced only so long as they purify the mind and make it pleasant (YS I.33, 34), but not to the extent of injuring health.

The second component is *svadhyaya*, which traditionally consists of three parts. The first is self-study. The second involves the study of scriptures that can lead one to liberation. And the third is repetition or *japa* of *mantras* like OM or one's *guru mantra* received through initiation, for the purpose of purification.

Finally the third component is *ishvara pranidhana* or surrender to God. One offers all these *kriyas* (Yoga practices and other acts) to the Supreme *Guru* (YS I.23, 26). Additionally one renounces the results of these practices and the fruits (*phala*) of other acts.

The second *sutra* expresses the twofold purpose of performing the Yoga of practices. The first is to bring about *samadhi* and the second is to thin down and then eliminate the afflictions (*kleshas*).

First, Kriya Yoga has the purpose of producing, developing, cultivating and nurturing *samadhi* (*samadhi-bhavana*: *bhavana* from the verb root "to be" meaning "to cause or bring into being"). This implies that the afflictions (*kleshas*) are not solid and strong, but have some gaps. One might use the metaphor of the sun and a cloudy sky. If the clouds are solid without breaks, the sun cannot be seen. But if there are breaks in the clouds, glimpses of the sun can be had more and more as the clouds begin to clear. Kriya Yoga is practiced without desire for its fruits (*nish-kama*) as a form of Karma Yoga. It purifies the mind of attachments and aversions by blocking negative thinking (*vrittis*) and also by increasing the strength of *sattva* in the mind field. The essence of the mind field is *sattvic*. It is the first constituent formed in the human personality as the *buddhi* (intelligence), which is its most *sattvic* component and the subtlest evolute of *prakriti*. As such it is the primary point of contact between *purusha* and the products of *prakriti*. The rising of *sattva* means that the *buddhi* is being purified. This leads to the mind field becoming progressively concentrated (*ekagra*). As this process proceeds the *kleshas* become attenuated naturally and effortlessly.

The second purpose of attenuation of the afflictions (*kleshas*) implies a reduction of their power and influence but not their extinction. One still has to perform one's duties appropriate to one's phase of life (*ashrama*) and so some *karma* remains. Attenuation blocks effects arising from causes, loosens and rarefies the *kleshas* so that they arise less frequently, and reduces and eliminates anything that can block the arising of discriminative wisdom (*viveka-khyati*). The words "knowledge" and "wisdom" here are used differently than in ordinary speech where they refer to mental content processed from the external world such as information, learning and erudition, experience, understanding, good judgment, discretion or sagacity. The word *khyati* has more the sense of awareness. Here it refers to an internal experience or direct awareness that the *purusha* or Centre of Consciousness is distinct and separate from the *sattva* of the mind field. In other words the Centre of Consciousness or Presence opens as a direct inner experience and is clearly distinguished for what It really is.

Referring to our metaphor above, the sun is no longer obscured by the remaining clouds in the sky of the mind. The process must continue even when the *kleshas* are thinned until they are burnt finally by the fire of this discrimination. For burnt seeds can sprout no further. The sky must be cleared of clouds and even of the capacity to produce more of them. When the *kleshas* are attenuated and finally eliminated this realized wisdom (*prajna*) of the experience of the Centre of Consciousness is no longer affected by them and one has crystallized and established one's awareness in the Presence. Now can begin the dissolution of the devolutes of *prakriti* in the reverse order of their appearance through the stages of *samadhi*. Note that to be effective, for Kriya Yoga to produce attenuation leading eventually to eradication of the *kleshas*, it must be practiced for a long time, without interruption and with care as described in YS I.14. No instant enlightenment here! This process is very gradual over many years of faithful practice.

It is important to note that there are two simultaneous processes at work here. One is attenuation of the *kleshas* through the practice of Kriya Yoga, which in terms of the chariot of *sadhana* comes under *vairagya* (detachment). The other is acquisition of discriminative wisdom, the opening of the Centre of Consciousness as an awareness distinguished from the *sattva* of the *buddhi*, the subtlest level of the mind – the cognition of the Presence as a direct experience. This is the *abhyasa* (practice) wheel of the chariot. Later we will explore in depth *ishvara pranidhana* as presented in the first *pada* of the *Yoga-Sutra* as a method of meditative absorption into the revealed Centre of Consciousness. This discriminative wisdom completes the removal of the ultimate causes of the *kleshas* in the mind field.

The metaphor is that of burning seeds so they can no longer sprout. These *samskaras* (residues, seeds, subtle causes) are dissolved into their causes and rendered ineffective. As long as the mind field continues to exist, its power or potency (*shakti*) to maintain the *kleshas* remains active. Each *samskara* has a potency inherent in its cause which remains as long as the cause does. This potency has to be "burned" by the discriminative wisdom. In this way the power of past *karma* to produce rebirth is destroyed, as is any future potential of the *kleshas*. Then liberation in life (*jivanmukti*) can occur. Thus Kriya Yoga attenuates the *kleshas* so that the awareness of the Centre of Consciousness can arise. This discrimination then burns the *kleshas* so that the mind field can no longer produce *samskaras* since they become like infertile burnt seeds. Going back to our metaphor of the sky, Kriya Yoga very gradually thins and disburses the clouds that cover the sun until it shines forth in a stable manner. Its heat then "dries" the sky until it loses its potential to even produce clouds.

The role of Kriya Yoga is in a sense indirect. It gradually wears the impurities of the *kleshas* down over a long time until the mind is subtle enough to be able to cognize the Centre of Consciousness. Kriya Yoga weakens the *kleshas* by reducing attachment and aversion to lessen the mind's reactivity, and thereby it weakens ignorance (*avidya*): i.e., it expands and deepens awareness. When the practitioner observes these gradual changes there is further impetus to practice and a virtuous cycle revolves.

The effects of Kriya Yoga are both experienced and hidden. One experiences increasing control of the mind, but at the same time the *sattvic* essence of the personality is progressively purified unconsciously below the level of experience. The mind gradually becomes subtle enough to reflect the Presence, the Centre of Consciousness, and that wisdom burns the seeds. As the impurities or opposites to *sattva* in the mind field are removed, *sattva* is strengthened in wisdom (*prajna*) and discriminating awareness (*khyati*) through *abhyasa* and *vairagya*, until it is no longer overcome and obscured by these impurities. Then a state of liberation in life ensues (*jivanmukti*). As one progresses through the lower *samadhis* there is a dissolution of devolutes of *prakriti* into their causes as the objects of concentration become subtler and subtler. A further virtuous cycle begins to function. The increasing realization of the Centre of Consciousness (*sakshat-kara*) dissolves more of the *kleshas* into their causes, which, in turn, increases the amount of the stream of discriminative wisdom that can flow uninterrupted by the *kleshas*. The resulting realizations and wisdom become more refined (awareness expands and deepens) until the discriminating wisdom of the separateness of *purusha* from the *asmita* (ego sense of the *sattvic buddhi*) is realized and the Presence awakens. Ultimately with the identity shift there is liberation while yet living (*jivanmukti*).

10

Kriya Yoga in the YOGA-SUTRA *2*

The text now elaborates the *niyamas* that make up Kriya Yoga in YS II.32 and 43–45.

> II.32 *shaucha-santosha-tapah-svadhyayeshvara-pra-ni-dhanani niyamah.*
> "These are the five *niyamas* (restraints and disciplines): mental purity, self-study of inspiring texts and *japa*, and surrender to God."
> II.43 *kayendriya-siddhir a-shuddhi-kshayat tapasah.*
> "From ascetic practice, through the elimination of impurities [there occurs] mastery over the body and the senses."
> II.44 *svadhyayad ishtar-devata-sam-pra-yoga.*
> "Through self-study and *japa* one attains concert with one's chosen deity."
> II.45 *samadhi-siddhir ishvara-pra-ni-dhanat.*
> "Through surrender to God accomplishment of *samadhi* [ensues]."
>
> Veda Bharati, 2001

Sutra 32 introduces the *niyamas* which turn the aspirant away from desires that lead to rebirths and by which he or she is moved in the direction of desireless actions that lead to liberation. Ordinary intelligence and common sense perceive these as right action. Traditionally each *niyama* is thought to depend on the other in sequence.

Shaucha (purity) is both external and internal. External purity involves cleansing the body with soap and water as well as the ingestion of pure foods, avoiding eating stale or rotten food. Internal purification refers to mental purification. It is a purification of sentiments and emotions such as frenzy, pride, intolerance, envy, niggardliness, jealousy, negative thinking, attraction or aversion. One washes these all off by cultivating the opposite positive sentiments. In external purification we think of avoiding the ingestion of stale or rotten food. But there is an analogy at the mental level where one takes care in terms of what one puts through the senses into the mind, especially vision and hearing. Violent or immoral television, movies, video games, books, or loud and raucous music would be examples to avoid. Indeed as one grows in sensitivity one will find these pursuits increasingly unpleasant and emotionally disturbing, and will have no difficulty letting them go.

Santosha (contentment) means to be happy and satisfied with what is received without desiring more than is absolutely necessary for one's life journey. It is the absence of the desire to grasp. The Centre of Consciousness provides a growing and perpetual sense of fullness that leads to non-desire for any undertaking. Here there is no desire, in contrast to *aparigraha* (nonindulgence) where desire arises, but is rejected because one sees the flaws in gaining the object of desire.

Now come the three *niyamas* that make up Kriya Yoga. *Tapas* is often defined as ascetic endeavor (ascesis). But here it does not equate with the grim rigors of strict asceticism as we might think of the word in the modern West. Rather it involves forbearance without aversion to the pains and discomforts of the pairs of opposites (*dvandva*) as long as this is conducive to Yoga. The word *dvandva* means "two by two" which refers to any pairs, of which only some are true opposites like heat and cold, and some are not like hunger and thirst. It includes standing versus sitting and implies resisting the discomfort of maintaining either posture absolutely motionless, such as the sitting meditation postures. *Tapas* includes other things. It includes worship and honoring of deities, priests, the twice-born, the *guru*, etc. Some authorities include the drying up of the body with special fasts which are done only as prescribed in the scriptures. It can include the practice of the *yamas*, *niyamas* and other limbs of Patanjali's eightfold yoga. It can also include the practice of one's *dharma* with its challenges like special fasts. Others include the practice of silence. Ordinary silence involves not speaking. But there is an extreme form referred to as wood-silence in which there is no communication of intent or desire even with physical or facial gestures. *Tapas* becomes effective even as one starts and is in the process of perfecting it.

Sutras II.43–45 not only describe each of the *niyamas* constituting Kriya Yoga, but like the *sutras* describing the other *yamas* and *niyamas*, also explain the accomplishment (*siddhi*) of each and its fruit. *Tapas* perfects the body and the senses and brings mastery when practice is stabilized leading to an unveiling of the *siddhis* (accomplishments, powers) and a perfecting of the senses which can then detect things which are subtle, distant or concealed (clairvoyance, clairaudience). It does so by removing *tamas* which acts as a veil of impurities (nonvirtue and sin as well as the afflictions (*kleshas*) of the mind). These block or veil the *siddhis* which are always ever existent. The *siddhis* are not something added that we lack, but potentials that we all have that are unveiled.

A better word to describe what is meant by the ascetic practice of *tapas* would be "discipline." Prolonged disciplined intensive practice is an essential undertaking for genius in any field no matter the level of intrinsic talent. This is true for musicians, mathematicians, surgeons, or Olympic athletes to name but a few examples, and it is also true for yogis. We live near a training facility for Olympic cross country skiers. Every day during the spring, summer and fall months athletes are out practicing on the roads in our area from dawn to dusk on their roller skis: back and forth, back and forth. Their presence challenges us with a constant reminder about the strength of our own commitment to spiritual practice. This continuous and intense practice gently but firmly pushes and expands the boundaries of one's capacities. It structures one's lifestyle. Above all, the practice of *tapas* should not be so extreme as to disturb the body's balance.

Svadhyaya refers to self-study (see also YS I.28, II.44). Traditionally the practice is twofold. The first involves the studying of scriptures like the *Upanishads* and reciting them. It also includes reciting laudatory hymns (*stotras*). This becomes a preparation for the second which is the *japa* (silent repetition) of the *mantra* of *saguna* deities (those bound by qualifications) or of OM. It includes cultivating and absorbing its meaning (*pranidhana*, equivalent to practicing the presence of God). Some authorities define *japa* as reciting the *Upanishads* for a period of three years in order to conquer the senses. Then the practitioner proceeds to the *japa* of OM.

Some further comments are in order regarding *japa*. The godhead is fundamentally *nirguna*: free of all conditioning, attributes or qualifications and beyond all qualification and manifestation, yet immanent in the universe. This *nirguna* Godhead has emanations which are *saguna* deities: qualified, delimited celestial beings who control and confer limited powers on a cosmic scale.

As above, so below. Some psychological theories ascribe parts to our personalities which are resident in the other-than-conscious mind, subroutines that carry out habitual actions like driving a car. They can be communicated with hypnotically and because they are brought to consciousness in this process they seem to behave like little people or subpersonalities within a person. The cosmic person can be thought of in the same way. It has "parts" which are the universal forces which carry out its activities, and because they share consciousness they behave like celestial beings.

Concentration and worship of these beings with *japa* of their *mantras* can liberate a *sadhaka* (spiritual practitioner) by bringing him or her through *samprajnata* to *asamprajnata samadhi*. This is the *siddhi* of *svadhyaya* and its fruit. Successful *japa* of the *mantra* or one's favorite deity (*ishta-devata*) leads to the deity showing itself to the devotee so that one can converse and receive grace directly.

Success means that the practice is carried out uninterruptedly, with intense feeling, for a long time, while contemplating its meaning (*bhavana*) by cultivating it and impressing it upon oneself until it becomes one's own nature. Indeed this can be done with more than just the *ishta-devata*, but with any higher order beings like *rishis* (ancient sages, the first mind-borne offspring of the Progenitor), *devas* (deities) and other celestial beings, *siddhas* (disembodied saints who are often seen at their abode in sacred places), saints and angels. Indeed one's worldly affairs may be taken care of by the grace of these higher beings to give one more time to practice.

It is worth emphasizing again that *siddhis* obtained through *tapas* or *japa* are not additions to or attainments by a personality. They represent an unveiling of what is already there by the removal of obstructing impediments like a blindfold removed from the eyes lets one see the sun which was always there.

Finally comes *ishvara pranidhana* or the practice of the presence of God. There are various interpretations of the term in this *sutra*. For Vyasa it is surrendering all acts to God or to the Supreme *Guru*. He specifically excludes the interpretation given in *sutra* I.28 which is equivalent to the practice of the presence of God. It is excluded here because the practice of the presence of God is a meditation. Swami Veda Bharati (2001) interprets it here as surrendering all acts to God, and not the contemplation of the Godhead. I take the position that I am not the doer and that God does the act with my mind. I Transfer to God all claims that I am the agent of my actions, I offer Him worship, and I surrender to Him all meritorious (and some would say both good and bad) acts, prescribed or unprescribed, without expectation of fruits – even the *yamas* and *niyamas*. It is in this sense that all acts are surrendered to God. The important point is the renunciation of all intent and desire for the fruit of action; one becomes desireless (*nishkama*). This is, of course, a core feature of Karma Yoga. It includes all of the practices of Yoga. Thus of the *yamas* and *niyamas*, *ishvara pranidhana* is considered to be the principal one.

This practice soon merges into the meditative practice of the presence of God. To be in good health (*sva-stha*) means here to dwell in oneself. In all conditions one maintains the awareness of the *Atman* and remains established in the Supreme Self (*parama-atman*) because the process of surrendering acts to God leads to union (*yoga*) with Him. Surrender done in this way leads to a constant remembrance of the Centre of Consciousness. "The yogi abides in the consciousness of the singular awareness of being full and blissful in himself as its witness, and sees that 'I am indeed that *Brahman* alone.'" (Swami Veda Bharati, 2001, p 501). This is *brahma-atma-pranidhana*: maintaining the self in *Brahman* from which various benefits flow. Worries and concerns (*vitarkas*) are eliminated without one's having to cultivate their opposites. The residues of actions in the mind (*samskaras*) as well as the actions stemming from them start to wane and the seeds of the propensities (*vasanas*) are eliminated. The yogi experiences the joy of liberation and is satiated and becomes desireless. Swami Veda Bharati (2001) points to a sequence for *ishvara pranidhana*. Surrendering all acts to God leads to union with God and the attainment of perfection. Then one realizes the life principle (*jiva-tattva*) and the impediments are removed. This, of course, is the core of Bhakti Yoga. We will have much more to say about this process later as the key to *abhyasa*.

But there is a catch. This is not about just doing what you please and then mentally tossing the activities in God's direction so you will be absolved of your intentional mistakes. To practice this way means that one commits always to carry out right actions in the right way and in the right place and time as best one can at one's level of awareness. One cannot ignore inner guidance and kill the conscience.

Sutra II.45 deals with the *siddhi* of *ishvara pranidhana* which is *samadhi*. There is much interpretive variation in the commentaries of this *sutra* (Swami Veda Bharati, 2001). As described here *ishvara pranidhana* is a special devotion (*bhakti*) that offers all one's acts to God without desire for their fruits. It means carrying out one's duty without having a hidden agenda and without seeking benefits as a reward or payment to oneself. The *sutra* says the result ultimately is *samadhi*. The grace of God and *guru* repels the afflictions (*kleshas*) and obstacles (*antarayas*) and fully awakens *samadhi*.

Samadhi as described here is awakened, manifested, but not created, because it is an already existing universal attribute of the mind field. *Samadhi* here means a resolution, harmonization and eventually integration and assimilation of mental conflicts and dualities first through the *guru's* teaching, and then resulting in a clear and pleasant mind field which is *samprajnata* with the full wisdom of the awakened intuition. Its accomplishment involves not only effort, but also loving devotion and eventually the grace of God through the *guru*. To be successful it needs a unified concentration (*samyama*) leading to meditation (*dharana* to *dhyana*) and then to *pranidhana* in which the *sadhaka* surrenders totally to the grace and presence of God in *samadhi*.

In the commentaries there is controversy over whether all the *angas* (the eight limbs of Raja Yoga of which the *yamas* and *niyamas* are the first two) are also needed or whether devotion alone is enough (Swami Veda Bharati, 2001). The opinion is that both can do it, but that they complement each other so that practicing them together reaches the goal more quickly. It is recommended that one practice all the *yamas* and *niyamas* to attenuate the afflictions (*kleshas*), and that neglect of any single one may render them all impotent.

As a prescription for behavior the *yamas* and *niyamas* may seem incomplete. But all the Yogas and other activities of practice are included under *tapas* (Swami Veda Bharati, 2001, p 503). Some authorities consider the *yamas* to be great vows (*maha-vratas*) which are universal and not constrained by either time or space. The *niyamas*, however, are not. The Yoga of practice (Kriya Yoga) is not a vow and its components are considered to be delimited by time and space. There is argument about whether *ishvara pranidhana* is the most important of the *yamas* and *niyamas*, or whether the *yamas* are the most important and the *niyamas* less so (Swami Veda Bharati, 2001).

There is an underlying idea in all of this discussion. It is not that the enlightened state is something that we lack and that we must acquire it through effort and grace. Rather the state of perfection is already ours, but it is covered up and obscured from our awareness by impurities in the mind field. Let us explore this idea a little further by an analogy that we might with a touch of humor call the floating cork metaphor of enlightenment.

Consider a cork floating in a vessel of water. Because of its buoyancy it floats naturally. Indeed to get it below the surface of water you have to actively push it under and hold it there. What if you were to attach to it some weights like the little lead weights that fishermen use? If you attached enough of these little weights eventually they would overcome the buoyancy of the cork and it would begin to sink as you added more weights. The level it reached in the water would be directly determined by the amount of weight that you added. A few weights and it would stabilize just below the surface. Many more weights and it would sink close to the bottom of the water before its level stabilized.

The weights are a metaphor for the obscurations and impurities that weigh down and slow the vibrational frequency of the mind field. The depth of the water is analogous to a vibrational spectrum with the highest frequencies at the surface and the lowest, slowest frequencies at the bottom. As the weights are gradually removed representing the beneficial effects of *sadhana* as well as grace, the inherent buoyancy of the cork exerts itself more and more and it rises up the scale of vibration from the depths of the water towards the surface. At some point it will come close enough to the surface that the surface even becomes visible and the water becomes clearer and more filled with light in contrast to the dim murkiness at the bottom of the water – perhaps a metaphor for the dawning of the Centre of Consciousness. When the weights are all finally removed the cork will burst through the surface into the air and the light of the sun above the water. One does not have to push the cork back up to the surface of the water. Its natural tendency is to do this itself through its inherent buoyancy. One need only remove the impurities that weigh it down.

This is why Yoga *sadhana* is often couched in words like "purification." There are other similar metaphors that are used for this same idea, such as removing obscuring shades from a lamp, or polishing away dust and impurities from the surface of a mirror until it can reflect perfectly. The underlying idea is always the same. What we seek is already there, we need only uncover it.

Samahita Yoga Includes Kriya Yoga

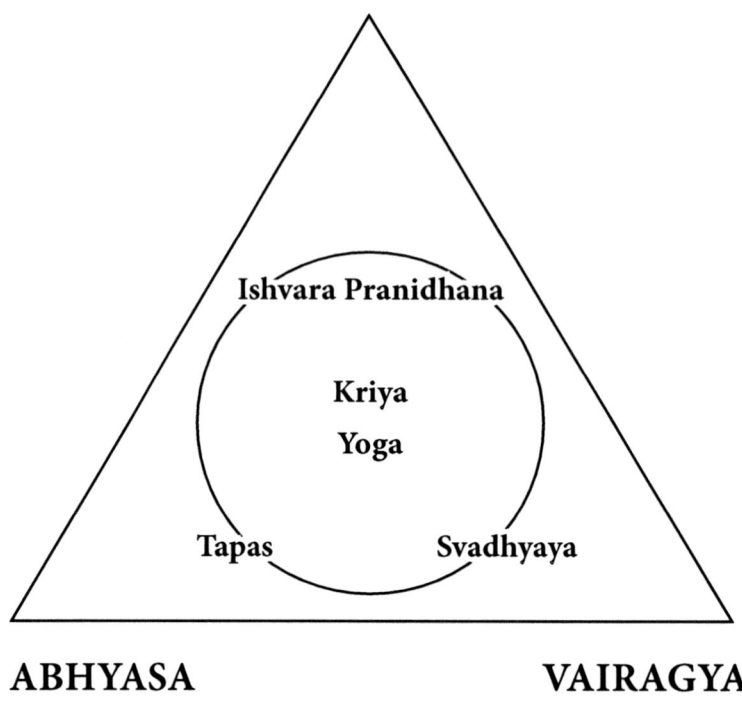

Figure 10.1 The Organizing Principle behind *Samahita* Yoga

We have spent some time discussing Kriya Yoga. The reason is that it lies at the basis of *Samahita* Yoga, the Yoga of harmony or equanimity. This idea is shown in figure 10.1. *Samahita* Yoga expresses the idea of the Chariot of *Sadhana* consisting of *abhyasa* and *vairagya* as described in the first chapter of Patanjali's *Yoga-Sutra*. This is represented by the triangle with the goal of the Centre of Consciousness at its apex. But this practice of the chariot is built on a foundation of two further levels. Kriya Yoga lies at a level in the middle and is a convenient organizing principle for our practice. We are all practicing the components of Kriya Yoga when one thinks of it as the map, the method and the goal. But *tapas* includes within it the basic level which is all of the practices that make up the eight limbs of Patanjali's Yoga discussed in chapters two and three of his *Yoga-Sutra*. This of course is the Classical or Ashtanga Yoga that makes up Raja Yoga. The diagram presents a way of organizing and integrating our thinking about our practice on all of these levels from the most basic to that of the most subtle, all directed toward the apex of the triangle, the Centre of Consciousness.

11

The YAMAS: *Moral Foundations of Yoga*

A major children's hospital calls a press conference to announce that they are trying to find over 2600 children who were operated on by a single surgeon since 1990. It was recently discovered that the surgeon was HIV positive. She became ill and died. She was turned in by a colleague as an "ethical issue."

A young female pop star marries her boyfriend and then has the marriage annulled after 55 hours.

A physician receives a research manuscript he knows nothing about from a drug company. The envelope contains a substantial honorarium for which he is asked to sign the paper so that it can be submitted to a peer reviewed scientific journal for publication under his name.

A local college introduces a regulation that students must submit all essays in every course to a web site that will analyze them for plagiarism (http://turnitin.com).

A major religious organization pays out close to half a billion dollars to settle claims of sexual abuse by priests.

After reviewing the American tragedy of 9/11, the ensuing Afghanistan and Iraq wars and the continuing attacks of suicide bombers worldwide, a television news commentator wonders if World War III will be waged against terrorism.

Today we live in a morally and ethically challenged world. Magazines and newspapers are filled with stories of corruption, sex and violence. Just flipping through the television channels for ten minutes on a typical evening will reveal physical violence and murder; explicit sexuality if not rape; endless commercials, all with a hard sell; soap operas, sitcoms and grainy reality shows filled with interpersonal manipulation and conflict; even the cartoons are often violent. People bemoan the growing incivility of modern society, especially of our youth, as well as the greed and commercialism that drive our economy. Enron, WorldCom, Vivendi and now Parmalat have become household words for corporate scandal. Many feel the world has entered a deepening shadow following the events of 9/11. A recent survey by Gallup International indicates that over 40% of people through-out the world, especially Canadians (57%), are remarkably fearful about the tenuous state of global security now and in the future because of terrorism, new disease epidemics and poor economic performance (Kennedy, 2004).

Setting the Context

The *yamas* and the *niyamas* constitute the first two limbs of Patanjali's Classical or *ashtanga-yoga*. The *yamas* are non-harming (*ahimsa*), truthfulness (*satya*), non-stealing (*asteya*), continence (*brahmacarya*) and non-possessiveness (*aparigraha*) (YS II.30). The *niyamas* are purity (*shauca*), contentment (*santosha*), austerity (*tapas*), study (*svadhyaya*) and devotion to the Lord (*ishvara pranidhana*) (YS II.32). Together they make up the "ten commandments" of Yoga. The *yamas* and *niyamas* have been called the "don'ts" and "do's," the restraints and observances of Yoga respectively. All major religions and all authentic spiritual paths assume a foundation of ethical behavior and moral discipline which for Classical Yoga constitutes the five *yamas*. These are moral obligations that make up the great vow (*maha-vrata*) that are to be practiced regardless of time, place, circumstance or social status (YS II.31).

The *yamas* have the purpose of controlling instinctual behavior, especially the survival instinct, and to rechannel it in service to higher purposes (Feuerstein, 2001, p 245). Relationships are the essence of worldly life. One wants to behave in a way that does not create external disturbances that interfere with one's spiritual maturation and progress by creating negative *karma*. By following the proscriptions of the *yamas* the yogi regulates his or her social interactions in a way that is beneficial and supportive of spiritual *sadhana*. They harmonize our relationships.

Our spiritual preceptor, Sri Swami Rama, would often say that we are each citizens of two worlds. The *yamas* deal with our outer world. But the *niyamas* deal with our inner world. They harmonize our relationship to transcendental Reality and help us with our inner transformation. As reviewed above, the last three: *tapas, svadhyaya* and *ishvara pranidhana*, constitute *kriya yoga*, the Yoga of transformative action (YS II.1). It should be practiced for bringing about *samadhi* and for minimizing the afflictions (*kleshas*) (YS II.2).

Although our emphasis here will be the *yamas*, both the *yamas* and the *niyamas* are to be practiced together along with the other limbs of Patanjali's Yoga in an integrated way. Initially one works with them as practices. The enlightened sage expresses them spontaneously as a natural state of being where they are totally trustworthy. Until one reaches that elevated state they are a means of "raising life to the level of your meditation," as so eloquently phrased by Swami Veda Bharati.

A further five moral precepts are described in later Yoga texts (Feuerstein, 2001, p 246). They include compassion (*daya*), moral integrity (*arjava*), patience (*kshama*), steadfastness in being true to one's principles (*dhriti*) and a meager diet (*mitahara*) since overeating can be considered as theft. Related to ethical practices are those put forth to define qualification (*adhikara*) in spiritual practice (Jerry & Jerry, 2001, p 38; Veda Bharati, 1986, p 66). Vedanta defines a qualified student as one who has practiced the "six treasures" (*shat-sampat*): *shama* (calmness, tranquility), *dama* (temperance), *uparati* (a spirit of renunciation), *titiksha* (fortitude, forbearance), *samadhana* (power of concentration of the mind), and *shraddha* (faith) (Veda Bharati, 1986, p 480).

In addition to these six, Johari (1986, p 9) adds an additional six for control over one's animal or biological nature: *daksha* (intelligence), *jitendriya* (sensory control), *sarva hinsa vinirmukta* (abstention from violence), *sarva prani hitata* (concern for universal welfare), *shuchi* (purity), and *astikya* (belief in truth as *vidya* (knowledge), *veda* (body of knowledge) and God).

He speculates that they coordinate the various phylogenetic levels of the brain: the brain stem (vegetative autonomic functions), Paul MacLean's R-complex (1984; Papez, 1937) now known as the limbic system (emotion) (LeDoux, 2002), and the cerebral cortex (consciousness, inspiration, abstract thinking, musical composition, reading and writing). This is consistent with the idea expressed above that the *yamas* rechannel our instinctual nature. Johari (1986, p 6) speculates further that, in general, purification practices which would include the *yamas*, energize the body by freeing psychophysical energy and creating electrochemical balance. With an integral practice of *ashtanga-yoga*, *pranayama* stimulates the brain stem, while ritual and discipline are thought to stimulate the R-complex. *Dhyana* including *mantra* and *japa* as well as visualization, stimulate the cerebral cortex. He proposes that together all of these factors coordinate all levels of the brain in all three states of waking, dreaming and deep sleep (Rama, 1982b; Nikhilananda, 1987a), leading the aspirant to superconsciousness or *turiya*.

Having defined and set the context we shall now examine each of the *yamas* in more depth. Our approach will be eclectic and will address four themes. 1) If they are taught at all, the *yamas* are often presented by teachers in a cursory manner like a set of rules, a laundry list of "don'ts," so that one can get on with more interesting things like postures. To try to follow them as mere rules for behavior without a substantial grasp of their psychophysiological origins is naïve. 2) The *yamas* and *niyamas* play an important role in emotional purification in the Himalayan Tradition of Yoga. 3) A blend of the ancient and the modern, of Classical Yoga and modern psychotechnologies are needed for effective practice of the *yamas* and *niyamas*. 4) Ultimately these guidelines must be applied by an individual in specific situations by following the expression of the Inner Teacher as the conscience as the best and true guide.

The *Yamas* in Daily Life

Ahimsa. Nonviolence lies at the core of all ethical and moral injunctions. The other *yamas* refine and polish this fundamental moral principle. The term is found in Jainism, Hinduism and Buddhism and perhaps more has been written about this *yama* than about the others.

The potential for violence is hardwired into our nervous system. To learn nonviolence is to rechannel that remnant of our animal nature. Nature itself is built on predator-prey networks. The phylogenetic remnant of the Darwinian struggle for survival is built into the limbic system along with the flight or fight stress response (LeDoux, 2002). The accompanying emotions of fear and anger direct our behavior daily whenever we feel threatened. With the advent of imaging and related techniques (MRI, fMRI, PET, SPECT, EEG, TCMS, evoked potentials, etc.) neuroscience is studying the neural basis of fear and aggression (Damasio, 1999; Goleman, 2003; LeDoux, 2002).

To behave nonviolently requires courage. Cowardice and violence are synonymous. Nonengagement from cowardice, fear or selfishness is not nonviolence. Only a very courageous person can go into a violent crowd and effect positive change. Despite our inbred instinctual aggressiveness the cultivation of nonviolence is possible as illustrated by the example of the saints. When one takes the vows of a swami in the Bharati tradition the vow of harmlessness is included: "May no living being fear me." Pandit Rajmani Tigunait (1991) has written eloquently on the Yogic approach to war and peace.

In our modern world one finds violence everywhere in business, family, everyday affairs, the media, sports, the arts and entertainment. We pour violence into our minds daily through books, art, theatre, radio and television, the print media and computer games. No one can seriously question the negative impact of such a steady diet on our youth. We have all experienced the frustrated aggressiveness of the type A personality. Will Durant is reputed to have said that no man who is in a hurry is quite civilized. It is encouraging, however, that serious violent and property crime rates (homicide, burglary and robbery) have fallen by over 40% in the U.S.A. during the 1990s, but for unknown reasons (Rosenfeld, 2004).

What is violence for one individual may not be for another and vice versa. We all have our threshold and for each of us that threshold is different. It is low for the suicidal terrorist and much higher for the average student of Yoga for whom the temptation to kill another human being would be unthinkable, but who might wage all out war on mosquitoes during a threat of West Nile virus infection. Each individual must work at his or her own level and take it one step at a time. Sri Swami Rama used to say that any society that has an army, police force, a legal system and an organized religion cannot be considered to be civilized.

Nonviolence must be practiced at the levels of thought, speech and action. At the **level of action** it involves not only not physically doing injury, but not inciting others to do injury nor allowing others to be injured. Actions range from war and suicidal terrorism through homicide to spousal and child abuse to vandalism, bullying and road rage. Swami Veda Bharati likes to gauge the spiritual progress of a student by watching how aggressively they drive or type at a computer. The practice leads one to take responsibility for the suffering of others. I am indeed my brother's keeper. It includes not plundering or despoiling the ecology and not harming nonhuman beings. Much has been written about the abuse to animals carried out by the food industry (Ballentine, 1987).

At the **verbal level** one avoids using words that inflict pain on others, like rudeness, insult, sarcasm, cursing, a nasty tone of voice, aggressive criticism, argumentativeness, judgementalism, negativity, putdowns, frightening others, and so on. Even the "silent treatment" is a form of abuse.

At the **mental level** one avoids cruel and violent thoughts, jealousy, negative evaluations or labeling of other people, excessive criticism, etc. The passive aggressive personality is included. People can often pick up on the "negative vibes" that such mental states put out. We all experience the lack of civility from our youth and government agencies daily. Nonviolence must also be practiced towards oneself. Self-abuse of body and mind is a common problem. The inner critic is alive and well.

All students of Yoga are advised to read the writings of Mahatma Gandhi (1983). He was the outstanding strategist of nonviolent action (Teixeira, 1987). His concept of *Satyagraha* (truth force) was designed to distinguish his style of nonviolence from others like passive resistance and civil disobedience. He recognized that *ahimsa* must be founded in *advaita*. Nonviolence was a means to actualize and express underlying unity. If all is one we must care for and not hurt others. Gandhi came to see *ahimsa* as the same as the Christian concept of *agape* which is the highest form of disinterested love. It is much more than nonviolence and nonaggression. It is also a matter of goodwill to others including one's opponents. For a yogi firmly established in nonviolence, in his proximity there is a loss of hostility in all living beings. It is said by his closest disciples that one could not be angry in the presence of Swami Rama if he so willed. Swamiji used the method to induce an uncaring government to provide aid to survivors of a devastating earthquake at Ginda near Uttarkashi in the Garhwal Himalayas. He began a fast to death on the front steps of a prominent government building in Delhi which soon resulted in an audience with the Indian Prime Minister. Swamiji castigated him severely for his lack of compassion. When asked afterwards about the dressing down the Prime Minister said, "What a blessing. I have waited my whole life to meet this man!" Thereafter the aid flowed in abundance. When a yogi is firmly established in nonviolence, in his proximity there occurs a natural loss of hostility in the minds of others (YS II.35).

Satya. Truthfulness is praised in ethical and yogic literature. Truthfulness is next to godliness, for divine Reality is ultimate Truth. It involves the proper use of the faculty of speech. Is my speech genuine and congruent with reality? Or do I lie or give false and misleading statements? Is there honesty and authenticity? The Laws of Manu tell us not to speak unpleasant truth or pleasant untruth. Indeed it requires a lot of energy and a very high level of intelligence to lie effectively and consistently. What a tangled web we weave when we decide to deceive! But our unconscious knows the truth and will express it through the autonomic nervous system as any lie detector will uncover.

Talkativeness and imagination are two enemies of truth. Through imagination one can lose track of what is real and unreal. We interpret external reality to conform to our inner constructs so that things become the way they should be rather than the way they are – the eye-witness fallacy. Silence is a great ally of truthfulness. If one cannot say anything nice, do not say anything at all. One must be aware of self-deception, the lies I tell about myself to myself. Can I break the habit of adjusting my story and finding excuses for myself with fibs that get me off the hook? "I was only speaking the truth." The principal of truth is expressed by *hitam*, *mitam*, *priyam*: cultivating a speech that is beneficial, measured, and pleasant (Veda Bharati, 1982).

Advertising, marketing, sales, advocacy all stretch the bounds of *satya*, sometimes with manipulation and a hidden agenda, and sometimes innocently. False claims in complementary and alternative medicine are a growing problem. One of us recalls our first encounter with this vividly. A group from Mexico visited our laboratory with an Oncodiagnosticator, a machine they had invented that could diagnose cancer from a blood test. They refused to tell us what was in the liquid used by the machine for the test. We tested a large panel of sera from normal and cancer patients in a blind study that showed quite clearly that the device was worthless. When we asked again what the liquid was one of them drank it down with a flourish and said it was distilled water. They chatted among themselves as we watched and decided it was the elevation of Montreal compared to Mexico City that was affecting the machine, and then got up and went away with their faith in the device quite unshaken.

It is common for people to believe that if there is a reasonable explanation for something then it must be true without any experimental test. This is a different lack of authenticity – the falsity of ignorance and confusion. Add a dash of advocacy and even reputable scientists can go wildly astray as the recent emotional debates around global warming have shown (Essex & McKitrick, 2003). And woe to anyone who tries to get the discussions back on track!

Truthfulness means both integrity and transparency. The aspirant must become harmless and transparent, as well as aligned with the spiritual core of the personality. Transparency means, "What you see is what you get." You "walk your talk." There are no hidden agendas; everything is on the table. You are as good as your word. You make no promises that you cannot fulfill. There is no hypocrisy. The phrase, "Do as I say, don't do as I do," does not apply. Transparency requires personal integrity which comes from an alignment of all parts of the personality with the Centre of Consciousness. Parts that create resistance, internal conflict and doubt indicate a lack of integrity. The power of will flowing from the core of the personality is diverted and disrupted so that thought, understanding, speech and action become confused. Producing this kind of internal integrity is the work of a lifetime. These qualities come first from the conquest of duality. As long as there is a perception of "other" then the issue of who or what is in control arises – me or that "other." Swami Rama so often urged his students and disciples to learn to be fearless. From fear flows anger and internal conflict. From attachment comes self-identified infatuation and involvement leading to pain, suffering and grief. Ultimately transparency flows from nonattachment. When a yogi is firmly established in truth his or her words always come true (YS II.36).

Brahmacharya. This subject, along with *ahimsa*, seems to attract most of the controversy, writing and discussion about the *yamas*. It is often presented only in terms of celibacy. But its meaning can be much broader – moderation and continence in all things of the senses.

One should maintain a balance in the normal behavioural pattern of emotion, consciousness or energy . . . [leading] to the expansions of our inner faculties. This leads to a developed awareness of the Self, which is *brahmacharya*. *Brahma* means supreme, divine, higher, and *Acharya* means knower of, or master. The absolute meaning of *brahmacharya* is not sensual abstinence; rather it is the merger of the individual with the higher consciousness and constantly maintaining that identity. Sexual abstinence came to be known as part of *brahmacharya* when evolved beings noted that passionless and desire free relationships with the opposite sex gave an insight into the transcendental awareness which is free of gross feelings. Therefore they said to abstain from animal passion so that the gross carnal desires evolve. Later in ignorance, man defined *brahmacharya* as total sensual and sexual abstinence to develop spiritual awareness.

Paramahansa Niranjanananda, 1992, pp 71–72

Like *ahimsa, brahmacharya* relates to the hard wiring in our nervous system at the base of the brain. Survival and reproductive function go together in the evolutionary process. Reproduction is essential to the survival of species and so it is no surprise that sexual experience is so compelling. Control of sexuality is a lifelong task and one takes it a step at a time within one's capacity. For the renunciate it may be complete celibacy, but the recent controversies over sexual abuse in the churches indicate how difficult a vow that can be. For the householder it can be monogamy. The nearly 50% rates of divorce in our society, never mind the high incidence of marital infidelity, show that this is an equal challenge.

Like violence, sexuality is everywhere in daily life, in business, the arts and the media. Sex sells everything from cars to cigarettes, from fashions to expensive vacations. Violence and sexuality often go together. Pornography is readily available. For some it is an addiction. Nearly half of Internet transactions involve pornography. Globally the sex trade, including sex slavery, is surpassed only by illicit drugs in profitability. The rates of sexually transmitted diseases are rising, and the most feared of all, AIDS, threatens to wipe out much of the population of Africa.

A young lawyer, Lisa Olson (2004) writes about "lesbian chic." It is now "cool" for young hetero-sexual women seeking attention to act gay in public displays of lesbian or bisexual acts, exemplified by the now infamous Britney Spears-Madonna open-mouth kiss. Olson opines that political correctness releases a barrage of content with no borders. We are asked to accept all viewpoints, every idea and all behaviors. "There are no lines, no right and wrong. Indeed, it is pushing many of us to compromise our beliefs and, perhaps, not form any in the first place as there is no room for disagreement, no allowance for criticism for fear of the label of 'intolerant' being thrust at you." There is freedom of speech only if that speech does not disapprove of the speech and actions of any other. "Accept everything, believe in nothing; it is the new age of ultimate tolerance." And we would add ultimate amorality.

But continence goes beyond into sensual control. This is the realm of addictions to drugs, alcohol, tobacco, gambling, etc. It is deeply rooted in attachment (*raga*) leading to addictive and compulsive behaviors in general: the workaholic, the information freak, the compulsion to play computer games, the shopaholic. The list goes on and on. Working with continence means overcoming not only the biological urges of sex and food but also the compulsion and obsession to reexperience pleasure in its broadest sense. One who masters *brahmacharya* gains strength, virility and capacity (*virya*) (YS II.38). Its ultimate perfection is the power to place knowledge into disciples, to impart *yoga-diksha*. "It is not for nothing that celibacy is called 'walking in God'" (Veda Bharati, 2001, p 538).

Asteya. Asteya is non-stealing. It relates to *ahimsa* since the victim of theft is injured thereby. Its usual meaning of theft or robbery is the common one of seizing someone else's possession by stealth or force and viewing it as "mine." Theft can create fear, defensiveness, isolation, dishonesty, and even violence.

Theft also has the meaning of accepting objects or services as gifts from another (Veda Bharati, 2001, p 482). This makes more sense when one realizes that much of gift giving and the giving of favors has a hidden agenda that can range from influence, persuasion or bribery to removing indebtedness or to gain recognition, a service or a favor from another.

The thought underlying theft is key and always precedes the action. One must resist covetousness, avarice and desire towards objects of the senses which have no intrinsic value. The attitude of possessiveness is to be put aside. There is a sense of entitlement sometimes: "The world owes me a living. Anything I want should be mine."

Asteya also overlaps with the next *yama*, greedlessness where I am motivated to take more than my share. I can steal what is not given or deserved and create socioeconomic disparity and failure to conserve resources of the earth and its people. Theft can breed deceit, cheating and loss of scruples with manipulative behavior. One can steal time. One can steal virtue with seduction ("date rape"). One can steal peace of mind, one's own or another's. One can steal an idea, a reputation or another's enjoyment. If I get something for nothing or at a bargain I say, "It's a steal."

Having goals are laudable, but when they lead to greed, obsessiveness and stealing they disrupt peace of mind. Obsessing over the desire disrupts meditation and the misappropriation of goals and goods ruins peace of mind. I can turn the borrowing of a book into theft by simply forgetting to return it. I can vicariously enjoy and identify with the qualities and achievements of another. If I do this as a parent I may vicariously live the life of my child by pushing that child into a sport, an art form or a vocation that the child does not want. I deny that child his own childhood and future. Do I do this for my benefit or for my child? Is this my secondary gain or is this what is beneficial for my child? This can be subtle and too easy to rationalize.

I can also steal another's creative contribution. Plagiarism is the obvious example and is a growing and serious problem in colleges and universities (vide www.turnitin.com and Ziegler, 2004). Copyright is a related matter (Boynton, 2004) and the Internet has pulled it from obscurity into the light of attention. Intellectual property law is at the center of major disputes in the arts, sciences and politics, and the 1998 Digital Millennium Copyright Act is quietly reshaping the culture. We hear the recording industry bringing lawsuits against those who download freely and share pirated music or movies. There was an attempt recently to force a prominent youth organization to pay royalties for singing songs around campfires. Can a private corporation patent human genes, living systems and genetically engineered animals? Opposition groups such as "Copy Left" are trying to create a "cultural commons" in the public domain as a shared stockpile of ideas where the majority of the world's music and literature would reside, from which anyone could partake without having to pay or ask permission. Information wants to be free.

At the base of all of this lie attachment and desire, a mix of greed and theft. I must acknowledge the feeling of lack that I do not have enough, and that I need to have more so that I keep seeking externals to satisfy me. This habit of wanting everything that I see is attachment. I need to learn that my wanting cannot be filled by objects in the external world. All things are transient and on loan for me to use to fulfill my purpose now during this journey of a lifetime. I may freely use them but I cannot own them. Conquest of this and the next *yama* is the result of gaining nonattachment (and nonreactivity in the broader sense) to all objects, both subtle and gross, ranging from actions and things to thoughts and ideas. One established in *asteya* attains all jewels and treasures at all times everywhere by his mere will (YS II.37).

Aparigraha. *Aparigraha* is non-grasping, non-grabbing or not greedy. It overlaps with *asteya* and much of what has been said above about non-stealing also applies here. It is sometimes rendered as non-covetousness and also non-acceptance of gifts for they can generate attachment and subsequent fear of loss. Virgil said, "I fear the Greeks, even when bringing gifts." (Aeneid, Book II, line 49). And beware the wrath of someone who is not recognized for their charitable gift or act of service.

In a broader sense it rejects all claims of "my" and "mine" over material means and possessions including the physical body (Veda Bharati, 2001, p 540). It is a rejection of the ego's claim of "mine" resulting in non-indulgence. As a mental attitude I do not possess or own material things, whether actually owned by me or offered to me as gifts, or presented to me as a sensory experience. In short, I learn not to indulge myself, my pleasures or even my body which is the means to experience, for such indulgence has its roots in attachment. These attachments pull the consciousness outwards and preclude the arising of inner wisdom and the inner knowledge of the Self (Veda Bharati, 2001, p 540).

Aparigraha is all about living the simple life, avoiding materialism, hoarding and possessiveness: not accumulating material baggage or becoming attached to belongings. The voluntary simplicity movement took off in the United States in the late 1980s. The concept encompasses both self-change aimed at bringing personal practice into alignment with ecological values, and cultural change that rejects consumerist values and careerism (Elgin, 1998; Grigsby, 2004; Vandenbroeck & Schumacher, 1996). As we go through the journey of life we carry only what is essential in our backpack. What we accumulate beyond that makes the backpack a burden. One has to work hard to be able to afford luxuries. Then one has to care for them, insure them and worry about them. One soon becomes attached to them. Things tend to accumulate like curios, magazines or books. It is easy to justify keeping them: one might need them some day; there are sentimental meanings, or "just in case." Life just gets more complex and becomes a hassle.

Swami Rama would frequently emphasize the importance of exhalation. One has to continually clean out the unneeded so that life can flow on and not stagnate. There is nothing more cleansing than a move to a new residence! Practice cleaning things out and keeping your belongings flowing. Do I need this in my backpack of life? What is my attachment to it? Can someone else use it? Can I recycle it or put it in a garage sale or donate it to the goodwill? Upon attaining stability in non-indulgence, one gains the knowledge of past and future incarnations (YS II.39).

12

The Principles and Practice of the YAMAS *in Daily Life*

Kleshas and *Karma*

To come to grips with the *yamas* and move beyond using them as mere rules and ritual one must address their causes and confront the problem of suffering in the world. First understand *karma*, the law of moral causation, and how the proscribed behaviors described in the *yamas* lead to negative consequences and to the production of *samskaras* (residues) and *vasanas* (propensities) in the deep unconscious mind. Then understand how these, in turn, under the right circumstances lead to the expression of more of these behaviors in a deepening vicious cycle. Learn the dynamics of dormant (*sanchita*), active (*prarabdha*) and potential (*kriyamana*) *karmas* and how these may be modified and prevented by practicing intense *tapas*, attaining *samadhi*, undertaking *mantra sadhana*, performing selfless service, being in the company of saints and sages, and obtaining the grace of God (Tigunait, 1997, p 9).

One must also understand the dynamics of the afflictions (*kleshas*) which are the causes of suffering (YS II.3). So much of unethical behavior flows from ignorance (*avidya*), in this case, defined as lack of awareness so the individual does not grasp the deep implications of his or her behavior. As a misapprehension about the real nature of things, *avidya* also leads to negative behaviors because of a lack of awareness of the Centre of Consciousness as a real experience. The ego or political self (*asmita*) preserves its own interests in separation from others. *Raga* (attachment) and *dvesha* (aversion) lie at the core of the emotional reactivity that can lead to proscribed addictive behaviors. Self-preservation as the fear of death (*abhinivesha*) can generate violence.

The Four Primitive Urges

The *yamas* rechannel the energies of our instinctual level. To practice effectively one must control what Sri Swami Rama called the four primitive fountains (Rama, 2002b, pp 15–33): food (*ahara*), sleep (*nidra*), sex (*maithunancha*) and self-preservation (*bhaya*). In some form they occupy most of the twenty-four hours of our day. Swamiji often talked about "hurry, worry and curry." The issues arising from food, sleep and sex fall under *brahmacharya* while self-preservation (which includes stress in modern language) comes under *ahimsa*.

We spend a third of our lives in sleep. Sleep medicine is now a recognized specialty and the toll in road accidents because of excessive sleepiness is on the rise. Think of the enormous impact of eating represented by the food industry in our social and personal life. While malnutrition is common in the developing world, America has an epidemic of obesity. Over half of North Americans are either overweight or obese, and at risk for hypertension, the metabolic syndrome, heart disease and type 2 diabetes, while 16% of children between the ages of six and eleven are overweight with an additional 14% at risk (St-Onge et al, 2003). We are now seeing type 2 diabetes, a disease of middle age or older, in young, preteen, obese children. In Western culture, sexuality is pervasive. From stress all the way to violence the issues of self-preservation lie at the base of the world's conflicts.

The world impact of the four urges is exemplified by the findings of the Global Burden of Disease Project, an ongoing collaboration between the World Health Organization and Harvard University (1990–2020) (WHO, 2004). In 1990 there were fifty million deaths globally. A third involved communicable, maternal, perinatal and nutritional (including obesity) diseases, all of which occurred in the developing world. The urges of food and sex apply here. A half of the deaths worldwide were due to non-communicable diseases, for which tobacco use and diet contribute upwards of two thirds of the risk. About 10% of the deaths were due to injury, both intentional (violence) and unintentional (accidents). Of the ten risk factors identified five are relevant here: malnutrition, unsafe sex, and the use of tobacco, alcohol and illicit drugs. Many of the behaviours proscribed by the *yamas* as well as the major emotions (Rama, 2002b, pp 87–94) flow from the four primitive fountains. For effective practice of the *yamas* one must learn to regulate, channel and control the expression of these urges without suppressing them.

Paramahamsa Niranjanananda (1993c, p 138) also writes of the four basic instincts which he describes as the four desires: for food; for progeny; for sleep and for property and wealth. He notes their interconnection. If the desire for food cannot be renounced then *brahmacharya* cannot be maintained. If these two cannot be controlled then sleep cannot be controlled. The issue is the control of consciousness within the state of sleep, which must be expanded until it penetrates through dreaming into deep sleep, which is *yoga nidra*. Otherwise one cannot be established in higher meditation such as *samadhi* because one must travel through the threshold of sleep without losing awareness to reach these higher states. A meditator knows the long struggle with both the flow of imagery and thought (dreaming) and with falling asleep in meditation. It happens so subtly and uncontrollably one is only aware that one has been asleep when one suddenly awakens. Individuals have mistaken this for *samadhi*. Thus paradoxically controlling the desire for food through practising dietary control, choiceless eating and occasional fasting helps with the control of sleep. Control one basic instinct and the others fall in line.

Models of the World

A practitioner should have a good working model of the mind and how it constructs one's experience of reality (Jerry & Jerry, 2001, p 63). The theory of Neuro-Linguistic Programming (NLP) is particularly helpful here (O'Connor & Seymour, 1990). It describes how the sensory-motor mind takes sensory inputs to create internal sequences of imagery, emotions and feelings that can initiate external behaviors. It also describes how the higher mind through the processes of generalization, distortion and deletion converts about 20% of this perceptual material into meaning as a cognitive map of experience or model of the world which is coded in language and stored in the unconscious as beliefs, values and attitudes; of these three, values have the strongest influence. We each live in our own personal virtual reality which creates not our world, but our experience of it. Along with instinctual and emotional factors as well as conditioning, one's beliefs and values play a critical role in thought, speech and behavior in relation to the *yamas*.

Our models of the world are obscured by ignorance (*avidya*), severely restricted by the self interest of the ego (*asmita*) which holds tenaciously to its beliefs, values and ideologies, and its likes (*raga*) and dislikes (*dvesha*) for its very survival (*abhinivesha*). Models of the world are homeostatic, for a change in their content means a change in the sense of self and hence a small death. Religious and political fundamentalisms are particular examples of how rigid these pictures of reality can be. Arguably over the centuries more suffering, death, war and persecution have arisen out of the clash of ideologies than from any other cause. The suicidal terrorist operating from political or distorted religious beliefs is our modern example. The postmodernist movement in qualitative research is another example of the rigidity of ideology. An anti-positivist if not anti-science ideology has grown up in the field of qualitative analysis (e.g., Lincoln & Guba, 1985) confusing a generation of students in the social sciences about the nature of truth (*satya*) as realized through experimental verification. Science is valid learning from experience. It is a way to reality-test creative imagination. A scientist's best ideas still have a 95% chance of being wrong.

We are talking here also about power. The terrorist uses power as violence in a survival world view that is consistent with the first *chakra* (Ajaya, 1983). But power has other forms (Greene, 2000). The use of power in the boardroom represents the model of the world from the third *chakra*. The tense and aggressive boardroom scenes from the current television reality show that showcases Donald Trump are an example. Control is another form of power and underlies social engineering and political correctness as well as the bureaucracies of governments and the military, and can be just as oppressive of human rights and expression in its own way. Husbands try to control wives; parents control children, even through cell phones. The latest is a global positioning system (GPS) attached to the family car or even as a subcutaneous implant!

Most of us believe that if there is a reasonable explanation of something that it must be true. In medicine this has been called the tomato effect (Jerry, 1985). In the early part of the 20th century people realized that tomato plants belong to the deadly nightshade (Solanaceae) family which include some of the world's most deadly poisonous plants, such as belladonna and mandrake, whose leaves and fruit can be deadly if taken in sufficient amounts. Hence only a fool would eat a tomato! A colloquial translation would be, "Don't confuse me with facts, my mind's made up!" It took large groups of people eating tomatoes without ill effect on the front steps of the Capitol in Washington to begin to change that belief. Now tomatoes are a major North American crop. The point is that when working with the *yamas* one must be able to understand and deal with the fundamental beliefs and values that drive these behaviors and make these ethical precepts very difficult to practice. The confusion is even deeper because so many people cannot distinguish between facts and their interpretation, often putting forth the latter as factual.

Recently people are realizing the impact of the Internet and virtual reality on how we construct our worlds. Schultze (2002) writes that the Internet is not just a neutral communications pipeline. It imparts its own code of conduct and is not morally neutral. The industrial revolution assumed that nature could be manipulated within limits by mechanical technology. But the postmodern information age now assumes that human beings can create their own "realities *ex nihilo,* out of nothing, just like the God of Genesis." Schultze refers to it as the chaotic world of cyber culture, which is not really a culture at all but dissolution of culture. The technology itself imparts a distinct set of values – complete personal control, unaccountable freedom, radical individualism, and above all, efficiency. By seizing control of more communication technologies we lose control of our moral imaginations. The cult of efficiency makes us impatient, angry, short-tempered and frenzied. As our machines become more "human," we tend to treat other humans like machines. There is self-fragmentation, a tendency to see reality as a series of isolated tasks. Soon our own lives become a sequence of isolated tasks and we begin to seek a foundation for our lives, some sort of meaningful goal. All of us know that eventually imagination must meet reality. But for the addicted, e-imagination is just another narcotic.

Kleshas, karma, models of the world, emotional reactivity, conditioning and instinctual drives represented by the four primitive fountains all combine to determine and influence thoughts, speech and behavior in the context of the *yamas.* Thus ritually practicing the *yamas* as a set of simple rules is naïve.

Ethics

The student should become familiar with ethics and morality as a branch of philosophy (for example, Edwards & Papp, 1973, pp 288–364). Medical ethics has become a specialty in its own right but unfortunately has evolved to obstruct and clog the everyday commerce of medical practice and research through substitution of rules for common sense. But one must become familiar with the moral faculty as the philosophers understand it and the principles of morals. Science and ethics, the objectivity of moral judgments and the undefinability of good are all issues. One must decide what position one will take with the situational ethics and moral relativity that characterize the secular humanism and pragmatism of our amoral society, how only winning is important, and how everything is fair in both love and war. While this may seem very abstract, the daily practice of the *yamas* evokes these principles over and over and challenges a too easy rationalization of convenient behaviors. To put it differently, Swami Rama emphasized that all students should have a philosophy of life to guide their thinking, speech and behavior (Swami Rama, 2002b, pp 1–13). Ethics is very much a part of this.

Capacity

To undertake a practice of the *yamas* can rapidly become an overwhelming challenge. Almost everything one thinks says or does seems to violate one or more of these principles all the time. Cut yourself a little slack! In the Tradition it is recommended that you work one step beyond your capacity so that your capacity can be expanded, but you are to take only one step at a time. The journey of 1000 miles begins with the first step. The expression of these virtues is never perfect. They are a work in progress until one becomes a sage.

If you were invisible and could do anything you chose without being caught, would you behave morally? This philosophical conundrum attributed to Plato has been the subject of much debate and of books, plays and movies. We recall it as the theme of one of the very early Star Trek television episodes. The answer is usually always no. If you need rules and must practice behaviors then there is the possibility of exceptions.

Ultimately the *yamas* must become *sahaja* – a spontaneous and natural aspect of one's being, an expression of who one really is. Then one is beyond rules and practices. Then one cannot but act in that way. This is the province of the sage. But start where you are and take it one step at a time.

Formulation

It was pointed out above that the *yamas* and *niyamas* are often poorly taught if at all. One reason may be their lack of interest and perceived irrelevance in our modern amoral Western society – something to pay lip service to. Or it may be that we need a better way of teaching them in an innovative curriculum. There is new material coming out that the practitioner could be aware of to help the process. The issue of bullying in schools and in the workplace is receiving a lot of attention (Coloroso, 2003). Research is occurring on the moral development of children (Damon, 1999), and new tools for brain imaging as well as new knowledge about the role of neuroplasticity in learning are creating a new neurobiology of morals (Jennings, 1999). In her study of moral intelligence, Michele Borba (2002) recommends empathy, conscience, self-control, respect, kindness, tolerance and fairness as seven essential virtues to build moral intelligence in children.

Family Life

Despite efforts to pass the responsibility to schools and religious organizations, the family still remains the primary source of moral education for children. In modern society, sadly, that trust has been deeply betrayed. Life is all about relationships. Swami Rama considered marriage and family life as a spiritual path (Rama, 1992b). The concept of marriage as holy matrimony between a man and woman is being threatened by gay activists in the United States, and especially in Canada. In addition to nonviolence, parents need the integrity and transparency of *satya* to educate children.

The most powerful influence comes from the example set by parents for their children. What I say and what I do must be congruent.

Husband and wife must dedicate their relationship and marriage to an overarching higher purpose that will transcend and sublimate their individual egos and desires. It puts in place a boundary beyond which selfish initiatives will simply not cross in order to preserve the union. To actualize that higher spiritual purpose they must be prepared to dedicate 25 or 30 years of persistent effort. In the process they will pass along those higher values to their children who ultimately copy their parents in these major behaviors. Yes, this is discipline, but is it any different than the discipline of the Olympic athlete, the surgeon, or the concert pianist?

Practice

The *yamas* can be practiced by focusing on one at a time over a week, a month, or preferably a year. The use of a diary to evaluate the day is helpful. One learns to view the day's activities through the filter of the chosen *yama*, such as nonviolence, and to be a witness of all that happens in the inner and outer world. This is a bit like making a diagnosis: it is difficult to solve problems of which one is not aware. Then analyze the day's experience in the diary. Can you see examples of violence, however subtle, in others, society, and yourself in action, speech, and thoughts? What were your feelings and reactions? What might you have done differently? Can you sense the whisperings of your conscience as the guide to right action in each situation? This is a discipline, a practice, and not a punishment.

There is no place for guilt. Indeed, Swami Veda Bharati has said that when he first came to North America he had no concept of guilt since it was not part of his training as a child in Yoga. If a mistake is made, correct it, do not repeat it, and get on with life without fussing over it. The key to this process is the ability to observe, to witness, to dis-associate and move into a meta-state. If you are fully aware you will sense the guidance of the conscience and you are less likely to act adversely. This process is very much the practice of *vairagya*, which can be intensified by complementary regular practice of Yoga, especially mindfulness and meditation.

Pema Chodron (1995) talks about practicing the three difficulties. When your "buttons are pushed" and you react, the first difficulty is to catch it when it first arises – that first sense of "Yes but . . . , No way!" The second difficulty is that even if you see it, it is difficult to do something different to interrupt the pattern, and likely anything different would do as a pattern interrupt. She uses Buddhist *tonglen* and we would use releasing (Dwoskin, 2003) or energy psychology (Gallo & Vincenzi, 2000). The third difficulty is to make this intervention a way of life. Our conditioning is so strong that even after a few successful interventions we fall back into the old habitual ways and forget again. We know we now have the skills to intervene but we do not do it.

Emotional Purification

Purification of thoughts and emotions is a key part of the Himalayan Tradition of Yoga meditation (Veda Bharati, 1998, p 3). It is done to prevent the internal disturbances arising from extraneous thoughts and feelings during meditation, but it also reduces the reactivity, both mental and emotional, that underlie behaviors proscribed by the *yamas*.

The practices of emotional purification include the *yamas* and *niyamas*; the four *brahma-viharas* or right attitudes (friendliness toward the happy, compassion for the unhappy, delight in the virtuous, and indifference toward the wicked (YS I.33)); and the use of antidotes or opposite thoughts to neutralize disturbing thoughts and to ward off thoughts opposed to the *yamas, niyamas*, and *brahma-viharas* (YS II.33, 34). These practices are said to produce ethical behavior which leads to loosening the bonds of *karma*; to mental purification that brings clarity and pleasantness to the mind field (*chitta-pra-sadana*); and to stability and steadiness of mind and body in life and meditation (*sthiti-ni-bandhana*).

An additional aspect of purification is the conquest of the nine obstacles or disturbances (*vikshepas*) in the path of meditation (sickness, laziness, doubt, lack of enthusiasm, sloth, sensory craving, false perception, despair caused by failure to concentrate and unsteadiness in concentration (YS I.30)), as well as their accompaniments (grief, despondency, trembling of the body and irregular breathing (YS I.31)). Unless these are conquered one remains bound to the disturbed states of mind (turbulent (*kshipta*), stupefied (*mudha*) and distracted (*vikshipta*)) which prevent progression to higher states of one-pointedness (*ekagra*) and then to totally controlled (*niruddha*) in *samadhi*. In addition to the above practices the Himalayan oral tradition adds additional methods such as certain *mantras* and meditating in the preceptor's presence to steady the *sadhaka*'s mind.

We recommend an integrated, two-pronged strategy that combines East and West, spirituality and science, the ancient and modern. The core is the practice of the eight limbs of *ashtanga-yoga* carried out in the context of *kriya-yoga* and the chariot of *sadhana: abhyasa* (practice) and *vairagya* (dispassion), to effect longterm transformation of the total personality. Ideally this would include *satsang* and the *darshan* of a master to provide the opportunity for initiation and grace. Then one uses modern Western psychotechnology to deal with acute situations and specific reactivities as the unconscious mind releases its contents during Yogic practice. Often students have to "tough it out" when dealing with this process of emotional purification, but with modern technology this kind of suffering is much less necessary. In addition to an organic overall fundamental growth and expansion of awareness and the personality, one aims at developing mental tranquility, a mind field that is so stable because of its high vibrational rate and energetics, that its reactivity to specific stimuli is lost, and even the capacity for it to be reactive in general is lost. Then one is in control, is able to follow the guidelines that the *yamas* provide for thought, speech and action, and is in touch with the guidance to right action that flows from the conscience.

A complete integrated Yoga practice is required, but aspects of *pranayama* are particularly helpful. Swami Rama used to prescribe long and intensive practices of *nadi shodhana* (alternate nostril breathing) for addictions and obsessions, for example. One includes all the elements of stress management which are rooted in Yogic practices such as relaxation, meditation and diaphragmatic breathing. Mindfulness is important. It is also taught in the Himalayan Tradition (Swami Veda Bharati, 1998, p 5) as referred to in YS I.20 as the practice of *smrty-upa-sthana* (Buddhist *sati-pat-thana*) (Buddhaghosa, 1975) which is taught by personal instruction. It takes many forms with full awareness of the states of the body, breath and mind in a very detailed methodology. It requires a very deep self-observation in all states of body, breath and mind. The student should have a regular practice of meditation which at a certain stage involves a prolonged process of "washing the mind" as unconscious material surfaces to the witnessing awareness. *Yoga nidra* (Yogic conscious sleep) is also helpful for purification of the unconscious, and the version taught by the Bihar School of Yoga is particularly designed for this purpose (Satyananda Saraswati, 1984).

There are also highly effective modern Western methods that can be used as adjuncts to Yoga practice. The Sedona Method of releasing is simple and effective in everyday life (Dwoskin, 2003). Neuro-Linguistic Programming (NLP) has many highly effective methods that one can use with oneself such as reframing, resolution of parts conflicts, submodalities, and especially visual-kinesthetic dissociation (O'Connor & Seymour, 1990). Eye Movement Desensitization and Reprocessing (EMDR) is also highly effective but not suitable for personal use without a therapist (Shapiro, 1995). But perhaps the best of all of these methods is Energy Psychology which has many versions. This process is easy to learn and to use by the student of Yoga (Gallo & Vincenzi, 2000). It is a recent development based on the hypothesis that negative emotions represent disturbances in the subtle energies of the acupuncture meridian systems. Each meridian is associated with specific emotions. Stimulation of the involved meridians (often by simply tapping a sequence of specific acupoints) restores energetic balance and resolves the emotional upheaval.

That negative emotions may represent disruptions in subtle energies is a completely new paradigm in psychology. Since students of Yoga are comfortable with the concept of subtle energy and *prana*, it makes a natural fit to yogic practice. In the hands of skilled clinicians it can have an effectiveness of up to 80% compared to traditional psychological techniques (30–40%). In anecdotal long-term follow-up the effects appear to be lasting. The methods work best with what used to be called neurosis as opposed to psychosis (with hallucinations and delusions that require professional assistance). It works also with obsessions and addictions, and can be used to change beliefs and enhance performance. Its associated concepts of neurological disorganization, over energy and psychological reversal which produces resistance to change, are all helpful for enhancing Yoga practice.

Ancient or modern, we believe that all of these methods have one thing in common. They all produce states of what is described in NLP as visual-kinesthetic dissociation, or in broader terms, sensory-perceptual dissociation. They split the link between internal thoughts or images and their associated feelings or emotions. The thoughts or images remain, but the emotional charge and the upset and suffering are gone. This is about detachment and forgiveness. In other words, all these techniques produce *vairagya* (dispassion) in specific situations and contexts. They neutralize suffering by dissolving attachment (*raga*) and aversion (*dvesha*) which are part of the *kleshas* (afflictions), the fundamental causes of suffering (YS II.3).

"Thou must be like a promontory of the sea, against which, though the waves beat continually, yet it both itself stands, and about it are those swelling waves stilled and quieted."

Marcus Aurelius

"In the physician or surgeon no quality takes rank with Imperturbability."

Sir William Osler

"The trouble with Archie is he don't know how to worry without gettin' upset!"

Television character, Edith Bunker.

Finally, if one is guiding a meditation group, one should have available the capability of ready referral to medical and psychological expertise that is sympathetic to Yoga. Students attend meditation groups over long periods, often for many years. They form deep and supportive relationships. As emotional purification proceeds, in our experience their burden of suffering becomes apparent at a level much deeper than one might see with students attending classes. One needs to be able to provide appropriate support, especially in times of personal crisis and when issues of spiritual emergence or spiritual emergencies arise (Nelson, 1994a, b). All of these can profoundly affect and even arise from intensive practice of the *yamas* in daily life.

Profit, sensory indulgence, prestige and power: all lie at the core of human frailty. It is fascinating how comprehensively the simple guidelines provided by the *yamas* encompass all of human fallibility. One starts with the discipline of practice and these moral guidelines, but ultimately duty (*dharma*) has precedence over following abstract rules. The ultimate guide is the Centre of Consciousness/ Inner Teacher in its aspect as the Conscience. In every situation learn not to kill your Conscience and to "follow your Spirit without hesitation." (Alarius, 1988). For those of us for whom this has yet to be perfected in every situation, a modern addition to the *yamas* might be the Rotary 4-Way Test created in 1932 by Rotarian Herbert J. Taylor as a statement of business and professional ethics. "Of the things we think, say or do: is it the truth? Is it fair to all concerned? Will it build goodwill and better friendships? Will it be beneficial to all concerned?"

Part Three
VAIRAGYA (*Dispassion*)

13

The Components of VAIRAGYA

In the last chapter we introduced *abhyasa* (practice) and *vairagya* (dispassion) as the wheels of the Chariot of *Sadhana*. We also pointed out that although Patanjali's Classical Yoga is usually associated with *ashtanga-yoga* some writers believe that the *kriya-yoga* described in YS II.1 more appropriately represents his own teaching. That *sutra* identifies ascetism (*tapas*), self-study (*svadhyaya*) and devotion/surrender to the Lord (*ishvara pranidhana*) as the constituents of *kriya-yoga*, the Yoga of ritual or transformative action. *Kriya* are sacred acts that fall under practice (*abhyasa*) and its complement is dispassion (*vairagya*), sometimes translated as non-attachment or detachment. The eight limbs can be thought of as subcategories falling under *tapas*. Together Patanjali presents practice and dispassion as the engine of spiritual *sadhana* and spiritual life. YS II.2 gives the objective of *kriya-yoga* as the cultivation of *samadhi* as well as the attenuation of the causes of suffering (*klesha*), and also as the prevention of future suffering (YS II.16).

Both Patanjali and the Buddha identify *avidya* (spiritual ignorance) as the primary source of all suffering, which then gives rise to the remaining four *kleshas*: *asmita* (I-sense), *raga* (attachment), *dvesha* (aversion) and *abhinivesha* (the survival instinct or will to live). These five *kleshas* together produce an innate pattern that motivates the ordinary life of the unenlightened and perpetuates the cycle of repeated births and deaths. *Kriya-yoga* counters and weakens this pattern to allow recovery of one's authentic identity as the Self. Only Self-realization can interrupt this *samsaric* (earthly) cycle of transmigration. In this chapter we will focus specifically on *vairagya*. Emphasis will be given to some practical methods for establishing it in daily life which take advantage of both ancient and modern technologies for producing detachment.

There are at least two basic aspects to dispassion: purification and dis-identification. The first refers to emotional and mental purification, to use the terminology of Yoga. Its purpose is to release attachments to the five *kleshas* (afflictions of body, mind and speech), which are the fundamental causes of suffering. Ignorance (*avidya*) as a lack of awareness lies at the core of all of them. It is the direct lack of knowing the Centre of Consciousness, a lack of direct awareness of Spirit. It is to live totally entrapped in time, space and causation as a separated being with no awareness of transcendental Consciousness.

The Components of *Vairagya* (Dispassion)

Purification. In the *Yoga-Sutra* (Aranya, 1981) the afflictions (*kleshas*) or causes of suffering are presented as fivefold: *avidya* (ignorance), *asmita* (ego; the sense of I as the doer), *raga* (attraction), *dvesha* (aversion; looking for something new) and *abhinivesha* (survival, fear of death; "May

I not cease to be"). *Avidya* is considered to be the chief of these. These five qualities ground the consciousness into the physical plane.

A similar concept for the *kleshas* is found in Tibetan Buddhism as we indicated under awareness in chapter 5 (Clifford, 1994).

Although *avidya* is usually translated as ignorance we indicated in chapter 1 that it really refers to limited awareness (Niranjanananda, 1993a), and that this limitation is the central cause of suffering. But as awareness deepens one's world view and its component beliefs will change naturally. Indeed, some aspects of one's pictures of reality will only be possible with deepening awareness.

In the Vedantic model of the personality, the five sheaths have also been conceptualized as three: the physical (*annamayakosha*), subtle (*prana-*, *mano-* and *vijnanamayakoshas*), and causal (*anandamayakosha*) bodies. The psychic body in Yoga is a deeper aspect of the subtle body (the subconscious) and the causal body (the unconscious) (Niranjanananda, 1993a). It is the approximate borderline zone between the subtle and causal bodies. The four states of consciousness (gross, subtle, causal and transcendental) are called the two experiences of Yoga. Gross and subtle represent the external experiences of mind. Causal and transcendental represent the inner experiences of mind or consciousness. Thus the psychic body is the zone from where both the inner and the outer experiences can be visualized and experienced. The psychic body is the link between the external physical and mental experiences and the deep internal energetic levels of the personality.

Kundalini Yoga having to do with the *chakras*, the *nadis* and the awakening of *kundalini* is based on experiences of the psychic body. Thus the *chakras* are known as psychic centres. *Muladhara*, *svadhisthana*, *manipura* and *anahata* are the four psychic centres belonging to the realm of outer experience, both gross and subtle. *Vishuddhi*, *ajna*, *bindu* and *sahasrara* belong to the inner dimension. The experience of the *chakras* and *kundalini* takes place in the psychic body which lies deeper than mental experience. The practices develop concentration, awareness and visualization of the psychic body. The *chakras* do not exist in the physical body, but this is where they are visualized.

> Muladhara represents self-identity and security, svadhisthana – deep samskaras, manipura – external or manifesting dynamism, and anahata – emotions and feelings. These four are the outer experience. Going beyond these four to the aspect of transcendence, purity, expansiveness and openness is vishuddhi. The intuitive faculty, pulling something from the unknown and translating it into the known is ajna. In bindu there is awareness of the source, the point where the microcosmic and macrocosmic experiences merge into one. Finally, in sahasrara, there is illumination. These four belong to the inner experience.
>
> Niranjanananda, 1993a

This is an area of great confusion, misinformation and complexity in the West. Unfortunately authentic descriptions and practices for awakening the *chakras* in Yoga are presented in highly symbolic language which is inaccessible to the casual reader without a knowledgeable guide. We will not cover the subject here, save only to make one point. We noted the importance of cognitive paradigms, models of the world or pictures of reality in creating personal experience. What is seldom understood is that each of the *chakras* embodies at the level of consciousness a particular model of the world (Ajaya, 1983). As Jung (1975) noted, "Each *chakra* is a whole world."

Each *chakra* has an archetypal drama that is enacted in real life. In the system of *chakras* these primary archetypes are organized into an evolutionary hierarchy from the primitive to the highly conscious. The manner in which consciousness evolves through these archetypal modes of experience reflects both phylogenetic and ontogenetic development as well as the structure and organization of the human organism. In Tantra the *chakras* relate to seven primary and distinct modes of consciousness and each has a corresponding physical centre. In its most primitive expression consciousness relates to the energy and physical processes at the base of the spinal cord. As consciousness evolves it localizes in progressively higher centres along the spinal cord and brain to culminate in the seventh *chakra* at the crown of the head.

> . . . the chakras of the Tantric system correspond by and large to the regions where consciousness was earlier localized, anahata corresponding to the breast region, manipura to the abdominal region, svadhistana to the bladder region, and visuddha to the larynx and the speech-consciousness of modern man.
>
> C. G. Jung, Collected Works 9, part 1, 467 n.12

These archetypal dramas at each level represent polarities as variations on a single theme. Each of us carries within us each of the archetypes with all the characters and enactments that unfold within each. Most of us are especially involved with a particular *chakra* and a specific part. Even though we may enact parts in dramas from other *chakras* we return over and over to our dominant role. The archetypal themes are impersonal and universal but a person identifies with the character assumed.

Ajaya (1983) summarizes these basic world views from the most primitive to the most evolved states of consciousness. Each *chakra* has an archetypal identity and an experienced polarity. *Muladhara chakra* deals with struggle for survival. The experience in *svadhisthana chakra* is sensory pleasure, and in *manipura chakra* – mastery, domination, power, control, conquest, competition, inadequacy and inferiority. Compassion, generosity and selfless loving service are experienced in *anahata chakra*, while devotion, receiving nurturance and unconditional love, surrender, trust, creativity, grace, majesty and romance are found in *vishuddha chakra*. In *ajna chakra* come insight, intuition and witnessing, but *sahasrara chakra* represents unitary consciousness beyond form with no archetypes or polarities experienced.

There are many ways to develop a typology of models of the world. They are not formed randomly, but seem to evolve in recognizable patterns in human beings everywhere. It is what makes us more alike than different despite our cultural, racial and linguistic diversity. The enneagram system of the Sufis is one example (Palmer, 1988); the metaprograms of Neuro-Linguistic Programming are another (James & Woodsmall, 1988). Whatever typology one uses the ancient wisdom points out that its origins lie with the *chakras*.

Both *Kundalini* Yoga (the Yoga of subtle energy fields) and *Laya* Yoga (the Yoga of dissolution) deal with the psychic body. *Kundalini* Yoga works primarily with the subtle energy structure with more emphasis on awakening the energy centres and channeling the flow of *ida, pingala* and *sushumna* energies. The related changes that occur with mind and consciousness are not the focus, and it is assumed that the energy changes will look after the necessary changes in consciousness. Whereas with *Laya* Yoga the techniques are more meditative in nature. Side by side with the awakening of energy one also observes the changes taking place in consciousness. These changes manifest as altered thinking and analytical processes, altered patterns of awareness and so forth. Consciousness is observed more intensely and energy simply becomes the tool or the medium through which changes in consciousness take place. While *Kundalini* Yoga deals with the seven major *chakras* and some minor *chakras*, *Laya* Yoga deals with the *lokas* (planes), here representing a progression of stages of awakening of finer states of consciousness – worldviews, if you like – that are experienced with the arousal of subtle energy and the *kundalini*. The *lokas* are seven in number and correspond with the *chakras* from the bottom (*muladhara*) as *bhu, bhvah, svah, mahah, janah, tapa* and *satya* at the top (*sahasrara*). This is another way to conceptualize Ajaya's model which is more than just a theoretical concept. Nelson (1994a, b) uses the *chakras* to conceptualize spiritual emergence and spiritual emergencies.

Thus the idea of *avidya* as ignorance in the sense of lack of awareness is rich with implication.

The ego or small self results from the tendency of Consciousness to identify Itself with one's mental model of the world. It is the sense we all have of individuality, the small "I" or self. The emotional component of the personality is embodied particularly in attachment (*raga*) and aversion (*dvesha*) reactions, in likes and dislikes. The process of detachment in the form of emotional purification particularly involves release from this *raga* and *dvesha*. While mental purification refers more to dis-identification of Consciousness from one's mental model of the world. The survival instinct, of course, relates to the small self and ultimately the identity shift of Consciousness from experiencing Itself as a separated individuality to a return or realization of Its transcendent state.

In the previous chapter we noted that the purification of both thoughts and emotions is central to the Himalayan Tradition of Yoga Meditation (Veda Bharati, 1998). Here it is used to prevent the extraneous thoughts and feelings that arise spontaneously during meditation from producing internal disturbances.

The Himalayan oral tradition uses special methods for the conquest of distractions that include emotional purification, the use of *mantras* and Tantric concentrations, initiation into *chakras*, etc. The whole integral system must be followed; reading a commentary on the *Yoga-Sutra* will not produce these states.

Dis-identification. The second aspect of detachment has to do with dis-identification of Consciousness from experiencing Itself in terms of a separated individuality, as an ego or small self, to realizing Itself as the Self or full transcendental Consciousness – called Self-realization in the Yoga tradition. The *Yoga Vasishtha* (Venkatesananda, 1993) looks at this issue of identity this way. It points out that if Consciousness entertains or holds a notion sufficiently long, that notion is experienced as reality, it manifests. By notion here is meant belief, idea, thought or imagination. If one imagines and believes as totally real oneself as a limited individuality or ego then this is experienced as reality. Beliefs are self-fulfilling prophesies since the experience of the world they engender seems to confirm the reality of the beliefs in a closed loop. This idea ties together beliefs, the experience of what is real and the identification property of Consciousness in a very profound way that lies at the root of the identity shift from self-realization to Self-Realization. Dis-identification is a process of releasing powerfully held beliefs about what is real, of disconnecting Consciousness from identification with thought, so that Consciousness shines alone and rests in Itself. Then the outpicturing of those thoughts or beliefs as the world is seen as the unreality of a dream.

> Whatever the inner intelligence [Consciousness] firmly believes in, that alone is experienced by it, as if it is obvious. . . . one realizes that this world is but a notion that arises in consciousness. . . . whatever notion arises in it is experienced as such.

> In this infinite consciousness it is a mere fancy that appears to be the created universe. It is like one's own dream-creation which is everybody's daily experience. Because the dreamer is a conscious being, the dream-objects appear to have an intelligence and a mind of their own; even so this non-creation known as the universe seems to possess independent existence and intelligence as if it had been created. . . . Whatever notion arises in this Brahman is experienced by Brahman as if it were an object of experience.
>
> Venkatesananda, 1993

Detachment involves a process of letting go, of releasing, even of surrender in the sense of letting go of what is not Self. Success in purification brings with it *chitta prasadhana*, a tranquil, even-mindedness with the disappearance of emotional and mental reactivity to external stimuli.

14

Dispassion (VAIRAGYA) *in the* YOGA-SUTRA

YS I.15 *drshtanushravika-vishaya-vitrshnasya vashikara-sanjna vairagyam.*
   "When the mind loses all desire for objects seen or described in the scriptures it
   acquires a state of utter desirelessness which is called detachment."

YS I.16 *tat parampurusha-khyater guna-vaitrshnyam.*
   "Indifference to the *gunas* or the constituent principles, achieved through a knowledge of the nature of *purusha*, is called *paravairagya* or supreme detachment."
                                                                    Aranya, 1981

We draw from the commentary by Swami Veda Bharati (Veda Bharati, 1986). *Vairagya* (dispassion,
detachment, non-attachment) means freedom from attraction and aversion to objects reflecting in
and colouring the mind. The word comes from the Sanskrit verb root, *ranj* meaning "to colour." It
refers to "the state of being devoid of, free from, *raga*, the attraction that accrues, as it were, from
the objects of attraction reflecting in and colouring the mind." (Veda Bharati, 1986, p 206). But this
is only the first of two levels. This absence of "colouring" presents as a freedom from attraction or
craving for objects, a dis-interest or indifference because one sees their faults or lacks the capacity
to enjoy them, perhaps because of illness. But in Yoga there is a second level of mastery or control
(*vashikara*) in which nothing can sway you.

Attractions can be both perceptible and imperceptible. The perceptible ones are perceived with
the senses and would include the opposite sex, food and drink, clothing, music, and so on. They
also include worldly success (*aishvarya*), affluence and power. The imperceptible attractions are
those heard of in spiritual scriptures or traditions, such as paradise, heaven, the angels or *devas*,
the subtle energy realms or astral planes, angelic music, and the like. They also include the eight
powers or accomplishments (*siddhis*) described in *pada* III (YS III.45) and the disembodied states
of advanced yogis.

There are two levels of *vairagya*: *para-vairagya* (*vairagya* that is transcending and beyond)
overcomes *rajas*, deals with the *gunas* and knowledge, and leads to *asamprajnata samadhi*. It is
dealt with in *sutra* 16. *Apara-vairagya* (*vairagya* that is not transcending) is explained in *sutra* 15.
It overcomes *tamas*, deals with worldly objects, and is part of *samprajnata samadhi*. *Apara-vairagya* is the means to *para-vairagya* and has four steps. The first step is the initial effort (*yatamana*)
which involves understanding the process, reducing desires, and gaining emotional maturity. One
learns from teachers and scriptures about the influence of attractions and aversions, about what is
important in the world, and about how action in the world can be flawed and leads to suffering. One
comes to understand what it means to be free of desires and what are the methods for developing

detachment. Emotional maturity comes as one sees that attractions and aversions have their source in the mind, producing emotions and pulling the senses towards worldly objects. At this stage one tries to reduce desires even if one cannot give them up completely.

The second level is ascertainment (*vyatireka*), an intermediate state in which one assesses what has been accomplished and what is left to do in the process. For which emotions and thoughts in the mind, for which of the senses, and for which attractions and aversions has dispassion been accomplished? For which is it presently maturing? For which has it yet to be perfected in the future? Beginning with the weakest of the attractions and aversions, one abandons them one by one until only the strongest attractions and aversions remain.

The third stage (*ekendriya*) pertains to a single sense (the mind) only. Having learned that involvement with the gross or subtle world leads to suffering, one's practice of dispassion has now matured so that attractions or aversions can no longer pull the senses towards external objects. Any remaining attractions or aversions in the mind have been greatly weakened and exist as objects of mere interest. The effort now is to work at the mental level with more abstract issues such as the desire for honour, name and fame, or aversion to dishonour, criticism, etc. In short, attractions and aversions are now mere interests, and the task is to work on mental states.

The fourth and final stage is mastery and control (*vashikara*). There is total neutrality even in the presence of former objects of attraction or aversion, and there is also discrimination between *prakriti* (nature) and the Self. The mind sees that being involved in the world with all of its defects and faults brings only suffering. Thus one becomes neutral to either attractions or aversions whether celestial or non-celestial objects are present. One is simply disinterested in these enjoyments and is unmoved. But there is a new factor. As the Centre of Consciousness opens, dispassion develops naturally through realizing the difference between even the subtle matter of the mind and the spiritual Self. The Centre is so fulfilling that worldly attractions are no longer of any interest.

All of this constitutes the mastery and control which is dispassion (*vairagya*) at the *apara* level. In the first three stages one still has a mental interest in worldly objects even though one has been successful in restraining the inclination of the senses to indulge. However, one must still avoid the temptation because that remaining interest could reawaken the senses and the practice would be abandoned. With the final stage of mastery and control comes total indifference and neutrality even though the objects of attraction or aversion are present. One is now in control and no longer at default. One no longer needs to control or avoid exposure to external objects for fear they will reawaken attachment or aversion. Both the awareness of the faults of worldly pursuits, and of the distinction between nature and the spiritual Self as more fulfilling make the dispassion sustainable.

The final step in this process is *para-vairagya* as described in YS I.16. It comes about through a double process of absorbing authoritative knowledge from the *guru* (*acharya* or realized teacher), the revealed scriptures (*agama*), and through one's own inference (*anumana*), as well as by the repeated practice (*abhyasa*) of realizing and seeing the spiritual Self, remembering the Centre of Consciousness, practising the Presence in all things. This latter process purifies the intelligence (*buddhi*) and fills it to satiety with discrimination. By discrimination here is meant the distinction between *purusha* and *prakriti*, between spirit and the mind field – the direct experience of the Presence or Centre of Consciousness and its qualitative contrast with our normal mental states. Only by dwelling within the Centre of Consciousness or spiritual Self can one experience that kind of satiety that will produce indifference towards knowledge and the means to it. The commentator Vyasa says, "One whose *buddhi* is filled, expanded and satiated with increased and strengthened discriminating wisdom because of the purification that occurs through repeated practice of realizing and seeing (*darshana*) the spiritual self is dispassionate towards the *gunas*, whether with manifest or unmanifest attributes." (Veda Bharati, 1986, p 215). This process of repeatedly practising the Presence purifies intelligence (*buddhi*) by washing off first *tamas* and then *rajas*.

Prakriti (nature) consists of the three *gunas*: *sattva*, *rajas* and *tamas*. *Sattva* is the principle of purity, luminosity, lightness, illumination, light, brilliance, calmness, balance, harmony, clarity, joy, tranquillity, peacefulness or pleasure, and is symbolized by the colour white. *Rajas* gives the qualities of activity, motion, movement, assertiveness, excitation, agitation, nervousness, aggression, anger, endeavour, energy, movement, pain, and is symbolized by the colour red. It impels and energizes, overcoming stagnation. *Tamas* brings inertia, stability, solidity, stagnation, stasis, torpor, stupor, heaviness, languor, dullness, darkness, depression, stupefaction, and is symbolized by the colour black. In the *Samkhya* system the three *gunas* are attributes or constituents of *prakriti* (nature, matter-energy) which evolve into all the various categories of existence. In unmanifest *prakriti* they are in equilibrium. Their disequilibrium produces the process of creation in which all material entities or evolutes including the mind are composed of the three *gunas* in various degrees and combinations in an evolving hierarchy (Veda Bharati, 1986, p 34). They bind individuals and are the basis of pain, pleasure and delusion, and paradoxically, they also serve to liberate them. This is not such a strange scheme when one realizes that only three primary colours combine to produce the whole visible spectrum of light with its infinite gradations.

The primary constituent of the mind field is *sattva*. It becomes smeared with *rajas* and *tamas*. *Apara-vairagya* deals with objects of the world and removes *tamas*. *Para-vairagya* deals with the *gunas* and with knowledge (*jnana*) and removes *rajas* (which also means "dust" and brings to mind the metaphor of removing obscuring dust and polishing the surface of the mirror of the mind field). Practising the eight limbs of Patanjali's *ashtanga* or Classical Yoga partially purifies the mind by removing *tamas* to the point that one begins to see the flaws in involvement in the gross and subtle (celestial) worlds, leading one to reach the lower or *apara-vairagya* until its level of mastery is reached (*vashikara*). But the dust of *rajas* still clings to the mind field and so *apara-vairagya* now becomes the means to the higher *para-vairagya* which removes that remaining dust of *rajas*. The knowledge of the faults of celestial or worldly involvement by itself does not lead to *vairagya*. Only by dwelling in the Self (the Presence or Centre of Consciousness) and becoming complete or filled to the point of satiety, can one become indifferent towards knowledge and the means to it.

Repeated practice (*abhyasa*), then, of realizing the Centre of Consciousness purifies the intelligence (*buddhi*) as *tamas* and then *rajas* are washed off the *sattvic* essence of the mind field. This results in a one-pointed concentration on *sattva* in a single, unbroken stream. The purified intelligence (*buddhi*) fills with the Presence, Being and Bliss of the Self and with the discriminating knowledge (*viveka*) that the *gunas* (i.e., nature, the world both manifest and unmanifest including the mind field) are quite separate from the spiritual Self. There results dispassion for the *gunas* – one no longer cares about the world. Although the *ananda* aspect of the Self is usually translated as bliss, it rather has the sense of fullness and completeness as a state in which our peace and equanimity are independent of a change in or maintenance of some external circumstance. We are full and complete and need no added condition because we are already full. Nothing can be added to us since we are the limitless (*ananta*).

> *Om purnam-adah, purnam-idam, purnat purnamu dachyate,*
> *Purnasya, purnam-adaya, purnam-evavashishyate.*
> *Om Shantih, Shantih, Shantih.*

> Om. That is full; this is full. This fullness has been projected from that fullness.
> When this fullness merges in that fullness, all that remains is fullness.
> Om, Peace! Peace! Peace!
>
> Invocation of Peace (*Shanti-Patha*), *Ishavasyopanishad*
(Nikhilananda, 1977b, p 200)

The *Upanishads* describe the Self as *sat chit ananda* (existence, consciousness, bliss) as well as *satyam jnanam anantam* (truth, knowledge, limitlessness) (Kaji, 2001, p 90). This accounts for the idea of the *buddhi's* satiety which then brings the final dispassion towards the *gunas* (nature) both manifest and unmanifest. In the *Yoga-Sutra* this state is called *dharma-megha*, the *samadhi* of the rain cloud of virtue and of the knowledge of the nature of all things.

Now that the mind is washed free even of *rajas* by practice (*abhyasa*) and dispassion (*vairagya*) it becomes clear (*prasada*) with a mental state of happiness, joyfulness and intense pleasantness, and flows like the image of clear flowing water. In meditation the mind no longer needs external objects for concentration. This is a state of perfection in which knowledge is at its clearest. This Self-knowledge constitutes the higher dispassion which brings permanent freedom from attraction to the manifest and unmanifest creations of the *gunas*. Once this ultimate Self-knowledge, which is itself dispassion, has been attained, the afflictions (*kleshas*) and the residues (*samskaras*) and propensities (*vasanas*) which they produce, have been eliminated, and the cycle of birth and death (*samsara*) has been broken. Liberation as *kaivalya* (isolation) immediately follows this highest dispassion. In other words, *asamprajnata samadhi* follows the *dharma-megha* state.

Swami Veda Bharati (1986, p 217) describes the process thus:

- A person receives authoritative knowledge from the *guru*.
- S/he develops discernment (*khyati*).
- By the practice of *khyati*, the initial stage of *dharma-megha* develops.
- This destroys the blemishes (*mala*) of *rajas* and *tamas* from the mind field, causing the mind to be purely *sattvic* and filled with *prasada*.
- The higher state of *dharma-megha* is then realized, which is the same as the dispassion towards *gunas*.
- The concomitant of this dispassion is the awareness that the reservoir of *karma* is cleared, all *kleshas* have been eliminated and total self-knowledge has been gained.
- Then the highest dispassion of *asamprajnata samadhi* ensues.

15

A Typology of Methods for Producing VAIRAGYA

Table 15.1 The Elements of *Vairagya*
Detachment as Purification of Subtle Energy Fields   • *Emotional Purification*   • *Raising the Energetic Set-Point of the Personality*
Detachment as Dis-Identification of Consciousness   • *From its Vehicles*   • *From the Five Kleshas*
Detachment as Releasing, Letting Go, Forgiveness

The methodologies for *vairagya* could be considered to act through three processes or elements:

• **Detachment** or nonattachment can be considered as a purification of the subtle energy fields at the mental and emotional levels in the personality. One aspect of this is emotional purification which ultimately eliminates emotional reactivity where situations or people trigger negative emotional outbursts as an automatic conditioned response. In Yogic terms they trigger the expression of residues (*samskaras*) from past action and experience (*karma*) resident in the unconscious mind.

Water is often used as a metaphor for emotion. When water streams over a window during a heavy rainstorm one cannot see through the window to the garden beyond. Similarly when the energies of emotion flow through and take over the mind field the Centre of Consciousness which lies beyond is obscured, and even the subtle rational intelligence of the *buddhi* is lost.

The methods for producing nonattachment appear to achieve this by breaking the kinesthetic (feeling) links of attachment and aversion that give the emotional coloring to personal history which produces reactive behavior in the moment to contextual stimuli from the environment. The process of visual-kinesthetic dissociation (V-KD) described in Neuro-Linguistic Programming would be a prime example of this kind of process (O'Connor & Seymour, 1990). The result is neutrality in the face of the stimulus which can rapidly become forgiveness. When asked to define forgiveness, the great sage Shankaracharya replied that if your worst enemy spits in your face your mental state remains completely unreactive. This is the kind of result that will be produced with a successful modern V-K dissociation or energy psychology intervention.

The second aspect of detachment is more subtle. Raising the energetic set-point of the subtle energy fields of the mind not only eliminates emotional reactivity of the mind field in a particular situation, it also eliminates the tendency of the mind field to react at all. In the first case the reactive tendency of the mind persists, even though particular examples of reactivity may be eliminated by a Yogic or psychotherapeutic intervention. But in the second case, the tendency of the mind field to be reactive at all is eliminated. Thus we add a preventive component.

So interventions may be combined, using modern psychological methods to remove specific reactivities in the acute situation, and then using Yogic techniques for the long term to eliminate any tendency for reactivity in the mind field at all. The Yogic technique for doing this primarily is meditation, but the other integrated practices of Raja Yoga, especially the breathing techniques, assist with this.

What do we mean by unreactivity of the mind field? Yogic practices harmonize the energy fields of the personality and align their parts with the Centre of Consciousness. The various components of the personality at every level are homeostatic (balanced), or more correctly, homeodynamic (dynamically balanced). Yogic practices balance the various levels of the personality and restore homeostasis. But the restoration of homeostasis refers only to the current average or set point of the vibrational levels of the energy fields of the personality.

The constituents that make up all the levels of the personality are energy fields arranged in a hierarchy of increasing vibratory levels, as we discussed in chapter 3. At the physical level modern physics has shown the equivalence of matter and energy. In Tantric terms a person is Consciousness (*Shiva*) enrobed in a hierarchy of energy fields (*Shakti*). The mind itself is considered to be a subtle energy field which at its extreme is so subtle that it may reflect spiritual Consciousness.

With the opening of the Centre of Consciousness and the beginning of alignment of the energy fields of the personality with that Centre, the vibrational set point of the personality begins to rise. With effective meditation this is experienced in the mind field as a stable, calm tranquility and equanimity, a detached pleasantness of mind that is unreactive in the face of any environmental stimulus. This state represents a very high state of vibration and energy.

The analogy is a spinning top. The top rotates so rapidly that it appears absolutely motionless. Yet it is not still but rotating very rapidly with high kinetic energy.

With this understanding it becomes clear how interventions like energy psychology can combine with Yogic practices like meditation to create progressive transformation of the personality that aligns its parts with the Centre of Consciousness and allows it to experience that Presence with increasing depth. The alignment itself might be analogous to tuning a radio to higher and higher frequencies or a television set to channels at higher and higher frequencies.

Here is another way to think of the process:

> Once somebody asked Paramahamsa Satyananda, "Is it possible to attain realization
> in one lifetime?" His answer was, "No, it is not possible to attain realization in one

lifetime." The questioner asked him, "Do you mean that our efforts to practice Yoga, or techniques of other spiritual traditions, and to follow the precepts of our religion, are in vain?" He said, "No, they are not in vain, but you have to understand one thing. A transcendental reality cannot be understood by an un-transcendental mind and personality."

So in order to understand that reality, you have to first convert this un-transcendental self into a transcendental being. The aim of spiritual practices is to convert the self into a transcendental being. Their aim is not to provide realization. Once your being becomes transcendental, the mind, the brain, the body, and the senses all become transcendental, then the transcendental awareness will merge with yourself. The practices provide the means to become transcendental.

Niranjanananda, 1993a

Yoga is not about enlightenment!

• The second basic process underlying methods that produce *vairagya* is **dis-identification** of Consciousness with the energy fields of the personality, beginning at the gross level of the physical body and moving progressively to subtler levels. It is this property of Consciousness to identify with the energy fields of manifestation that results in the formation of the ego, small self or the sense of individuality. The sensory-motor mind (*manas*) captures the form, color and movement of a horse in a pasture. The intelligence (*buddhi*) identifies it as a horse. The I sense or ego (*ahamkara*) owns it as "my horse" and the residues of the experience are stored in memory and as *samskaras* in the unconscious mind (*chitta*).

This dis-identification can be thought of as two types. One is dis-identification from the vehicles that make up the personality and the other is from the five afflictions or *kleshas* at the mental level. The former can be conceptualized as the practice of the eight limbs of Patanjali's *ashtanga-yoga* with gradual withdrawal of identification with the sequence of evolutes of *prakriti* (nature) based in *Samkhya* philosophy. Progressive relaxation, for example, can be done as a process of detachment step by step from bodily identification through a witnessing stance and a letting go at each point. The series of exercises for *yoga nidra*, such as 61 points, moves the awareness from the physical into the subtle body. Another way to conceptualize the process is the *via negativa*, the *neti neti* (not this, not that) of Jnana Yoga, dropping the identification with the layers of the personality one by one from gross to subtle (Brunton, 1935). Ramana Maharshi's method of "Who am I?" is an example (1988).

Dis-identification from the *kleshas* is the second aspect. To review briefly, in the *Yoga-Sutra* (Aranya, 1981) the afflictions (*kleshas*) or causes of suffering are presented as fivefold: *avidya* (ignorance), *asmita* (ego; the sense of I as the doer), *raga* (attraction), *dvesha* (aversion, repulsion; looking for something new) and *abhinivesha* (survival, fear of death; "May I not cease to be"). *Avidya* is considered to be the chief of these and their foundation. These five qualities ground the consciousness into the physical plane. *Vairagya* particularly addresses the emotional reactivity of *raga* and *dvesha*.

This process of dis-identification creates *vairagya* by gradually severing the effects of *raga* (attachment) and *dvesha* (aversion); in other words by attenuating emotional reactivity with the development of mental equanimity until the mind field becomes still and unshakable, and of very high energy. The idea of raising the set point of the mental energy field applies here as well. External events simply cannot shake you out of your awareness of the Centre of Consciousness. Just as water flowing over a glass pane obscures it, the watery element of emotion obscures the clarity of the mind field and obstructs spiritual awareness. Likewise, just as throwing a stone into the glassy still surface of a pond disrupts its clarity with the waves and ripples so produced and prevents one seeing the bottom through the still surface, likewise emotionally-driven thought forms, called *vrittis*, obscure the clarity of the mind field and cover the Centre of Consciousness just as surely as clouds cover the sun.

• Finally the third process implicit in *vairagya* is one of **release or surrender**, a letting go, another aspect of forgiveness. A modern technology for this has been developed by Lester Levenson and two versions are available: the Release Technique (Crane, 1998) and the Sedona Method (Dwoskin, 1991; 1999a, b; 2003; Dwoskin & Levenson, 2001). These represent the processes that Lester Levenson described using to produce his own enlightenment after being diagnosed with a fatal disease (Levenson, 1998). They are remarkably simple and surprisingly effective. They also resemble the self inquiry of Jnana Yoga as epitomized in the *neti neti* (not this, not that) or "Who am I?" process of Ramana Maharshi (1988). We have found that they can be used in meditation to release subtle obscuring thoughts just as they originate in the mind field, thereby bringing a further clarity to the awareness of the Presence. Their effectiveness shares the witnessing and dis-associative states that make Visual-Kinesthetic Dissociation (V-KD) so effective in Neuro-Linguistic Programming, and that give some meditative techniques in Yoga their quality also of V-KD that allows thoughts and feelings to come up and disperse – a process called washing the mind.

Some Technologies of Detachment

With this map of *vairagya* we can now summarize how some of the Western technologies of detachment as well as Yoga may produce their effects. Some of them are gathered together in the table below. It is not our intent here to present these methods in detail, but rather in summary form to show how they may work in this context as agents for producing detachment. Some such as meditation and *yoga nidra* are discussed in later chapters.

For producing detachment both the Yogic and the Western technologies have similar effects. They may act in one of two ways. The first is through producing *dissociation or dis-identification*. In Neuro-Linguistic Programming the word "dis-association" is used rather than "dissociation" in order to distinguish this normal process of detachment or dispassion from abnormal dissociated identity disorders (like multiple personality disorder and related psychiatric dissociated states), which is not what is meant here. Alternatively Yogic and Western methods may act by *purification of subtle energy fields* at both the mental level and at the level of the subtle energy body. The word "purification" is a Yogic term. Alternative terms in this context might be harmonization, alignment or coherence.

Table 15.2 Some Technologies of *Vairagya*
Producing Dissociation/Dis-identification • *Kaya Sthairyam* • *Antar Mouna* • *Yoga nidra* • Meditation, *pratyahara, sushumna,* mindfulness • Release Techniques (Sedona Method) • Power Therapies   Neuro-Linguistic Programming

Producing Purification of Subtle (Pranic) Energy Fields
• *Pranayama*
    Balance or Homeostasis (*Nadi Shodhana*)
    Quieting the mind field
• *Bhuta Shuddhi* (The Subtle Elements)
• Power Therapies
    Meridian or Energy Therapies

16

Detachment: Dissociation or Dis-Identification 1

For producing dissociation or dis-identification, all three categories of methods can be used: Yoga, release techniques and the power therapies.

Kaya Sthairyam. The ability to sit absolutely still with the head, neck and trunk straight is essential for meditation and the attainment of transcendent states. In learning meditation, Swami Rama recommended spending the first month learning to sit absolutely still with the posture erect. To keep the mind occupied he suggested letting it travel as an observer through the body. This becomes the progressive relaxation which begins a meditation session. For those who prefer a more formal process, there is a Tantric method called *kaya sthairyam* that is used to train the body into stillness in a proper meditative posture. It can help a student adapt to a meditation *asana*. The term means body (*kaya*) steadiness (*sthairyam*). It is like a witnessing meditation in which the attention is drawn to any aspect of bodily discomfort. This takes advantage of the natural agitation of mind. If necessary one lets the mind wander but keeps the body awareness. When the mind is focused on something its natural restlessness soon takes it elsewhere like a rebel. When forced to focus through concentration on bodily sensations and discomfort in a meditative posture the mind soon becomes bored and its natural restlessness moves it elsewhere. This is exactly what is wanted, since "elsewhere" in this circumstance is in the direction of internalization and leaving behind bodily consciousness. In summary form the process is done as follows:

Kaya Sthairyam

- Sit in a comfortable meditative asana with the head, neck and trunk straight.
- Close the eyes and do a complete progressive relaxation.
- Become aware of the body and imagine it immobile like a tree rooted into the ground, a huge rock or a mountain. Feel that absolute stillness.
- Create a mental image of the body. Move through it concentrating for a few minutes on its sensations, or on any aches or pains until the mind is bored.
- Make a mental image of the right foot and feel its sensations, concentrating for a few minutes. Continue this process in sequence for the left foot, right leg, left leg, the whole back, abdomen, chest, right arm, left arm, neck, head, and end with the whole body again. This completes one round. Do two or three rounds. Intensify the awareness with each round.

Swami Satyananda Saraswati, 1981, p 169

Resolve to be absolutely still like a statue, resisting any impulse to move or to scratch. With time one will detach from the body as something separate from oneself with less and less inclination to move it. The body will feel stiff and rigid (psychic stiffness), and as though it is weightless.

Maintaining a witnessing state during this exercise is essential for producing the desired dissociation from bodily sensations that distract the mind. Thereby the posture becomes absolutely still allowing the mind to go inward into *pratyahara* leaving body awareness behind. If the Presence is available as an inner experience, do the exercise with the awareness immersed as much as possible in It. The witnessing state is automatic since the Presence is the Ultimate Witness. If surveying the body finds areas of pain or discomfort, pause for a few moments, breathing through the area of pain or discomfort while being fully present as a witness or immersed in the Presence if available. Accept the discomfort and allow it to be there with no resistance. Be fully present to it during this observation. And then move on. This kind of body scan can also be incorporated into the progressive relaxation that precedes meditation. Kabat-Zinn (2002) uses a similar body scan in the context of guided mindfulness meditation to assist individuals with the pain and discomfort of chronic disease.

A variant to the process has been suggested by Tolle (2005, p 52) as "feeling the inner body" which can be added as an extra step to *Kaya Sthairyam* or to a progressive relaxation. By "inner body" he means the life or subtle energy experienced as an intensely alive energy field. Begin with the hands by feeling their subtle energy as aliveness. It may start with a mild tingling sensation and then intensify as a feeling of aliveness with continued attention. After starting with the hands for a minute, move on to the feet, and then to both together. Progressively add other body parts as in *Kaya Sthairyam* until one can feel the whole subtle body as a generalized sense of aliveness. Tolle believes that this awareness of the subtle body breaks identification with both body and mind – a dis-identification and moving away from form into formlessness and Being that is the Presence. It is an escape from the ego and it is alleged to strengthen immunity and the body's healing ability (Tolle, 2005, p 53). He recommends doing the practice at every moment possible throughout the day.

Antar Mouna. Another method from Tantra called inner (*antar*) silence (*mouna*) is used to deal with mental restlessness and sensory distraction. Again it is an observational or meditative technique that produces profound dissociation through the witnessing of the arising of mental contents. A silent and peaceful mind is a very powerful mind. It becomes a perfect instrument to receive the bliss and wisdom of the Centre of Consciousness. But the everyday ongoing stream of disturbing thoughts and emotions pouring through the mind prevent this inner Silence from ever arising. All of this turbulence has to be removed before one can experience the inner Silence. *Antar mouna* eradicates mental noise and induces calmness in the mind through its dissociative ability (Satyananda Saraswati, 1981). It is very similar to Buddhist mindfulness meditation which could be used for the same purpose (Salzberg and Goldstein, 2001).

The principles underlying *antar mouna* have profound significance for psychology. It may underlie the catharsis of modern psychiatry. It can address directly neurosis and emotional disturbances, and can release the oppressive mental tensions that we are all subject to as a byproduct of modern living. From childhood we have learned the habit of forgetting painful experiences by suppressing negative thoughts and desires. These mental impressions or *samskaras* are subconscious residues in seed form. They must be removed to stop them from re-expressing to produce more pain, unhappiness or frustration. When used by people with mental disturbance *antar mouna* can gradually harmonize the mind and prepare it for meditation.

Antar mouna systematically creates a dispassionate resistance to external disturbances in the first stage. In the next stage subconscious thoughts and suppressed negative emotions are allowed to gradually surface into witnessing consciousness so that emotionally disturbing contents of the subconscious mind are confronted directly. Thoughts and feelings that have been hidden for years rise to the surface into conscious awareness where they are released and exhausted. As the mind empties over time it is gradually harmonized, becoming progressively tranquil and one-pointed.

Eventually subconscious thoughts and emotions remain as remnants, a mere nuisance. Because they are minor they can be dissolved back into the mind field to induce a state of thoughtless stillness and silence which eventually leads to meditation and perception of the Self. This direct perception of Being is uniquely and powerfully transformative for one's understanding of existence and one's place in the universe.

Antar mouna is a progressive set of exercises in six stages. Swami Satyananda Saraswati (1981) summarizes the six stages of *antar mouna* as follows:

Stage 1: Awareness of sense perception
Stage 2: Awareness of spontaneous thought process
Stage 3: Conscious creation of thoughts
Stage 4: Awareness and disposal of spontaneous thoughts
Stage 5: Thoughtlessness
Stage 6: Psychic symbol awareness
  Pratyahara leads to *dharana* and then to *dhyana.*

Each stage of *antar mouna* prepares for the next and one spends a month or longer perfecting each stage before proceeding to the next. Moving to the later stages 3, 4 and 5 without mastering the earlier ones is a waste of time. For our purposes here we are concerned only with the first two stages.

The first stage produces sensory withdrawal or *pratyahara*. The later stages work with the arising of thoughts in the mind field itself, progressively emptying the unconscious that feeds those thoughts until the mind is still and concentrated. It is analogous to the mindfulness process of meditation (*vipassana*) in Buddhism. Indeed the deliberate practice of mindfulness as a form of self-observation and witnessing, a meditation in action, can be a powerful practice for producing dissociation and detachment.

It is often not realized that mindfulness is taught usually by personal instruction in the Himalayan Tradition where it is called *smrty-upa-sthana* (described in YS I.20) and is the same as the Buddhist *sati-patthana* (Veda Bharati, 1998, p 5; Bhikkhu Nanamoli, 1999). It has many forms that involve a full awareness of the states of the body, breath and mind. Swami Veda Bharati (1985) has discussed its use for the practice of *asana* with deep self-awareness and self-observation of all states of the body, breath, and mind.

In Tantric *antar mouna* the first stage as taught in the Bihar School involves awareness of external sense perception; sound is the most influential. It can be practiced at any time and place by cutting oneself off from external stimuli so as to calm the mind even in the presence of intense noise and unpleasant surroundings. Its essence is awareness and the ability to witness (*sakshi bhava*) with intense alertness. If the Presence is experientially available internally one does it from that Centre. One avoids becoming involved with any experience of external sense impressions. Stage one has the purpose of inducing a state of introversion in preparation for stage two which works with emotions and thoughts. We are conditioned to remain extroverted with a strong attachment to outside stimulation. It is impossible to begin exhausting negative subconscious residues from the mind or to meditate until we are able to become introverted. Stage one neutralizes responses to external stimulation allowing us to be detached and unaffected by the external world.

One can try to force the mind to be introverted and to ignore sensory inputs. This leads to fighting the mind and is ineffective. Because it creates tension it also prevents meditation. In stage one, one moves from trying to suppress external awareness to becoming intentionally aware of the outer world. This paradoxical process involves attending to external stimulation until the restless mind becomes bored and spontaneously loses interest in the outside world. At this point the mind introverts automatically. When this process has been mastered one then moves on to stage two to deal with thoughts and emotions. The method is summarized as follows, and the reader should refer to the original for details (Satyananda Saraswati, 1981, p 635).

Antar Mouna Stage One
Awareness of Sense Perception

- Sit absolutely still in comfortable meditative *asana* with the head, neck and trunk straight, and the eyes closed. "Now I will start the practice of *antar mouna.*"
- Focus intensely on all the sensations of touch all over the body until the mind loses interest.
- Become aware and receptive without resistance, to all external stimuli from your surroundings. Use choiceless, detached awareness. Sound will predominate. Hear only the sound without interruption as though for the first time. Continue for a few minutes. "I am the seer unaffected by these sounds."
- Choose a sound for exclusive attention for about a minute, and then choose another, and repeat over and over. Do not sleep; no thoughts. Then be aware of all sounds that arise at the same time. Expand your perception to its limits to hear even the slightest sound.

- Then breath awareness for a few minutes with no external perception, and no thoughts.
- Again be aware of general noise and then move to individual sounds as above.
- Alternate between awareness of the external sounds and breath awareness until the exercise is finished.

Swami Satyananda Saraswati, 1981, p 635

While stage one deals with outside stimulation, stage two of the process is practiced to deal with negative emotions like guilt, worry or fear and with the pressure of thoughts that arise from inside the mind. The point of the process is to exhaust negative thoughts and feelings from the subconscious mind which represent *samskaras* (residues). One allows them to bubble to the surface without suppression, accepting their presence, letting them evaporate or pass through the space of the mind like moving clouds. In this way these thoughts, memories, visions and images, and emotions are exhausted and the mind is purged. Although we allow positive thoughts into awareness we have a habit of suppressing negative ones back into the subconscious. These emotionally charged, unexpressed residues can create continual disturbance, depression and dissatisfaction with unhappiness and mental tension as they act as a block in the mind.

The process of *antar mouna* allows all thoughts, both negative and positive, to arise into the mind without suppression. It is a passive awareness of the thinking process. There is no attempt to create thoughts or to try to think; it is a state of allowing combined with intense and present witnessing and alert awareness, centered in the Presence if It is available. Thoughts are allowed to arise and disappear naturally and spontaneously. The practitioner remains a witness to these thoughts, a disinterested spectator of everything that comes up in the mind. In the beginning breath awareness can be added to anchor the awareness. The mind needs a support (*alambana*) and we find that mindfulness of the breath makes this process easier. There may be times when the mind seems blank and without thoughts. One does not try to create thoughts to fill that space. Strong suppression can prevent thoughts from arising, so one simply watches the mind and waits for the spontaneous flow of thoughts to start again. One may experience thoughts that one did not think existed in the mind, like childhood memories, phobias, beautiful or frightening visions, all from the deeper layers of the subconscious – a kind of conscious dreaming. One simply observes them as an impassive witness, letting them come up without suppression, and without like or dislike. Gradually the mind is purged of suppressed thoughts. The result is a state of mental tranquility and one-pointedness.

The practice can be done at night just before sleep to release disturbances from daily affairs so that one can have a good night's sleep. The practice can also be done in the early morning after awakening. At this time thinking is more subtle for grosser thoughts have been partially exhausted in dreams. This is a good time to release deeper negative thoughts from the subconscious. Their elimination can have a positive effect on the personality. Again the essence is Awareness and the adoption of the witnessing stance. The alertness is intense and one avoids becoming involved with any experiences or feelings, thoughts or images that bubble up. One is the seer, the detached observer and not the thinker. Suppressed thoughts can then bubble up from the subconscious quite freely and be exhausted. Practice this spontaneous thought awareness twenty-four hours a day. Practicing breath awareness as much as possible throughout the day can help keep the witnessing focus of awareness in the present and not let it associate into mental content and be swept away into the past or future with their unconsciousness and conditioning. Swami Veda Bharati is fond of prescribing an exercise to meditation students to find out how many breaths it takes them to travel from the class back to their homes. One should always be aware, a witness of one's thoughts, allowing them to arise and then dissipate and vanish. Any buildup of emotions is prevented and tension is released. One should not avoid unpleasant thoughts, feelings and experiences by suppressing them. Allow them to bubble up, emptying the mind of its impurities and removing the blocks that veil intuitive knowledge. This process along with meditation is ideal for emotional purification in this stage of the path. The method described in the Bihar School is summarized below. The reader should consult the original for details (Satyananda Saraswati, 1981, p 658).

Antar Mouna Stage Two
Awareness of Spontaneous Thought Process

- Sit absolutely still in a comfortable meditative asana with the head, neck and trunk straight and the eyes closed. "Now I will start the practice of *antar mouna*."
- Practice *antar mouna*, stage 1 on external sounds for a few minutes.
- Focus all awareness on and observe thoughts arising spontaneously from the subconscious, freely and without restriction, whether they are pleasant or unpleasant. Accept whatever comes without judgment or analysis. Remain alert. Do not sleep. Observe the thoughts as though they were occurring outside you. "I am different from these thoughts."
- Now allow all emotions to arise in the same way.
- Remain a witness, a seer, separate from emotions and thoughts.
- After five minutes shift the awareness to the *chidakasha* (the inner screen of awareness behind the eyes and forehead). Witness and observe whatever arises on that inner screen of consciousness with no resistance and no expectations, whether visions arise or whether nothing arises.
- After five minutes go back to watching the thought process and the emotions again.
- Alternate between watching the thought process and watching the *chidakasha* at five minute intervals until the exercise is done.

Swami Satyananda Saraswati, 1981, p 658

One should note the importance of detached observing or witnessing to the success of the method as mental and sensory content flow through the mind. Thus one way in which it likely acts is through visual-kinesthetic dissociation. One can also see the potential for combining modern Western methods such as VK-D from Neuro-Linguistic Programming or Energy Psychology with a practice like *antar mouna* for enhancing and accelerating the progress to meditation. In *antar mouna* the process during stage two could also be appreciated as a form of surrender, and as such, can benefit from the Sedona method of Releasing.

Releasing. Lester Levenson developed a series of practices for releasing negative thoughts and emotions based on his own experience with transcendental states of consciousness (Levenson, 1998).

These have been developed further by Crane (Crane, 1998) and Dwoskin (1991; 1999a, b; 2003). The methods are very simple, but to our knowledge there is no research validation as to their effectiveness beyond anecdotal reports of seminar participants. Nevertheless, they are worth mentioning briefly here. They are subtle, and easily and quickly used within a meditation practice. They are also easily used at any time during the day to deal with mental negativity. But how powerful they are as an intervention is unclear.

The art of releasing or letting go has been formulated in four steps. The first is releasing by simply choosing to release. One just drops whenever one is holding on to in the moment emotionally or mentally. This may resemble the detachment that is achieved by mentally stepping back from a problem as in the dis-association of Neuro-Linguistic Programming.

A second version employs allowing. One allows whatever is to be in this moment in the mental field from an observer or witness position. One treats the mental content with AWE – Allowing it to be, Welcoming it fully, and even Embracing it. And then one releases with the paradoxical questions (which one does not try to answer), "Could you just let it go? Would you? When?" One treats the thought or emotion as an energy in the mind field and allows it to pass through in the same way that clouds pass through the sky automatically, needing no changing, correction or fixing.

A third version of the process involves confronting the emotion or negative thoughts directly. One dives into the core of whatever the feeling is. One may discover it is empty inside or even full of goodness. There is not the darkness one assumes will be there. Sometimes a metaphor is used of drilling into the energy form or inserting a pipe into it that allows it to release as though under pressure. The head may rest bowed on the chest for kinesthetic access, and release with an exhalation can be helpful.

Finally, there is a holistic releasing which can deepen the other three procedures. It involves the deliberate and repetitive juxtaposition of positive and negative versions of a statement in order to bring the two sides of the polarities together so that they can neutralize each other. One focuses on both sides of the polarities by going back and forth between the two with persistence until a neutrality or feeling of inner expansion occurs as a sense of limitation dissolves. With practice one begins to notice how frequently one creates artificial polarities in life and one learns to bring the two sides together as one goes. Eventually just noticing them is enough for them to start to dissolve.

From our perspective, if one side of the coin of surrender is releasing the negative, the other side is acceptance of the positive. Allowing and releasing move the student to loving acceptance.

Releasing	**Acceptance**
"Could you just let that go?	"Could you just accept that?
Would you?	Would you?
When?"	When?"

Dwoskin, 1991

Acceptance of the positive then unfolds a sequence of positive attitudes from praise through appreciation, gratitude to reverence and love which raise the vibrational set-point of the subtle energy fields of the personality. Loving reverence then opens the personality to grace. Here is a brief summary of Releasing. The reader should consult the original texts and tapes for details (Dwoskin, 2003).

Releasing
(The Sedona Method)

- Bow the head, and insert an imaginary pipe into the negative feeling usually felt in the chest or abdomen, and let (imagine) its pressure release with an exhalation. Repeat until the feeling is exhausted (Crane, 1998). OR
- Treat the negative feeling with AWE:
  Be fully present to the feeling by
>> Allowing it,
>> Welcoming it, and even
>> Embracing it.
  Then, "could you just let it go?"
>> "Would you?"
>> "When?"

Repeat until the feeling is neutralized, usually about five times (Dwoskin, 1991). Alternative statements to "Could you just let it go?" that can be used are:
>> "Could I let go of wanting/needing to change this?"
>> "Could I let go of wanting/needing to control this?"
>> "Can I let go of wanting to understand or figure out this situation?"
>> "Can I let go of wanting to change this as best I can?"

- In both methods be fully focussed and present as a neutral observer or witness. This detached stance is crucial for the success of the method.
- An interesting parallel from the Yoga tradition comes from M. Govindan (2000, p 4):
>> "As various disturbing thoughts, emotions or sensations arise, ask the question: 'Could I let it go?' Cultivate detachment towards them."

17

Detachment: Dissociation or Dis-identification 2

Pratyahara. The Sanskrit word *pratyahara* is made up of two root words: *prati* ("opposite," "in opposition to") and *ahara* ("to fetch," "bring back," also "to take food"), which gives a literal meaning "to oppose the bringing back" or "to oppose the taking of food." In Yoga it means that sensory perception is opposed. We receive input about the external world through the five senses continuously. This flow of perceptions can be thought of as feeding the mind. If we do not choose carefully what we put into the mind, what we "feed" the mind, so that perceptions flow in indiscriminately, they will keep the mind extroverted and continuously agitated. *Pratyahara* implies that incoming sensory data are opposed, that the mental intake of "food" for the senses is blocked, that inner perception is cut off. The senses are disconnected to produce a state of sensory withdrawal. This is another aspect of detachment at the level of the cognitive senses.

During the waking state perception is directed mostly towards the outside world through the senses. *Pratyahara* prevents external perception, allowing our awareness to remain within the mind where it is available for introspection. The first stage of *antar mouna* described above has the purpose of cutting off external perception.

During dreaming we are aware of the various layers of the subconscious mind. We experience similar alpha states in reverie, daydreaming and hypnosis, and during certain stages of meditation. Stage two of *antar mouna* described above is a similar state. But the important difference is that in dreaming and sleep there is only slight or no awareness, while the essence of methods like *antar mouna*, mindfulness and meditation is a high level of awareness. Like a safety valve dreams release tensions from the mind. The process of confronting the inner mental tensions arising from the subconscious is enhanced when there is detached awareness. It is the dissociation and witnessing that allow these methods to work by releasing thoughts and emotions in a kind of ongoing catharsis of the stream of consciousness. Dreams generally lack awareness as we define it here (excluding lucid dreaming). Thus a technique like stage two of *antar mouna* is essentially a process of "conscious dreaming" that accelerates the release of mental tension.

Cutting off external sensory perception is only the first stage of *pratyahara*. When perfected, both external sensory perception and the flow of thoughts and emotions from the subconscious as the stream of consciousness are transcended. Then *dharana* (concentration) arises and eventually leads to the state of *dhyana* (meditation).

The whole point of mindfulness methods like *antar mouna* is to induce *pratyahara* as a means to meditation and to make the mind one-pointed. The application of *sushumna* also produces a tranquil and pleasant mind and is a method for producing *pratyahara*. Sri Swami Rama used to say humorously that gaining enlightenment was very simple – learn to apply *sushumna* and then raise the *kundalini* to *sahasrara*; that's all there is to it! In Raja Yoga *pratyahara* is a rung preceding concentration and meditation. Without it meditation is impossible. *Pratyahara* is not easy to attain and so few people actually experience true meditation. The approach must be correct and systematic otherwise meditation will not arise even if one practices twenty-four hours a day for twenty years. First *pratyahara*, then *dharana* and then *dhyana*. *Yoga nidra* is also an aspect of *pratyahara* and we shall discuss it below.

Meditation itself has been described as washing the mind. It is a powerful method for producing detachment and for bringing the mind field to tranquility. It is preceded by the practice of *pratyahara* or sensory withdrawal, which is effectively detachment at the level of sensory input. Indeed, the progressive relaxation that is a part of proper meditative practice effectively dissociates the awareness from the physical body. The application of *sushumna* as part of the breathing techniques associated with meditation is an essential aspect of *pratyahara*. Mindfulness with breath awareness is a powerful technique to purify the mind. We will discuss some of these methods in more detail in Part Five and try to show their similarity to visual-kinesthetic dissociation as it has been described in Neuro-Linguistic Programming.

Yoga nidra. There are many related practices that produce profound relaxation that come under the grouping called *yoga nidra*, or conscious Yogic sleep, which takes the awareness into the *anandamayakosha*, the deepest layer of the personality. It is here that the awareness extends into deep sleep. The practice of *yoga nidra* allows one to access this sheath and the state of deep sleep with full awareness.

Yoga nidra is a series of profoundly effective relaxation techniques that can take the state of relaxation far beyond anything that the West has yet to discover with progressive relaxation. It has many practical applications. It can induce a deep relaxation of the whole human personality. Some consider it as a technique of meditation and others consider it only as a process for relaxation. It is also a dissociative method like the various techniques considered above for producing detachment. It is an ancient Tantric process for exploring, deconstructing and disidentifying from the levels of the personality. It takes the awareness into the *anandamayakosha* or *karana sharira* (causal sheath) – the *karmashaya* or field of *karma* with its *vasanas* (propensities, deep desires) and *samskaras* (residual impressions of actions), which Western psychology knows as the unconscious. It can be beneficial for psychosomatic ailments (for example, the treatment of hypertension). It can eradicate deep rooted psychological complexes, and in this sense is an advanced psychiatric tool. *Yoga nidra* can induce and improve deep sleep and relieve insomnia. It can recharge and rejuvenate the physical, *pranic* and mental levels of the personality. It can be used to explore the mind and awaken its potential, including intuition. *Yoga nidra* has been used in education for accelerated learning, especially of languages (Suggestopedy: Lozanov, 1978). The absorption and retention of information from external sources is enhanced as well as access to one's own knowledge.

The words *yoga nidra* mean "Yogic sleep." By ridding the mind of chronic tension and bypassing rational thought it induces physical and nervous tranquillity and brings inner peace, which, in turn, induces meditation and brings forth the inner knowledge of intuition.

We discuss here two methods which are really two different, if not unrelated, practices that happen to share the same name. The method taught by the Bihar School of Yoga is a systematic method for inducing deep relaxation with inner awareness (Satyananda Saraswati, 1981; 1984). It involves a great deal of guided imagery that takes one to an alpha threshold state between sleep and wakefulness called the hypnagogic state, or what Swami Satyananda has called the hypnayogic state (Satyananda Saraswati, 1984: p 6). He describes it as essentially a method of *pratyahara* (Satyananda Saraswati, 1984: p 33). In this state contact with the subconscious and unconscious occurs spontaneously which can be used to clear the mind of *samskaras*, for accelerated learning, and for enhanced creativity and problem solving.

Swami Satyananda developed the method himself from personal experiences and the study of Tantric scriptures: "I began studying the tantric scriptures . . . I came across many important but little known practices . . . After practising them myself, I decided to construct a new system called *yoga nidra* which would incorporate the essence of these practices without any of the complicated ritualistic drawbacks." (Satyananda Saraswati, 1984: p 3). Initially he called it psychic sleep or yogic sleep and later *yoga nidra* (Satyananda Saraswati, 1984: p 4).

It includes as a central feature the systematic rotation of consciousness through the body based on the Tantric practice of *nyasa* ("to place; to take the mind to that point"). It is a means of consecrating the physical body by instilling higher awareness or divine consciousness into body parts during Tantric ritual practices. In this practice specific *mantras* are placed and felt at different parts of the body. The external (*bahir*) form involves physically touching parts of the body, while in the internal (*antar*) form *mantras* and the awareness are mentally placed. A large selection of different *mantras* can be used and rotated throughout the six *chakras* and the various parts of the body. The chanting of *mantras* and rotation of awareness is said to harmonize the nervous system, balance the *pranic* flows, and render the mind one-pointed. Each part of the body is systematically charged with the energy of the *mantras*, thereby purifying body and mind which are then prepared for meditation. Although *mantras* can be used, modern-day versions of *yoga nidra* are devoid of *mantras*. In the Bihar system rotation of awareness with *mantra* is *nyasa*, while rotation of awareness without *mantra* is *yoga nidra*.

Swami Satyananda modified the process as described in the ancient texts, including removing the *mantras*. He correlates the order of the sequence of rotation of consciousness throughout the body parts with the motor homunculus mapped to the precentral gyrus of the brain (Satyananda Saraswati, 1984: p 42). With the recent availability of fMRI and PET scanning it should now be possible to test whether this working hypothesis is actually correct.

The Bihar method describes three specific states of *yoga nidra*. While the objective of *yoga nidra* is to acquire the ability for conscious sleep, someone who is tired, exhausted and constantly under stress and worry will find that the practice induces a refreshing, beneficial DEEP SLEEP. For others the practice will induce conscious dreaming with a stream of imagery from the subconscious mind, called PSYCHIC SLEEP, which lies between sleep and wakefulness where one confronts subconscious problems, suppressions, fears, and conflicts. Regular practice like this slowly purifies and washes the mind to create detachment. The deepest state of *yoga nidra* is SLEEPLESS SLEEP. Here one treads the borderline between introversion and extroversion. Some consider this to be the path of *sushumna* corresponding to the awakening of the *kundalini* (Satyananda Saraswati, 1981: p 768).

Here there is some confusion of terminology. The *Mandukya Upanishad* describes three states or layers of mind as *jagrat* (waking state; conscious mind; *sthula* or gross dimension or body; surface thoughts and perceptions of the external world), *svapna* (dream state; subconscious mind; *sukshma* or subtle dimension or body; individual memory and mind), and *sushupti* (deep sleep state; unconscious mind also containing memory; *karana* or causal dimension or body, cosmic mind) (Nikhilananda, 1987b; Rama, 1982b). Beyond these three lies the superconscious state of *turiya*, the blissful and mystical state of Yoga that corresponds to superconsciousness.

> When *sankalpa* (desires) and *vikalpas* (fancies and imaginations) are rooted out then one is influenced no more by *karma*. When *sankalpa* and *vikalpa* are removed by constant Yogic practice the ever-blissful state of *yoga nidra* dawns.
>
> Shankaracharya, Yogataravali

> Beyond these three states (*jagrat, svapna* and *sushupti*) there is *turiya*. It is a state that is spontaneously experienced by yogis. It is real *yoga nidra* in the form of pure, illumined consciousness. This *yoga nidra* is not part of *prakriti* (nature) but it is the manifested form of *purusha* (consciousness).
>
> Shankaracharya, Yogataravali, v.26

Here *yoga nidra* is identified as *turiya*, whereas usually the state of conscious deep sleep (*sushupti*) is meant by the term.

Yoga nidra starts from the *svapna* state with an exploration of the subconscious mind. With increased mastery perception deepens until one contacts and explores the *sushupti* or cosmic mind. Those who master Yoga transcend the mind to enter the state of superconsciousness, which is called *turiya* (the fourth dimension of being) in the *Mandukya Upanishad*, the highest state which few attain.

There are many varieties of *yoga nidra* that can be practised (Satyananda Saraswati, 1981, 1984; Miller 2000; Rama, 1982b). We have used the Bihar version extensively with cancer patients, who enjoy the great deal of visualization involved (Satyananda Saraswati, 1981, 1984). It uses nine sequential stages and evolves progressively through many increasingly complicated variations on these stages. They include:

1. Preliminary adjustment of the body.
2. Preliminary relaxation of the physical body.
3. Preliminary relaxation of the mind.
4. *Sankalpa* (resolve).
5. Rotation of awareness throughout the different parts of the body.
6. Visualization.
7. Reflection and symbol awareness.
8. *Sankalpa.*
9. Return to external awareness.

The visualization and symbol awareness use archetypes for unburdening the unconscious.

The method used in the Himalayan Tradition is a more abstract series of breathing and relaxation exercises as taught by Sri Swami Rama (Rama, 1982b; 1988). It originates from the oral and textual tradition of the Himalayan Masters and is grounded in the *Mandukya Upanishad*. There are some seven versions of it that are taught depending on personal circumstances. It has the following basic structure:

YOGA NIDRA

Shavasana
Withdrawal from place, space and time
Deep progressive relaxation of muscles and joints

Shavayatra
32 point exercise, progressing to
61 point exercise, progressing to
blue star exercise and/or
nyasa with a personal *mantra*

Shithali Karana
breathing successively between toes, ankles, knees, and the crown 10× each, then
breathing successively between perineum, navel, heart, throat, upper lip (*sushumna* point),
    between eyebrows, and the crown 5× each. In some versions one breaths through the
    bridge of the nose between the *sushumna* point and *ajna* and then reverses the process
    back down to the toes.

Yoga nidra
breathing through eyebrow centre ×3
breathing through throat centre with visualization of a moon ×3
breathing through heart centre – rest, no *mantra*

Gentle exteriorization at completion

The posture and first two stages through the relaxation are identical with meditation in the Himalayan Tradition. Then come two deeper, more advanced relaxations. *Shavayatra* is a process of travelling with the awareness through the body. One begins with 32 points in sequence beginning with the point between the eyebrows, the pit of the throat, and then the right shoulder, elbow, wrist, tips of each of the fingers and then back up in reverse to the pit of the throat, followed by the same sequence for the left arm and hand. Then one moves to the nipples and heart *chakra* to complete the 32 points. Each point is a *chakra* in the subtle body which is stimulated by the process. When this procedure can be done consistently without losing concentration or falling asleep one moves on to the full 61 points, by proceeding to the navel, the perineum, and then the hip, knee, ankle and toes of the right leg. One reverses up the leg again to the perineum and then the same sequence down and back up the left leg to the perineum. One concludes with the navel, heart centre, pit of the throat and point between the eyebrows to complete the 61 points.

The points are mentally counted in sequence. When this can be completed without losing concentration or falling asleep, one moves on to the next stage of the blue star exercise in which one visualizes placing a blue star at each of the 61 points. One's personal *mantra* can also be placed in each of the points at a later stage. The points represent *chakras* in the subtle body (*pranamayakosha*) which makes this part of the process an exercise with the energy body.

Now comes *shithali karana* which is a further deep, advanced relaxation. It involves point to point breathing linking the crown with the toes, ankles, knees, hips, the first, third, fourth and fifth *chakras*, the *sushumna* point where the bridge of the nose joins the upper lip (*nasagra*) and the sixth *chakra* – inhaling from each point to the crown and exhaling back down. Once this is mastered without losing concentration or falling asleep, one then goes on to the *yoga nidra* proper, breathing in turn through the eyebrow centre (centre of waking consciousness), the throat centre while visualizing a full moon (the centre of dreaming), and finally the heart centre (centre of deep sleep). One rests in the heart centre with only breath awareness, no *mantra*. During deep sleep there is no content and one rests in the void. A deep spontaneous sigh from the body is the signal that the session is complete.

The Bihar version of *yoga nidra* is strongly recommended for its psychotherapeutic uses in purifying the subconscious as noted above. What about the Himalayan version which takes one to the state of deep sleep and the unconscious? As the awareness expands with the practice through the levels of the conscious, subconscious and unconscious mind one gains insights about how the mental and emotional processes operate within the personality structure. One has a direct experience in both *yoga nidra* and meditation – which complement each other – of the latent impressions contained in the unconscious which contains the *karmashaya*, the storehouse of *karma* as *samskaras* and *vasanas*. As consciousness touches them we see how it causes these latent impressions to stir from this causal level. They rise into the subconscious as invisible thought processes which are experienced initially only in dreams – what in psychology is called "primary process." Then they come forward into the waking state and we see how they engage the cognitive and active senses for expression in the external world and how the four primary functions of the mind interact with these levels: the sensory-motor mind (*manas*), the ego (*ahamkara*), the *chitta* (memory or storehouse of impressions), and the *buddhi* (the knowing, deciding, judging and discriminating faculty as well as the source of intuition from its higher levels).

There is a transition state between waking and dreaming called *unmani,* which is the hypnogogic state mentioned above experienced as the pleasant alpha daydreaming state as one comes out of a good sleep yet is not fully awake or externally aware. There is also a transition state called *aladani* between dreaming and deep sleep which is not normally experienced. This very subtle state is a transition of which we are not normally aware, where latent, formless unconscious impressions (*samskaras,* the source of our *karma*) begin to stir and then take form in the subconscious as dreams. This is the transition in which the subconscious subtle world and subtle thoughts are born from the deeper causal level.

As the complementary processes of meditation and *yoga nidra* progress, awareness expands progressively into these levels and one begins to be aware of how consciousness permeates and holds all of these levels and transitions, and that our essential nature is consciousness and not the forms of its content. As we witness immersed in Awareness the rising contents of impressions as they bubble up from the bed of the unconscious through these levels and let them go, the mind is progressively purified. We can do this at two levels: at the transition between dreaming and wakefulness as both methods of *yoga nidra* do along with meditation, and the Bihar method with its guided imagery is specialized to do, and also at the transition between the unconscious and subconscious which the Himalayan method can address.

Although not the primary goal of the Himalayan practice, it can address the very bed root of the *karmashaya* where the stirrings first begin and are released at a deeper and more fundamental level by allowing them to dissolve back into the mind field. The deep sleep state is the bed that has the roots of our habit patterns, desires, attractions and aversions that express themselves in dreams or become actions and speech in the external world. These are the *kleshas* or afflictions (spiritual ignorance, egoism, attachment and aversion, and fear of death). At this deep level one begins to see how the subtle and material realms manifest and how they can be manipulated. By letting them come and then go through witnessing and detached observation non-attachment results and the colouring of the mind by the *kleshas* attenuates. The *samskaras* lose their potencies to bind and thereby drive thought, speech and action in habitual behaviour, and become mere memories. The direct access to these deep impressions provides the *yogin* with mastery over thought, speech and action through control of *samskaras* and allows him or her to create new habit patterns that do not conflict with the old which are attenuated and burned.

Meditation, contemplation and *yoga nidra* in the Himalayan Tradition complement each other in allowing the *yogin* the ability to address the roots of habits and the afflictions directly. It is no accident that meditation has been called the highest therapy. The attenuation of the potencies of *samskaras* also is a natural outcome of the deep introspection of *yoga nidra.* The end result is the progressive development of dispassion or detachment (*vairagya*).

Karma Yoga. Karma Yoga has been described as among the best methods for developing detachment (Paramahamsa Niranjanananda, 1993a, p 160). Niranjanananda defines it as mindful action. Action is to be done mindfully and with full consciousness and awareness rather than habitually and mechanically. When thought, speech and action are done in perfect awareness detachment develops quickly and one becomes immune to external influences like success and failure or pleasure and pain. Thereby one becomes tranquil and peaceful. To act mindfully is to be aware not only of the action but that you are doing the action. When one acts without mindfulness one's actions are *karmic*. Practice breath awareness and/or remembering one's personal *mantra* as often as possible during the day's activities to stay present and detached. If the Presence is available, let action flow from that Centre. Karma Yoga is action flowing from the Centre of Consciousness. It does not produce *karmic* reaction as does action originating from the ego.

Power Therapies. The remaining group of methods for producing dis-association are the power therapies, so-called because of their high efficacy as psychotherapeutic tools. They are relatively recent developments from the latter part of the twentieth century and include three categories: Neuro-Linguistic Programming (NLP) (O'Connor & Seymour, 1990), Eye Movement Desensitization and Reprocessing (EMDR) (Shapiro, 1995), and energy psychology (EP) (Gallo, 1999; 2000) also known as (subtle) energy meridian therapies or acupressure for the emotions (Gach and Henning, 2004). In this book we will concern ourselves only with NLP and EP, the practical elements of which an aspirant can learn to use quite easily. They nicely complement Yogic approaches to producing detachment through emotional purification, especially in the face of emotional reactivity due to attachment and aversion.

NLP is relevant to our discussion here. There are many patterns in NLP that produce dis-association and detachment. Hall and Belnap (2000) should be consulted for details. They classify 77 of the most used patterns as:

- Basic or foundational patterns
- Patterns for incongruity of parts
- Patterns for identity and self
- Patterns for Neuro-Linguistic states
- Patterns for languaging
- Patterns for thinking patterns and cognitive distortions
- Patterns for meanings and semantics
- Patterns for mental strategies

Visual-kinesthetic dissociation is foremost among these groups of patterns for producing dis-association. It serves as a model for how detachment may be produced by Yogic processes. But other useful patterns for producing detachment include reframing algorithms, submodality and swish interventions including compulsion blow out, resolution of internal conflicts through parts negotiation and integration, belief changes and value hierarchies, time-line interventions, the meta-model of language, meta-program distinctions, and mental strategies including the new behaviour generator as examples. All of these dissociate the emotional charge from the memories of personal history.

18

Detachment by Purification of Subtle (PRANIC) *Energy Fields*

Pranayama. As shown in Table 15.2 in chapter 15, detachment can also be produced through purification or alignment of subtle energy fields. The breathing exercises of *pranayama* act not only to quiet the mind field itself, but also to produce homeostasis and realignment in both the subtle energy body and the physical body, the latter through the psychoneuroimmune system of host resistance (Jerry, 1996; Jerry & Jerry, 2001). Two exercises in particular are important here. *Nadi shodhana* (channel purification or alternate nostril breathing) balances the sympathetic and parasympathetic divisions of the autonomic nervous system and the corresponding *pingala* and *ida nadis* in the subtle body respectively (Jerry, 1996) thereby re-establishing homeostasis. The application of *sushumna* quiets the mind field, making it peaceful, pleasant and ready for meditation.

Bhuta Shuddhi. The Tantric exercise called *Bhuta Shuddhi*, (purification of the elements) uses visualization, breathing and *mantra* to purify the five elements that underlie the structural foundation of the subtle body (Rama, 2002c; Satyasangananda Saraswati, 1984; Goswami, 1999, p 319). The following summary gives an idea of the process; the original should be consulted for details (Rama, 2002c). The Himalayan Institute in Honesdale, Pennsylvania, provides a practice tape and chart of the *chakras* to assist in learning it.

Bhuta Shuddhi
(Purification of the Elements)

- Exhale with *Hum* to 1st *chakra* visualizing the uncoiling and awakening the *kundalini*
- Visualize *kundalini* rising up *sushumna*, absorbing each *chakra* in turn:
  Visualize 1st chakra; 4 petals; earth (*prithivi*); repeating *lam* at least 16 times
  Visualize 2nd chakra; 6 petals; water (*apas*); repeating *vam* at least 16 times
  Visualize 3rd chakra; 10 petals; fire (*agni*); repeating *ram* at least 16 times
  Visualize 4th chakra; 12 petals; air (*vayu*); repeating *yam* at least 16 times
  Visualize 5th chakra; 16 petals; ether (*akasha*); repeating *ham* at least 16 times
  Visualize 6th chakra; 2 petals; mind; repeating *so'ham* at least 16 times
  Visualize 7th chakra; 1000 petals; repeating *hamso* at least 16 times
- Inhale left nostril repeating *yam* (16 counts) into the heart centre; retain (64 counts of *yam*); exhale right nostril (32 counts of *yam*), visualizing drying the impurities.
- Inhale right nostril repeating *ram* (16 counts) into the heart centre; retain (64 counts of *ram*); exhale left nostril (32 counts of *ram*) visualizing burning the impurities.
- Inhale left nostril repeating *vam* (16 counts) now from *ajna* into the heart centre; retain (64 counts of *vam*); exhale right nostril (32 counts of *vam*) visualizing the inflow of *mantras* to divinize the whole personality.

- Visualize *kundalini* descending through *sushumna*, manifesting each purified *chakra* in turn:
  Visualize 7th chakra; 1000 petals; repeating *hamso* at least 16 times
  Visualize 6th chakra; 2 petals; mind; repeating *so'ham* at least 16 times
  Visualize 5th chakra; 16 petals; ether (*akasha*); repeating *ham* at least 16 times
  Visualize 4th chakra; 12 petals; air (*vayu*); repeating *yam* at least 16 times
  Visualize 3rd chakra; 10 petals; fire (*agni*); repeating *ram* at least 16 times
  Visualize 2nd chakra; 6 petals; water (*apas*); repeating *vam* at least 16 times
  Visualize 1st chakra; 4 petals; earth (*prithivi*); repeating *lam* at least 16 times
- Visualize the *kundalini* coiling again 3 ½ times around the *lingam* of the 1st chakra.

The essence of Yoga is the purification of body, breath and mind until the light of the Self can shine through. Thoughts are removed from the mind field which is then made one-pointed and turned inwards towards the Centre of Consciousness. Detachment is the key to this kind of purification. The *asana* and *pranayama* used in combination with meditation in Raja Yoga cleanse the body and strengthen the nervous system so that the mind can be controlled. *Bhuta shuddhi* is not described in Patanjali's *Yoga-Sutra* but the practice is compatible with Raja Yoga. *Bhuta shuddhi* comes from Tantra and *Kundalini* Yoga.

Bhuta shuddhi is a technique to purify body, breath and mind while awakening the *kundalini shakti* by purifying the basic elements of the subtle body (earth, water, fire, air and ether) and their corresponding *chakras*. It uses visualization, *pranayama*, and the repetition of the seed (*bija*) mantras of the seven major chakras thereby purifying the subtle being with the fire of the *kundalini*. It prepares the aspirant for *kundalini* awakening. Tantra regards the body as a living shrine for the indwelling Divinity. *Bhuta shuddhi* renders the body pure and wholesome. It is practised after channel purification (*nadi shodhana*) and before meditation into which it provides a smooth transition to turning the mind inward. The method trains the mind to concentrate and helps with the mastery of *pranayama*. The inclusive combination of seed *mantras*, breath retention and intense visualization unblocks subtle energy channels more effectively than other methods, and Swami Rama (2002c) writes that it activates auditory and visual brain centres and coordinates their linkages to speech and thought.

Power therapies. The meridian or energy therapies are also useful here for realignment of the turbulence of subtle energy fields and for correcting related imbalance in the meridians. These approaches include not only the tapping procedures but also the methods for treating neurological disorganization and psychological reversal. If the personality is analogous to a radio receiver, the energy therapies might be imagined to remove static and to tune the receiver by aligning it with transmissions from the Centre of Consciousness. Here there is room for research and an integration of Yogic breathing techniques with energy therapies. Energy interventions are beginning to use diaphragmatic breathing, but there is much more that can be explored.

19

How Is Detachment Produced?

Sensory-Perceptual Dissociation: A Model for *Vairagya*

In Neuro-Linguistic Programming (NLP) there is an algorithm that is used to produce visual-kinesthetic dissociation (V-KD) to remove the emotional charge from past (and even future) severe traumatic and phobic experiences of all kinds. An external stimulus triggers feelings associated with a past or even a future projected traumatic experience. The feelings are overwhelming and produce a phobic response. V-KD is a rapid and highly effective intervention that can neutralize such overwhelming responses. An effective application of V-KD leaves the subject in a state of neutrality when remembering the traumatic event and the emotional reaction or phobic response no longer occurs from either the memory or the external triggering stimulus. One of the many versions of V-KD is called the Fast Phobia Cure. For a severe trauma it should be done only under the guidance of an experienced professional therapist. The original references should be consulted for details (Cameron-Bandler, 1985, p 151; Hall & Belnap, 2000, p 112). The metaphor of a theatre is used to set up a double dissociation. In summary the method is done as follows:

Visual-Kinesthetic Dissociation

- Imagine being in a movie theatre seeing yourself on the screen (first dissociation step) in a still, black and white snapshot doing something neutral or pleasant. (Black and white dissociates while colour associates.)
- Now imagine floating up into the projection booth behind and above the audience. Watch yourself in the audience watching yourself on the screen (second dissociation step). Here the therapist uses various anchoring procedures (conditioning) to maintain this second dissociation step. For the subsequent procedure to work the subject must maintain this double dissociation while reviewing the trauma without falling into the events on the screen (association). Reviewing the events from a dissociated state is the key to making this procedure work by erasing the emotions and feelings from the events.
- The subject now imagines a black and white, still, silent snapshot on the screen of him/herself just before the first encounter with the phobia. (Stillness versus movement and silence versus sound are dissociating.)
- The subject then runs a black and white movie without sound from the beginning to the end of the traumatic event out past the end to a place of safety and holds it there, taking as long as is needed. The anchors are used as needed to maintain the dissociation throughout.
- The subject now associates into the still snapshot at the end with all sensory modalities, then turns the picture to colour. S/he then runs the movie backwards fully associated in colour

and sound to the starting point just before the phobic event. This is done as fast as possible (1 to 4 seconds), the faster the better. This is rapidly repeated five times one after the other.

- One tests the result by running the direct memory fully associated. If there is any reaction at any point the whole V-KD procedure is repeated again as needed until one can review the traumatic memory two or three times without any reaction. If possible one should also test in a real situation.

With a successful application of the method the emotional reaction or phobic response will completely and permanently disappear in the face of the triggering stimulus. The memories remain along with whatever the subject learned from the experience, but the trauma is gone. The subject may wonder why s/he was ever upset by such a trivial thing or even deny s/he ever had the problem. This is a state of dispassion, detachment, non-attachment or forgiveness in relationship to the event.

Meditation Technologies for Detachment

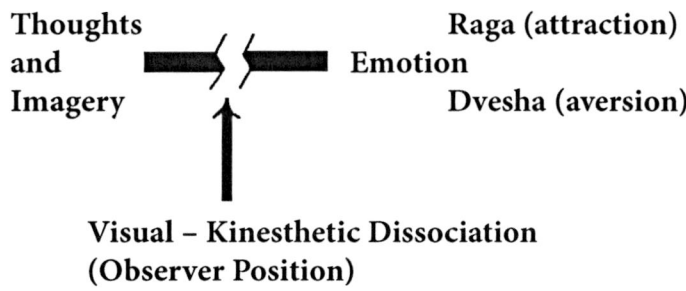

Figure 19.1 Sensory-Perceptual Dissociation Models the Production of Detachment in Yoga

We propose that this phenomenon of V-KD is a model for how states of detachment might be produced by Yogic methods. Witnessing and mindfulness are obvious examples because such states are dis-associated observer states. The dis-associated observer states in *yoga nidra* or *antar mouna* are further examples. Meditation has been described as a process of "washing the mind." Its ability over time to clear the subconscious of *samskaras* involves a similar process. The posture, flow of the breath and *mantra* together anchor the awareness in a dissociated state of witnessing with the mind one-pointedly focussed on the flow of breath and *mantra*. Images and feelings that bubble up from the subconscious pass through the mind field like clouds across the sky and are released without shaking the witnessing state. If the Presence of the Centre of Consciousness is also part of the experience then the cleansing effect of the dis-association is even more powerful.

If one of these images is powerful enough the meditator can suddenly be pulled to associate into feelings. The state is lost without the meditator even realizing the lapse. The posture sags, the breath becomes irregular, and the concentration and flow of the *mantra* are lost. Indeed, there are some who believe that "participating" in the memory with its feelings in an associated state simply strengthens it and sends it back to the subconscious again rather than releasing it. The awareness is caught up in the flow of the memory, perhaps for some time, until the meditator "comes to" and suddenly realizes the witnessing state has been lost. At this point one reapplies the posture, and brings the awareness back to the sound and the breath flowing together to re-establish the one-pointed, dissociated, witnessing state. V-KD deals with the visual and feeling aspects. We propose a more general term of "sensory-perceptual dissociation" to describe the process producing detachment in meditation and allied methods.

Vairagya as Elimination versus Transcendence

As the subconscious mind is emptied with meditation or any of the purification methods described above to bring about *vairagya*, the serious aspirant may find the process rough going.

> If you're doing meditation correctly, you're in for some very rough and frightening times. Meditation as a "relaxation response" is a joke. Genuine meditation involves a whole series of deaths and rebirths; extraordinary conflicts and stresses come into play. All of this is just barely balanced by an equal growth in equanimity, compassion, understanding, awareness, and sensitivity, which makes the whole endeavour worthwhile.
>
> Comments from an interview with Ken Wilber
> Combs (1995), p 231.

Lacking a knowledge of alternatives, teachers may helplessly advise students to just "tough it out." Fortunately the advent of the power therapies in psychology, especially energy psychology or meridian therapies, mean that this kind of pain and suffering need not occur. The acquisition of dispassion takes consistent, persistent and discriminating effort, but it no longer needs to be so psychologically painful.

Aziz Kristof (2000, p 188) identifies a linear assumption that most aspirants have about Self-Realization: it can be reached only by eliminating negativity, even eliminating the mind. Rather the Ultimate is reached not through elimination but through expansion. Purification and the resulting levels of dispassion are not about emptying the mind of its content and leaving a person mindless. Instead it is about severing the emotional reactivity to that content which is the source of our bondage, conditioning and habitual behaviour that prevents our consciousness from expanding into the Presence. The emotional pressure drives the upsurge of the *vrittis* of the stream of consciousness that block out the Centre just as clouds block the sun. Being or non-doing does not arise from the elimination of doing; it arises from expansion into the Presence, the Silence, the Centre of Consciousness that is Existence, Consciousness and Bliss. Purification breaks the bondage to temporality that holds us back, but in so doing it does not destroy the manifest. Aziz (2000, p 187) quotes the sage Hui-Neng:

> . . . any concept of meditation which speaks about the elimination of thoughts is very dangerous and incorrect. This concept is called the "heretical view" in Zen. Hui-Neng said that the real no-mind includes everything – mountains, rivers and oceans.

Why should it not include also thinking? This vast space contains everything and is all-inclusive. This master used to say that "the essence of mind does not increase in Samadhi, nor does it decrease in agitation." Not only is your mind included but also your difficulties, your desires and your longings. You as a human being cannot fully avoid negativity. Negativity is a part of this dimension, but through the inner expansion it is fully embraced.

20

Meridian Energy Interventions (Energy Psychology)

We wrote about modern power therapies above as powerful ways to produce detachment. One group of these make up what is now called energy psychology, meridian energy therapies or acupressure for the emotions. These are very powerful tools for emotional purification in *sadhana*, and are a natural complement to Yogic practice since both deal with the subtle energies or *prana*. We refer the reader to the end of this chapter for a list of resources for further study and practical exploration. At the present writing energy psychology is still very new and not yet accepted by mainstream psychology. This is partly due to the lack of proper research in the area, although studies are beginning. But it is more because of the subtle energy paradigm that currently underlies the subject. While Yoga is quite comfortable with subtle energies which it calls *prana*, traditional psychology definitely is not.

The key idea underlying energy psychology is that thoughts and emotions are subtle energies. Emotions are thought to be linked to the subtle energy meridians of Traditional Chinese Medicine. Specific emotions relate to specific meridians and points of the Oriental acupuncture system. This is why these are called meridian energy therapies. Students of Yoga are familiar with the subtle energetic anatomy of the *pranamayakosha* with its complex systems of *nadis* and *chakras*. It is said that the *nadis* and *marma* points may be the origin of the Traditional Chinese Medicine acupuncture system (Lele et al, 1999). But these are not well known in the West. The acupuncture meridian system is better worked out and so is used in energy psychology.

The theory is that negative emotions predominate when meridians are disrupted. Positive emotions predominate when meridians are balanced. Perturbations in subtle energy fields, some would say thought fields (in Yoga the mind is conceptualized as a subtle energy field), are said to be the basis of emotional disturbance. This would implicate the *pranamayakosha* and to some extent the *manomayakosha* as their source. The concept is quite Yogic because emotional disturbances are visualized as warps in the personality's *pranic* fields, and their purification is thought of as a smoothing out of those warps: the idea is somewhat similar to turbulent versus smooth or laminar flow in a moving fluid. Thus perturbations disrupt normal subtle energy balance.

The idea behind the therapy is that stimulation of meridians via specific acupoints (usually by tapping them) while attuning the problem thought field, rapidly collapses the perturbations to restore subtle energy balance in the affected meridians. The result is a rapid release of the disturbing emotions and the development of lasting dispassion to the underlying traumatic events. As explained above this and other interventions work by producing sensory-emotional dissociation analogous to the visual-kinesthetic dissociation procedure described in Neuro-Linguistic Programming (NLP). It is about raising the energy or vibrational level of the mind field to create a stable state of equanimity.

Extensive clinical experience indicates that the procedures are fast, lasting, and 60–80% effective, a major improvement in efficacy over traditional psychotherapies.

Energy psychology has arisen over the past decade or two from very heterogeneous origins. It has a strong base in kinesiology, Traditional Chinese Medicine and several practice paradigms in modern psychology (behavioral-environmental, cognitive, systemic cybernetic, neurological and biochemical). Concepts have also been borrowed from NLP, EMDR (Eye Movement Desensitization and Reprocessing), Yoga and acupressure, as well as modern physics (quantum mechanics and thermodynamics), cognitive neuroscience, information theory and mimetics (Gallo, 1999; Furman & Gallo, 2000). There are over forty variants, each with a unique name and acronym.

Energy psychology is touted as a paradigm shift in psychology because of its enhanced efficacy and for its underlying energy paradigm. From the point of view of Yoga, emotional purification need no longer entail suffering or prolonged work. Energy psychology can be thought of as a modern Western technology of detachment. It is also a modern application of *prana vidya*, the science of *prana*. Thus it has the potential for wide applicability to Yoga as an adjuvant and complementary support to traditional Yogic technologies, and this is why we introduce it here.

Some Key Concepts in Energy Psychology

- Thoughts and emotions are subtle energy.

- Specific emotions relate to specific meridians.
    Negative emotions predominate when meridians are perturbed.
    Positive emotions predominate when meridians are balanced.

- Perturbations in thought fields are proposed as the basis of emotional disturbance.

- Perturbations disrupt normal subtle energy balance.

- Stimulation of meridians collapses perturbations to restore energetic balance and homeostasis.

- Blocks to treatment effectiveness:
    Psychological reversal
        Psychological resistance and self-sabotage that block healing.
    Neurological disorganization (switching)
        Left-right brain disorganization; misconstrued neural inputs.

- Subtle energy diagnosis:
    Muscle testing from kinesiology
    Therapy localization to acupoints
    Use of subjective units of distress (SUD) to quantify responses.

- The apex problem: subjects deny they ever had a problem after its successful resolution.

- Energy toxins: Blocks to treatment efficacy by certain drugs, foods, allergies, electromagnetic fields, etc.

Applications of Energy Psychology to Yoga

There are many possibilities for integrating the processes of energy psychology with the practices of Yoga. This has the potential to be a rich field of research and exploration at the leading edge of psychospiritual development for decades to come. Indeed, if the many New Age predictions of a planetary transition into higher consciousness come about in this new millennium, there will be a great need for processes coming from such an integration to assist people with the birthing of this new consciousness. For some it will come gently and easily, but for many it may come as a spiritual crisis.

Applications of Energy Psychology to Yoga

Principle: Yoga *sadhana* for longterm spiritual transformation combined with energy psychology for short term problem solving as a technology of detachment.

Emotional Purification – Diagnosis and Treatment of Emotional disorders
    Trauma and Post-traumatic Stress Syndrome
    Anxiety disorders: stress, anxiety, panic
    Addictions: e.g., smoking, alcohol, drugs, gambling, sex, workaholism
    Phobias: e.g., insects, small animals, claustrophobia, flying
    Depression
    Anger and Rage
    Obsessive Compulsive Disorders
    Guilt, Shame, Embarrassment, Jealousy
    Physical Pain and Functional Disorders
    Emotional Components of Physical Disease
    Dysfunctional relationships

Diagnosis and Elimination of Resistance and Blocks to *Sadhana*
    Psychological Reversal
    Neurological Disorganization

Diagnosis and Change of Beliefs, Values and Attitudes

Performance Enhancement
    Hatha Yoga, *Pranayama* and Meditation

Diagnosis and Treatment of Energy Toxins

Basal Energy Analysis and Maintenance of Energy balance

Handling Spiritual Emergence and Spiritual Emergency

Training Spiritual Guides in Yoga

But for the most part, we expect that energy psychology used as an adjuvant will complement the methods of Yoga. Yoga creates a longterm foundation for personal transformation. Energy psychology provides crisis and acute interventions to address the many short term emotional and psychological problems that arise as unconscious residues (*vasanas* and *samskaras*) surface during the purification process. Some represent the exigencies that we all face in everyday living. Others may be precipitated by intense spiritual *sadhana* itself. Serious personal transformation is challenging enough at any time. It would be very beneficial to have access to effective and powerful rapid methods to ease these transitions. Emotional purification is a central aspect of Himalayan Yoga (Veda Bharati, 1998). As a powerful technology of detachment, energy psychology is an ideal tool to use.

Acu-yoga (Gach & Marco, 1981) is a blend of acupressure and Yoga that results in enhancement of both. Yogic *asanas* are combined with acupressure of meridian points, and the *asanas* are analyzed in terms of their effects on the meridian system and *chakras*. More recently Gach and Henning (2004) have written in detail about the use of acupressure for emotional healing. There is room for much research here on the well-known effects of Hatha Yoga on *prana* and the subtle energy body from the newer perspective of energy psychology. The use of energy psychology for enhancing performance of physical skills is another area for research with *asanas* (Veda Bharati, 1985)

Let us take meditation as a specific example and look at the interaction with energy psychology. What follows for meditation also could apply to any Yogic practice like *pranayama* or *yoga nidra*.

Although meditation has had, and still has ongoing extensive research validation of its many effects, research into energy psychology is only beginning. The evidence to date for its efficacy is impressive, but still largely anecdotal based on case histories where one tends to see the successes but not the failures reported. Longterm follow-up is still unavailable to know how long the effectiveness of the interventions lasts. The change is claimed to be permanent, but there are indications in some cases that the beneficial effects are not long-lasting.

There is no experience of which we are aware of combining energy psychology with meditation. But intuitively they should complement one another. Both are technologies of detachment. Both cleanse the mind through release of emotional reactivity. We would see energy psychology as useful for the management of specific reactivities while meditation might be used as a long-term way to reduced mental reactivity itself – a kind of prevention strategy. Here is a field for practical research. Can the addition of energy psychology to a practice of meditation ease the emotional purification process, and enhance performance and efficacy of meditation itself? Can the addition of meditation and related techniques, especially breathing exercises, enhance the efficacy of energy psychology interventions? As to the former, we can think of several specific areas where energy psychology could assist a meditation practice.

- Performance protocols applied to meditation itself, the ability to sit still, and adjustment to a comfortable posture.
- The relief of resistance and blocks to meditation practice.
- The relief of fear.
- Releasing attitudes like boredom, impatience, not wanting to do it, not having time to establish a practice, feelings that the procedure is useless or does not work, etc.
- Addressing the list of problems encountered in meditation as described in the *Yoga-Sutra*.
- Resolution of negative beliefs about meditation.
- Dealing with the emotional reactivity and other problems that face the average person in an ordinary day, and which if not resolved, disturb meditation.
- Dealing with problems that arise during the practice of the *yamas* and *niyamas*.
- Stress release.
- Realignment and balancing of subtle energy fields.
- Management of psychological reversal and neurological disorganization.
- Relief of mental restlessness.

The Challenge of Spiritual Emergence and Emergencies

- A young woman experienced over several weeks recurrent episodes lasting several hours of profound deepening of consciousness, expanded awareness and a sense of oneness with all things, feelings of bliss and Presence, and deep intuitive insights. Then as suddenly as they began, these experiences stopped. For the ensuing ten years she wrestled with frequent episodes of severe depression and feelings of unworthiness, convinced that God had abandoned her.

- A single 45 year old male psychiatrist and Yoga student began to have almost continuous experiences of profound deepening of consciousness with feelings of bliss and oceanic expansion and oneness. These states were intense enough to interrupt his clinical work which then drew the attention of his colleagues and partners in their joint psychiatric practice. They diagnosed him as an acute manic psychosis, committed him to a locked psychiatric ward, and persuaded him to accept antipsychotic medication. The drugs shut down his altered states of consciousness which never returned. After discharge from hospital he was left bereft and was unable to get any help from his Yoga teacher. He felt that his career as a psychiatrist and his credibility with his partners in the joint psychiatric practice had been seriously impaired. He now wondered what to do with the rest of his life, much less where to turn for help.

- A 50 year old woman experienced repeated and often prolonged experiences of deep spiritual Awareness accompanied by guidance that expressed itself in exquisite channeled poetry and written teachings. These were mixed with periods of extreme emotional turmoil which she interpreted as emotional purification and clearing. She was diagnosed as manic-depressive, but thus far she has refused to take antipsychotic medication and her spiritual experiences continue. Her experiences include hearing the internal unstruck (*anahata*) sounds of the *chakras* and the universal sound of AUM. Her physician diagnosed this as tinnitus.

- At age 23 as a medical student, a physician began to experience periods when he felt an invisible Presence in the room and a sense of being perpetually watched by an invisible Witness. The experience created a sense of anxiety for which he consulted another physician. He was placed on stelazine which reduced the anxiety, but at the expense of side effects and a feeling of emotional dependency on needing the drug for support. Eventually he was weaned off the drug after two years. But he was left for many years thereafter with some mild agoraphobia and phobic reactions to closed spaces like elevators or seats in the middle of a row in a theater. It was well into his forties before he eventually received guidance from an accomplished spiritual adept and learned that this was the opening of the Centre of Consciousness, which by then had become a stable and welcome part of his inner experience and awareness. However, the phobic reactions persisted and were eventually resolved only many years later by NLP and energy psychology.

As the above vignettes indicate, there is a dark side to spiritual practice in the West. With its materialistic foundation modern western psychiatry tends to classify major spiritual transformations, spontaneous or induced by *sadhana*, as evidence of psychological dysfunction or even psychosis. A few progressive psychiatrists have tried to distinguish the two and to bring the understandings of transpersonal psychology to practical application for this problem. The relationships among madness, creative genius and spiritual experiences have fascinated scientists and philosophers for centuries. For people in emotional crisis, it is important to distinguish among intractable psychoses, temporary breakdowns in the service of healing (spiritual emergence) and psychotic breakthroughs (spiritual emergency).

With spiritual emergence, spiritual growth and awakening may be accompanied by emotional and mental turmoil as well as unusual physiological effects at critical developmental points. These can be misdiagnosed and treated with potentially damaging psychiatric or medical intervention. Frequently certain mental or physical effects are called *kundalini* arousals, but these are in fact very rare. In most cases they represent an arousal of life force (*prana*), known in Yoga as *prana-vyutthana*. This is an area where there is much confusion and misinformation in the West (e.g., Sannella, 1992).

Stanislov and Christina Grof (Grof & Grof, 1989; Grof, 2000) coined the term "spiritual emergency" to refer to a dysfunctional state or phase within the process of spiritual emergence. The individual is overwhelmed in a true crisis by disturbing emotions, thoughts, occasionally suicidal ruminations and disruptive behaviors that need external help. Neither traditional nor alternative and complementary medicine (despite its holistic paradigm) is able to assist for lack of theoretical and experiential knowledge of the mechanisms involved in spiritual emergence and spiritual emergency.

Psychospiritual healing is an approach that goes deeper to work with the subtle energy structures of the personality – *prana*, the *nadis* and the *chakras*. The approach is also referred to as "Tantric medicine." It addresses the imbalances present in spiritual emergency at the level of the subtle energy field, since this is the link between mind and body which can therefore act on both. The deeper causes of spiritual emergency arise in the mind and express first in the subtle energy field before they manifest later in the body. Firsthand knowledge of the *kundalini* process and the *chakras* with their attendant states of consciousness is essential to deal effectively with these problems (Nelson, 1994a, b; Harrigan, 1996).

A Spiritual Emergence Network has been established through the Institute of Transpersonal Psychology at Menlo Park, California. Nelson (1994a, b) has written knowledgeably on the management of spiritual emergencies from the point of view of transpersonal psychology and psychiatry as have others (Grof & Grof, 1989; Grof, 2000; Bragdon, 1990). The approach addresses healing at the physical, emotional, mental, spiritual and social levels, but is for the most part only supportive. There is a great opportunity here for research into the application of energy psychology methods for more effective resolution of the distressing emotional components of spiritual emergencies.

Mention might be made here of holotropic integration developed by Stanislov and Christina Grof (Grof & Grof, 1989; Grof, 2000) for releasing long-buried emotional traumas. It uses a mixture of modalities centered on hyperventilation to induce mild acute spiritual crises that trigger a cathartic release of long-repressed emotions. Holotropic therapy is appropriate for people in mild spiritual emergencies and for nonpsychotic people with stubborn emotional barriers to spiritual emergence. It is unsuitable for people in chronic psychosis or with paranoia. Very frequently such emergencies are confused with schizophrenia. But we have also seen instances in which they have been confused with manic-depressive illness (bipolar disorder) in manic crisis. McFetridge (2004a, b) has recently reviewed the field of peak states of consciousness which can further confuse the recognition of spiritual breakthroughs.

Guiding from the Centre of Consciousness

In Part One we have discussed in detail the opening of the Centre of Consciousness into direct awareness and its spiritual significance. It is worth mentioning that conscious access to the Centre adds the spiritual dimension to guidance. When the Inner Teacher awakens, especially in a professional therapist, that individual's skills are greatly enhanced. One learns to do therapy and to guide naturally from that Centre, intuitively. Indeed one cannot hide that Light within; one's very presence becomes therapeutic. This is spiritual counseling which cannot begin until that Awareness has blossomed and can be easily and reliably accessed at will. The Masters and the sages are natural healers at every level by virtue of their access to transcendent Awareness.

Does that mean that one needs no technical training? Yoga teachers are often approached by their students for support and counseling for personal problems. Unless professionally qualified, yoga teachers are generally not properly qualified to provide counseling or therapy. But many submit to the temptation and provide bad advice anyway, sometimes making matters worse or getting caught up in their students' melodramas. We strongly advise that any yoga teacher, especially of meditation, who is not a health care professional, should have access to sympathetic qualified medical and psychological help to refer their students. But for the qualified professional, the Centre of Consciousness uses the therapist's personality and knowledge as a skilled instrument – the more skilled the better. But those skills are used so much more effectively. This is yet another aspect of Karma Yoga – action flowing from the Centre of Consciousness through a skilled and surrendered instrument.

The perennial philosophy uses a lovely metaphor of the Lord as Krishna playing enchanting music on a flute, so enchanting that those who hear it cannot resist, but must follow. The story of the Pied Piper in the West is a similar metaphor. Krishna represents the Inner Teacher. The flute is the surrendered (i.e., hollow) instrument of the disciple's personality. The enchantment of the music bespeaks its profound healing qualities.

The actual process is quite simple. One accesses the awareness of the Presence or the internal *nada* (sound of *Aum*) and follows Its intuitions without hesitation within the therapeutic situation. Note that this is not a trance nor is it elegant hypnotic work with the unconscious mind as Milton Erickson used to do. Clearly a similar process will provide for intuitive diagnosis and treatment for energy psychology, adding a natural spiritual influence to the process.

The Importance of Intuition

It is important to understand what is meant by intuition in Yoga. If the sun is a metaphor for the Centre of Consciousness, then its light would represent intuition which illuminates everything on which it falls with understanding. In one sense the sun and its light are different, and in another sense they are one and the same.

Mastering intuition is key to working with the Centre of Consciousness. The process is both an art and a skill. It comes gradually from long practice and training. The whisperings of intuition are available to us all. But in Western culture we often confuse intuition with instinct. Moreover, the tyranny of reason persuades us to dismiss intuition as unreliable. Although scientists would never admit, in fact the march of real discovery in science is led by intuition with the rational faculty working out the practical implications of the insights given.

With true intuition one gains a direct perception of Truth. The mind is used as though it were a sixth sense. The Truth is perceived directly without any intervention of language, reasoning or calculating in the same way that physical reality is perceived directly by the five physical senses. In a particular context one simply knows instantly and directly what needs to be known.

One is surprised to learn that language is not necessary for knowing or thinking. This is contrary to current scientific thought and popular belief, which hold that one needs language to think. Intuitive knowing is holistic and instantaneous. It may come as a continuous gentle flow of knowing or as an injection of knowledge into the mind as an instantaneous gestalt which can be accessed over and over for its rich content. One soon learns that language is a clumsy and inadequate representation of such a gestalt and much too slow. It cannot capture all of the knowledge nor can it capture its richness.

One realizes that the mind is a subtle energy field, and indeed all the universe of energy is not a thing. Rather, it is a perfect process. Through ignorance one may use the process to create for good or ill. But whatever the result, the process for manifesting it always works perfectly.

One must learn to distinguish the flow of intuition from "everything else," the contents within the mind. That "everything else" lies in time, space and causation. Intuition, however, comes from the Centre of Consciousness beyond, but it is introduced as content into the spatiotemporal energy field of mind.

What are these contents? They are rich and complex. They include an almost infinite range of feelings, which must be distinguished from emotions arising from the subtle body. They include the kinesthetic sense produced by the neuromuscular structures of the physical body. They include all of the imagery that comes from the five physical senses. In this regard, it is helpful for the student to learn about the modalities, and submodalities that characterize sensory imagery as well as concepts such as sensory dominance, the sequencing of internal imagery in strategies, eye and body accessing cues, etc., as described in a discipline such as Neuro-Linguistic Programming (Cameron-Bandler, 1985; Hall & Belnap, 2000).

Other content would include thoughts which often occur as internal dialogue. The products of reason must also be distinguished. One must particularly avoid the common process of *post hoc* rationalization. So much of human action flows from instinct, habit and conditioning as a reaction to stimuli arising within a certain context. In other words action is so often simply reaction. These conditioned responses act so quickly and below the conscious awareness that they are barely noticed. Then the rational faculty rapidly comes into play to provide a reason for the behaviour. The latter occupies awareness to the exclusion of the former and the individual genuinely feels that he or she has acted rationally when in fact the action has come from conditioning, instinct or emotional reactivity.

There are other mental contents which must be distinguished that play out their action in time. They include memory and particularly material coming up from the unconscious and subconscious minds, as well as imagination and related states such as reverie or conscious dreaming. One must also become familiar with altered states such as trance, dream, sleep, etc. None of these constitute the whisperings of intuition and one must learn to distinguish.

What are these whisperings like? They are not like any of the contents of the normal mind noted above. There is no reason, no imagery, nothing to infer, and nothing to figure out. The experience is closest to a flow of pure knowing into the mind. There is no language, although at times a few words may appear. The source is the Presence, the Centre of Consciousness. Sometimes there is an instantaneous, total gestalt that seems to sit high in the mind field like a wispy cloud of energy existing in no space and no time. It would take books of language to portray the content of this intuition, and yet its full meaning would still be inadequately expressed. You simply know, and you know that you know, and you know with absolute certainty that what you know is true.

Swami Rama often emphasized the self-evident knowing and certainty of such intuitions. There may be glimpses of direct perceptions such as clairvoyance. The psychologist may have instant and direct perception of an individual's life history and problems without asking. The physician may know intuitively a patient's diagnosis. The writings of Barbara Brennan describe the remarkable insights that can be received from intuitive diagnosis (Brennan, 1987). Swami Rama was a master of intuitive diagnosis. Indeed, one can know anything that one needs to know. One simply needs to ask and to be able to "hear" the response. But "need to know" is the operative phrase here; idle curiosity draws a blank.

One learns that spirit communicates through subtle feelings, and sometimes emotions if strong guidance is needed. There are no voices in the head. Energy fields carry information in their vibrations. Communications from spirit are sensed as subtle feelings, "vibes" in popular language. We normally have many internal states that are sensed the same way. We know we are secure because of how we feel. We know we are free because of a feeling. So one learns to read the meaning of subtle transmissions of feeling, of subtle vibratory energy fields.

> What is Truth? A difficult question; but I have solved it for myself by saying that it is what the "voice within" tells you.
>
> Mahatma Gandhi

In this day of New Age writing the reader will have heard of channelling. Individuals who have this ability to channel consciously learn to translate into language the ongoing subtle energy transmissions that come to them from the channelled source in the form of whole blocks of meaning and knowing. Effectively what we are talking about here is channelling the Centre of Consciousness in all things: in teaching, studying and reading; in action, writing and speech. This is truly what makes one a spiritual guide. But the instrument, the personality, must be skilled and well-grounded.

> Until the first step has been taken in this development, this knowledge, which is called intuition with certainty, is impossible to man. And this positive and certain intuition is the only form of knowledge which enables a man to work rapidly or reach his true and high estate, within the limit of his conscious effort. To obtain knowledge by experiment is too tedious a method for those who aspire to accomplish real work; he who gets it by certain intuition, lays hands on its various forms with supreme rapidity, by fierce effort of will; as a determined workman grasps his tools, indifferent to their weight or any other difficulty which may stand in his way. He does not stay for each to be tested – he uses such as he sees are fittest.
>
> Collins, 1976, p 34

This little manual, *Light on the Path* (Collins, 1976), has much more to say about the importance of the development of intuition. It emphasizes that the development of intuition in no way disparages the scientific method. The latter is applicable only to matter and to the physical universe. The advance of scientific understanding and technology is a major accomplishment of this century and before. But intuitive knowledge is an entirely different thing. It is not acquired, but rather is more like a faculty of the divine soul, a manifestation of the Centre of Consciousness. It is up to the student to gain awareness of this intuitive faculty by a resolute effort of indomitable will. In this regard faith plays a key role. The engine of faith can accomplish all things. It is like a covenant between the Centre of Consciousness and the ego in the personality. Faith is necessary to obtain intuitive knowledge, for a student must believe that such knowledge exists before he or she can claim and use it.

Simply put: without intuition the student is lost! In the West we worship rationality and the intellect. There is no doubt that these are powerful tools – witness our science and technology. Unfortunately, however, any position can be rationalized or argued. It takes intuition to show what needs to be given to the tools of rationality so that they may play their proper role. Even though it is ridiculed and confused with instinct, good science uses intuition first.

Kashmir Shaivism proposes a model of intuition in the context of the expression of language into manifestation. The source of language is described as being experienced as a flash of light (insight). The technical term is *pratibha* which means a "flash" or "flash of intuition." This *pratibha* emerges into awareness as though from elsewhere (beyond the sense of "I") and manifests itself in three stages. It unfolds from "flash" to unformed ideas and images, then to images and ideas formulated only partially in language, and finally to spoken and written word. One experiences the process as beginning with a tiny flash, which becomes ideas and then words. It takes many, many words to embody the "flash" whose content cannot be captured no matter how many words are used. It is a process of manifestation that evolves from the subtlest to the subtle to the gross.

In the *Shiva Sutras* (Singh, 1979), a major text of Kashmir Shaivism, three important points are made about this process. This process of manifestation of language is the same as that for manifestation of all reality. The source of the "flash" is Divine – to be understood as a non-dual, all pervading consciousness that acts as a "ground" beyond which the ego perceives the entry of the "flash." This is described in detail in the *Spanda Karikas*, a related text also from this tradition. Finally, the method for transcending manifest reality is to follow the path of linguistic manifestation in reverse. This becomes a theoretical basis for Mantra Yoga. As a linguistic manifestation, a *mantra* is repeated and refined, allowing it to become an idea/image which is then coaxed back through the veil of the ego into the ground of the Divine. The meditator's intent is to allow the individual consciousness to follow the *mantra* as it dissolves into the beyond (Singh, 1979; Dyczkowski, 1987).

Resources for Meridian Energy Interventions (Energy Psychology)

Over forty variants have been described, each with their own name and acronym, and some are listed at http://www.integrativehelp.com/healing_techniques.html .

An extensive listing of Internet networks and links, discussion groups, downloads, instruction videos, audiotapes and DVDs, manuals, newsletters and practitioners has been compiled by Debbie Vadja at http://www.the4dgroup.com/DebbyVajda/default.htm .

Start by downloading Gary Craig's manual for Emotional Freedom techniques (EFT) from www.emofree.com . His site has a tutorial and an excellent collection of DVDs to illustrate the process.

Books for the beginner include:

Arenson, Gloria, *Five Simple Steps to Emotional Healing*, Simon and Schuster, 2001.
Callahan, Roger J. with Richard Trubo, *Tapping the Healer Within: Using Thought Field Therapy to Instantly Conquer Your Fears, Anxieties, and Emotional Distress*, Contemporary Books, 2001.
Gallo, Fred and Harry Vincenzi, *Energy Tapping: How to Rapidly Eliminate Anxiety, Depression, Cravings, and More Using Energy Psychology*, New Harbinger, 2000
Lambrou, Peter and George Pratt, *Instant Emotional Healing: Acupressure for the Emotions*, Broadway Books/Random House 2000.

Books with a more advanced treatment:

Feinstein, David, *Energy Psychology Interactive: Rapid Interventions for Lasting Change* (integrated CD-Rom and companion book), Innersource, 2004 – also available from http://www.Energy PsychologyInteractive.com .
Feinstein, David, Donna Eden and Gary Craig, *The Promise of Energy Psychology: Revolutionary Tools for Dramatic Personal Change*, Tarcher/Penguin, 2005.
Gallo, Fred, *Energy Diagnostic and Treatment Methods*, Norton Professional Books, 2000.
Gallo, Fred, *Energy Psychology: Explorations at the Interface of Energy, Cognition, Behavior and Health*, CRC Press, Second Edition, 2004.
Nims, Larry and Joan Sotkin, *Be Set Free Fast*, 2003. Available through http://www.BeSetFreeFast. com or http://www.ProsperityPlace.com .

Part Four

ABHYASA (*Practicing the Presence*)

21

ABHYASA (*Practice*) *and the Chariot of* SADHANA

It is said that in Yoga there are only three rules for success. The first is practice. The second is practice. And the third is also practice! But one must understand what is meant here by practice. It is something much more subtle than the more structured practices of Raja Yoga. As practices advance they become increasingly more subtle and more internal. *Abhyasa* is most frequently translated as "practice." The Monier-Williams Sanskrit Dictionary shows it as "*abhy-√as*: to concentrate one's attention on, practice, exercise, study." But practice of what? In *Yoga-Sutra* I.13 *abhyasa* is taken to mean the endeavor towards stillness and stability (*sthiti*) of the mind field so that it flows peacefully without *vrittis* (thoughts; mental content). Stillness implies a one-pointed mind field when it is without *rajasic* or *tamasic vrittis*. But one-pointed on what? On the Centre of Consciousness. The mind field becomes filled with the Presence which some commentators also refer to as the Silence or Stillpoint.

Swami Veda Bharati (1986) proposes that "practice" is not a direct translation of *abhyasa*. He points out that the verb root *aas* (to sit) is the same as in the word *asana*, which is both the seat to sit on as well as the posture. It is closely connected with the root *as* (to be), and both suggest the sense of "abiding." The prefix *abhi-* means a facing towards, with a goal, repeatedly. The idea conveyed by the word is that of repeatedly facing the *Guru* or God with a certain goal. It is in this sense that we use the word here as referring to the unceasing awareness and remembrance required to invoke the Centre of Consciousness within, with the unfolding of its qualities of Presence, Wisdom and Bliss.

We will meet these three words, *rajas*, *tamas* and *sattva* frequently in what follows. Swami Veda Bharati (1986, p 456) defines them in this way. They are the three *gunas* (qualities), "the attributes of unmanifest *prakriti* (nature), which are in equilibrium before the creation of evolutes and whose disequilibrium constitutes the process of creation. All material entities (evolutes) including the mind are composites of the three *gunas*: purity and illumination (*sattva*); activity (*rajas*); and inertia (*tamas*). They are the seats of pleasure, pain and delusion."

Abhyasa as practice is enshrined in *ishvara pranidhana* or surrender to God. It is called practicing the presence of God in the Christian Meditative Tradition. This is what we mean here by "practice" when we use that word to translate *abhyasa*. The core of *abhyasa* is the practice of meditation, re-membering that the word *pranidhana* has the meaning of "placing the mind in," in this case *Ishvara* or God in Its expression as the Centre of Consciousness or Inner Teacher. Indeed, if one describes Yoga as the science of spirituality, then meditation is its core method to explore inner space. Meditation bridges the wheels of the chariot of *sadhana* in our metaphor. Thus practice becomes a process of surrender to that Centre and gradual absorption into It.

The Hill of *Sadhana*

In understanding the interaction between nonattachment and practice one might consider the metaphor of the "hill" of *sadhana*. One starts by climbing the hill in a process that emphasizes "away from," to use one of the metaprogram distinctions of Neuro-Linguistic Programming (NLP) (Hall & Belnap, 2000). The emphasis is purification with a moving away from what is not wanted and from what blocks realization. The practices actively create nonattachment and require effort at every level of the personality. This emphasis on "doing" embodies the quality of *rajas* or activity in the personality's energy fields. One is reminded of the tale of Sisyphus from Greek mythology. He was a shrewd and greedy king of Corinth who was doomed forever in Hades to roll uphill a heavy stone which then always rolled back down again. We talk about a Sisyphean labor or task, one that is endless and difficult. Often this prolonged phase of *sadhana* feels like this to the aspirant who seems to make no or little progress, and may become discouraged and even leave the effort and the path. The seed has been planted, and one works endlessly watering, fertilizing, weeding, and yet nothing appears above the ground.

However, when the top of this metaphoric hill is reached and one starts to descend the other side toward the goal, there is a shift in the metaprogram distinction to "towards." With the beginning opening of the Centre of Consciousness into direct experience which marks the top of the hill, the spiritual aspirant increasingly experiences a moving towards what is wanted. The process of purification becomes more spontaneous. Attachments and aversions simply start to fall away by themselves. The activity of "doing" now flows into states of "being" (*sattva*), and effort dissolves into surrender, releasing and forgiveness.

This whole process describes the identity shift from small self to transcendental Self. What do we mean by an identity shift? We invite the reader to take a moment to do a metaphoric visualization with us to illustrate the idea.

Focus your attention for a moment on one of your big toes. Either one will do. Really concentrate on that toe. Associate your awareness so closely with the experience of that toe that it is as though you become that toe. Be that toe. Feel yourself as that toe with all your senses. See what you see, hear what you hear, feel what you feel as a toe. Imagine that you were so powerful that you could truly become that toe in your experience, that you could put your whole identity, your whole awareness inside that toe. Imagine yourself so powerful that you could shut the door, as it were, and completely exclude any awareness of your larger and higher self as a full human being. (And fortunately you cannot do this so you can release any sense of panic or anxiety that such a situation would induce.) And with the passage of time, even the memories that might remain of yourself as a full human being fade and vanish.

Your experience as a toe would entail much suffering. You would be in default. Life would simply happen to you completely out of your control. You would spend much of your time in the dark, encased in a sock, or worse, a hard shoe, jostling with other separate toes for space. Sometimes space would be so scarce that you would develop painful blisters from friction, or worse, suffer the pain of a stubbed toe – you are that toe. You might get some fresh air in summer but you could get sunburned. In winter you could be numb with cold. One could go on. But the point is that the very restricted identification of being a toe is a metaphor for being that small self identified as the ego personality, while your larger awareness as a full human being continues unaffected and completely outside of your limited awareness as a toe.

Now bring your awareness back to your full self as a human being. What a comparatively expanded feeling this is! Yet from this larger awareness, you can still choose to be fully aware of your toe, and many other things besides. And as you think about your toe you do so from the perspective of your larger awareness as a full human being, retaining that expanded awareness always. Your sense of your toe is contained within your larger human awareness. Clearly this latter state is a metaphor by comparison for the expanded awareness of being the true Self. What operates here is an identity shift. Who am I? Am I a toe, or am I a full human being? How my consciousness is identified defines who I think I am, my experience. To move my awareness from toe to full human being, from small self to Self, is a shift of the identification of Consciousness, an identity shift. This is a trivial if not silly metaphor but we hope it will give the reader an experiential idea of what is meant by identity shift and why we think of an aspect of detachment as a dis-identification of awareness and Consciousness from the psychophysical personality.

It has been said that we are all masters (Alarius, 1988). To be fully identified as a toe is a metaphor for being a master of limitation. As small selves, as egos, we are all masters of limitation. One needs only to look at the daily news or television programming to see this mastery of limitation by the "political self," the ego, in full action. One has to admit that it takes real mastery to be able to consistently make a mess of one's life and of the lives of others on a daily basis! The spiritual path is about turning us back into "Masters of Divine Expression." A fully realized spiritual master or *Guru* is by definition a "Master of Divine Expression." Such a being expresses fully from the Centre of Consciousness in all thought and action. This is Karma Yoga, the direct ongoing experience of action flowing from the Centre of Consciousness through the personality as a surrendered instrument.

Thus this whole process symbolically describes the identity shift from small self to Self. But metaphors like this have limits. This metaphor implies a journey from a beginning to an end. In actual fact there is no goal. There is nowhere to go and nothing to attain. Thus acceptance lies at the base of this identity shift, this shift from "away from" to "towards" – simply a fundamental acceptance of the reality of the Self as It has always been. It answers the question, "Who am I?" in the sense of unfolding, of who have I always been, not "Who will I be?" as some future state to be attained.

What Is *Abhyasa*?

Abhyasa is defined in Patanjali's *Yoga-Sutra* in *sutra* 13 of *pada* I:

> Exertion to acquire *sthiti* (tranquility) or a tranquil state of mind devoid of fluctuations is called practice.
>
> Aranya (1981)

In this and the next *sutra* (YS I.14), Patanjali makes the following points about *abhyasa*:

- Meditation brings the mind to stillness and stability (*sthiti*), by which is meant one-pointedness with the mind flowing in a calm, pacific, smooth stream.
- Effort to achieve *sthiti* must be vigorous, heroic (*virya*) and enthusiastic, as well as persevering (*utsaha*). It is a heroic, intense concentration to bring the mind to stillness.
- Practice (*abhyasa*) is the observance of the means to gain *sthiti* as well as the will to achieve its fulfillment.
- Practice (*abhyasa*) is to be carried out for a long time, without interruption, and with a positive and devout attitude.
- Practice (*abhyasa*) reaches firm ground when it cannot be distracted by pleasure or pain, when one can reach the depth instantly, at any time, and under any condition or situation, and when that depth becomes a natural plateau of awareness in which one remains at all times.

Let us examine these two key *sutras* in more detail (Veda Bharati, 1986).

> YS I.13 *tatra sthitau yatno'bhyasah.*
> "Between these two, practice and dispassion, the endeavor towards stillness and stability (*sthiti*) of the mind field is called practice."
> (Veda Bharati, 1986, p 198)

What is meant by *sthiti*? The word can be translated as "stillness, stability, settling down, coming to rest, or steadiness." (Veda Bharati, 1986, p 198). The commentator, Vyasa, says that stillness or stability (*sthiti*) means that the mind field is flowing pacifically when it is without thoughts (*vrittis*). Indeed there is no *samprajnata samadhi* possible until this stillness (*sthiti*) is experienced. It does not mean the total absence of mental content (*vrittis*). Rather through meditation it means bringing the mind to stillness or stability so that there are no thoughts, images, emotions or sensations that constitute *rajasic* or *tamasic vrittis* which produce turbulence. The mind has a one-pointed concentration (*ekagra*) on a single, *sattvic vritti* (i.e., object of concentration like a *mantra*). That concentration is uninterrupted so that the mind flows in a calm, pacific, smooth stream. The mind field is free of any *vritti* other than the object of concentration. Thus stillness is one-pointedness of the mind field when it is without the *rajasic* and *tamasic vrittis*. This is the state of *dhyana* (meditation). When the Centre of Consciousness opens into awareness that Presence, into which the *mantra* dissolves in deep meditation, becomes the object of concentration. Thus absorption into that Centre is a meditative phenomenon. In this sense the devotional focus (*Bhakti*) of *ishvara pranidhana* becomes a process of meditation. Swami Veda Bharati (1986) comments further on the meaning of "pacific" or "calm" (*shanta*) with a quotation from the Mahopanishad IV.32: "One who upon hearing, touching, seeing, tasting or smelling whatever pleasant or unpleasant is neither pleased nor displeased is called pacific, or calm (*shanta*)." Clearly this is a simultaneous state of dispassion (*vairagya*). Here the two wheels of the Chariot of *Sadhana* turn together.

The effort to achieve this state of *sthiti* is called both *virya* and *utsaha* (Veda Bharati, 1986). The word *virya* denotes virility, vigor, strength, energy, potency, the qualities of a hero. The word *utsaha* refers to enthusiasm, perseverance, fortitude, firmness, exertion, or vigorous pursuit. Since the mind naturally flows outwards, this process of achieving calmness is a heroic and intense concentration to bring the mind to stillness. This is an active rather than a passive process and stance. Some commentators go further and make the Centre of Consciousness the object of meditation. "On this *sutra* NTC says stability (*sthiti*) means one-pointedness (*ekagrata*) upon the transcendental self (*para-atman*) whose nature is essence (*sat*) and consciousness (*chit*)." (Veda Bharati, 1986, p 200). In addition to the practice of the *yamas* and *niyamas*, the effort involves *utsaha* (zeal and enthusiasm), *sahasa* (courage), *dhairya* (steadfastness and patience – if not in this lifetime then in some future one), *adhyatma-vidya* (the pursuit of spiritual science: the mind field (*chitta*) is extinguished like fire when no more fuel is provided. One sees the lack of purpose in and the falsity of objects, as opposed to a true purpose in *atman*, and *maha-seva* (service to the *Guru* or Master).

What then is practice (*abhyasa*)? The commentator Vyasa writes that practice is the observance of the means thereto (*sthiti*), with the will to achieve its fulfillment. What are the means toward *sthiti*? What is the practice?

- YS II.29ff: the eight limbs of Raja Yoga.
- YS I.20: the preconditions of *samadhi* are listed by Vyasa as faith (*shraddha*), strength (*virya*), intentness, meditation and the awakening of wisdom (*viveka*) in *samprajnata*. By the practice (*abhyasa*) of that and through dispassion (*vairagya*) concerning it, the *samprajanata samadhi* occurs.
- YS I .35–39: other objects of meditation to achieve this stability of the mind field include:
    I.35: direct experience or perception of subtle or celestial objects;
    I.36: the natural mental state which is free of grief and is called lucid;
    I.37: the sages who are free of attachments;
    I.38: observation, awareness and knowledge of dream and sleep states; and
    I.39: meditation in whatever way or on whatever object that is agreeable.

How is the practice done (. . . with the will to achieve its fulfillment)? The point is made that unless there is a definite resolve and exertion of will the effort will not bear fruit. The practice must be done with the attention and awareness. It is not done passively. It does not involve daydreaming or sleeping. It is work, but work with attention that is not performed mechanically or as a ritual. The practice is to be done with will and intent to fulfill the purpose, which provides the motivation to undertake the observance of the means and methods of Yoga. These are pursued with heroic perseverance, vigor, power and virility so that the mind becomes one-pointed on a *sattvic vritti* (like a *mantra*) alone. And then the mind flows in a calm, pacific, unturbulent, smooth stream. Swami Veda Bharati (1986) points to an alternative translation: "the effort to remain there is practice." Usually a practitioner reaches a depth and then tends to fall back. Or s/he cannot maintain that depth in daily life. But through the use of will and constant practice eventually one is able to remain at that depth during meditation and later to maintain that depth in daily life (YS I.14).

YS I.14 *sa tu dirgha-kala-nairantarya-satkarasevito drdha-bhumih.*
"That practice when continued for a long time without break and with devotion
becomes firm in foundation."

Aranya, 1981

Practice (*abhyasa*) must be firm, because it has to counter and overpower the force of residues (*samskaras*) in the unconscious mind of worldly involvements (*vyutthana-samskaras*) which have accumulated since beginningless time. It must also counter the impressions of *rajasic* and *tamasic* thoughts (*vrittis*).

Thus there are three aspects to practice. First, it must be done for a long time. This means it must be done for years, if not for lifetimes.

Reaching accomplishment after many life spans, one then arrives at the transcendental
state.

Bhagavad Gita VI.45

Second, it must be done without interruption. This implies frequent, consistent practice repeated every day, without interruption. There must be practice in every moment. An interruption in the practice permits the accumulation of opposite mental content (*vrittis*) which again overpower the residues laid down by the practice of Yoga (*yoga-samskaras*). The practice must be done with awareness and not absent-mindedly or as a mindless ritual. One receives the benefit of Yoga practice only when it is done with full awareness. This, in turn, means that the practitioner must be interested in the practice, fully committed to it, and single-mindedly obsessed with obtaining the Centre of Consciousness. At this stage, this is hard work! Ultimately the Presence is to be progressively crystallized as a stable background to everyday awareness in all things.

The practitioner, however well-intentioned and dedicated, soon learns how powerful the pull of worldly involvement, of desires, of emotional reactivity from attachments and aversions really is. He or she begins to collect the toolkit of tricks and practices that keep the momentum of awareness on this chosen task despite demands of the external world. Indeed, it will seem sometimes as though the whole universe rises up to block and divert the aspirant from this task. It takes great patience for a practitioner in the face of such obstacles to stay with the program and continually return the mind over and over again to the contemplation of the Centre without struggling with these obstacles and interferences. In part this means developing gradual detachment (*vairagya*) to the turbulence of worldly influences.

The whole process gradually develops the strength of will (*sankalpa shakti*) which is the key to success in the endeavor. Only this practical experience can teach the *sadhaka* what this will power really is. There comes a quiet sense of the rightness of the task, and that it *shall* be completed (indeed is already completed in the fullness of time), under the guidance and protection of the Centre of Consciousness, and that nothing can prevent this. It would remind one a bit of the gradual inexorability of flowing water to wear down the hardness of rock.

Finally, the practice must be done with due respect. It is done with deep interest and reverence, with devotion and with positive feeling. Without this attitude meditation becomes disturbed by sleep, distractions and worldly attractions. The mind is noisy. One must constantly affirm this positive attitude of reverence for the path.

Sutra I.30 on the obstacles is relevant here. If one does not practice for a long time, or if one breaks it many times over a long period, then one lacks sufficient faith and devotion for the task. Then distractions (*vikshepas*), attachments, aversions, disrupting emotions (*kashayas*), etc. arise which the practice does not counter.

What is meant, then, by a positive attitude? Swami Veda Bharati (1986, p 203) describes it as having it four qualities. First it involves *tapas* (ascetic practice or austerity) which reduces material and physical pleasures and luxuries as well as the dependence of the body on objects (see YS II.1, 32). Life is voluntarily simplified to reduce distractions. One is reminded of Duane Elgin's philosophy of voluntary simplicity (Elgin, 1998). Second it has the quality of *brahmacharya* (celibacy) which maintains control over sensual passion (YS II.30). It involves control over the four urges (sleep, food, sex and self-preservation). Next it has *vidya* (knowledge) which means proficiency in the tradition as well as the texts and proper systematic methods of practice. The student knows the proper way to practice and can do it correctly. Finally this positive attitude is immersed in *shraddha* (faith). It is the "faith and devotion that *samadhi* is the only worthy goal, the path I am on is the correct one for me, the lineage of my *Gurus* is authentic, I shall certainly reach *samadhi*, and I revere, honor, adore, have faith in my goal, my path, my *gurus*, and myself." (Veda Bharati, 1986, p 203). This attitude of faith expresses itself in service to the *guru*, a stance of humility towards all, constantly examining and curbing the ego, and expressions of devotion.

But this practice must also be firm of ground. This means first that one cannot be distracted or moved from it by even the strongest pain or adversity or even by the subtlest pleasure or most powerful attraction or desire. One's practice cannot be overpowered suddenly by a worldly residue (*vyutthana-samskara*) erupting from the unconscious mind. Secondly, it also means that one recognizes and attains the greatest depth of experience that particular practice is capable of providing. One achieves a mastery that allows one to go to that depth instantaneously at any time and under any condition or situation. Gradually that depth becomes the natural plateau of awareness in which the practitioner remains at all times. Then one reaches to gain a higher ground using the same process. This is another way of describing the progressive process of crystallizing the Presence.

Table 21.1 The Elements of *Abhyasa*

The Inward Arc Absorption into Being	*The Outward Arc* Manifestation into Doing

• Sat: Being – Rest, Silence, *Shantih*
• Conversation → Friendship →
  Communion → Absorption
• *Bhakti* – Devotion, Reverence
	• The Yogas of Life:
	  Wisdom (Intuition) – *Cit*
	  Bliss – *Ananda*
	  Will – Action
	• Co-creative Process Between self
	  and Centre
	• Attunement and Alignment of Parts
	  with the Centre

Practice (*abhyasa*) in the *Yoga-Sutra* (I.13), then, is the effort to acquire a tranquil state of mind (*sthiti*) devoid of fluctuations (*vrittis*). This is not an empty or blank mind, but a tranquil mind filled with the effulgence of the Presence. It is essentially *dhyana* – meditation. As we think about *abhyasa* or practice and its methodologies, the situation is a little more intricate. With *vairagya* one is releasing what blocks access to the Centre of Consciousness. But with *abhyasa* one is looking directly at that communication. The communication or communion is two-way. There is an INWARD ARC that involves progressive absorption into Being. And there is also an OUTWARD ARC of manifestation into activity or "doing." The latter includes intentionality or will, wisdom as the function of the Centre of Consciousness as the Inner Teacher, and co-creative action in the world.

22

The Inward Arc 1

There are three aspects to be considered for the inward arc. Its essence or core is surrender with absorption into Being. First there is the *sat* aspect which refers to an experience of profound Existence or Being, an experience of total and Primordial Rest or Silence, as well as the quality of *Shantih*, known as the Peace that passes all understanding. We equate this to the experience of Being described in the model of Aziz (Kristof, 2000) which was reviewed in Part One. He refers to It in Its purest form as the Absolute. It also refers to the *sat* of the *saccidananda* (existence-knowledge-bliss) of *saguna* (with qualities) *Brahman*. In Advaita Vedanta this *saccidananda* is the very essence of *Brahman* and not just attributes of It.

The second and associated aspect is Bhakti which manifests as an experience of devotion and reverence, mixed with praise and gratitude directed to the Centre as well as to the *guru* whose consciousness is one with that Centre. A persistent attitude of gratitude is one of the most powerful and healing states of mind that one can hold. Speaking metaphorically, the "universe" responds by providing more of what one is grateful for in a virtuous circle.

Finally there is the aspect of the relationship between the student and the Inner Teacher. This begins as a kind of conversational exchange between the two which then blossoms into a friendship as the relationship forms. It then moves to a state of communion which leads to the absorption of *samadhi*.

The practice of Silence is an important discipline in the Himalayan Tradition (Veda Bharati, 1979a). It is widely misunderstood as not speaking in a retreat setting. This often results in the passing of notes among people which defeats the purpose of the practice. For many of us just keeping verbal silence can be a challenge and after two or three days can induce emotional upheaval in some people. But the deeper practice of Silence is the practice of the Presence in all things, putting aside all distractions, even of reading the texts. This is the practice of stillness (such as *kaya sthairyam* and *antar mouna*) with one-pointedness (*dharana*) as a support to the all-important meditation. Such a tranquil mind is filled with the Centre of Consciousness. The Centre becomes the object of meditation at a certain stage. In his book, The Secret Path, Paul Brunton has this to say about the practice of mental quiet.

> The sovereignty of nature has been allotted to the silent forces. The moon makes not the faintest echo of a noise, yet it draws millions of tons of tidal waters to and fro at its bidding. We do not hear the sun rise nor the planets set. So, too, the dawning of the greatest moment in a man's life comes quietly, with none to herald it to the world. In that stillness alone is born the knowledge of the Overself. The gliding of the mind's

boat into the lagoon of the spirit is the gentlest thing I know; it is more hushed than the fall of eventide.

Only in deep silence may we hear the voice of the soul; argument but beclouds it and too much speech stops its appearance. When you have caught your fish you may share it, but while you are angling for it, talk breaks the spell and frightens the fish away. If we could occupy ourselves less with the activities of the larynx and more with the activities of the deeper mind, we may arrive at something worth saying. Speech is an adjunct, not an obligation. *To be* is the prime duty of man.

Life teaches us silently while men utter their instruction in loud voices.

The treasure-trove of the real self is within us, but it can be lifted only when the mind is still.

Brunton (1935, p 45).

The Art of Unceasing Worship

The core practice at this stage of the path is what the Christian literature calls practicing the presence of God. Here we might call it practicing the Centre of Consciousness, or practicing the Presence. The task is to hold that awareness of the Presence for twenty-four hours a day without a gap in all circumstances and activities until It becomes natural (*sahaja*), stable, continuous, effortless and unshakable in all circumstances. This is the process that Aziz calls crystallizing the Presence (Kristof, 2000). Although simple in principle, it is very difficult in practice. Indeed, it is a challenge to even remember to do it in the midst of the daily flow of thought, speech and activity. It can take a long time, even years, to achieve. Recall that in Patanjali's *Yoga-Sutra* I.14 that practice must be carried out consistently over a long time. (YS I.14: "That practice when continued for a long time without break and with devotion becomes firm in foundation."). As this process proceeds there is a very subtle shift of the centre of identity from the ego to that Still Point within.

This is the beginning of the identity shift. Initially one experiences one's individual self against the deepening and increasingly continuous background of Light, Stillness and Presence at the very core of the mind. This Background is experienced like an object by the individual sense of small self which plays out its role against that Background. Gradually and subtly the executive sense of self identity begins to shift its centre into that Stillness or Still Point. One begins to sense will and action as beginning to flow from that Silence once the sense of identity begins to centre in that Silence and Presence. It is as though one had shifted from the roar and chaos of the periphery of the hurricane of daily life to its still centre from which one can experience that movement whirling around the periphery. Instead of being solidly within the mind and body as a vehicle from which to experience reality, one begins to experience the mind and body contained within one's sense of self as this larger Presence and Silence. Swami Rama often said that while the body is within the mind, the mind extends far beyond the body.

Right in the Center of every wheel there is a point which is absolutely motionless. This is also true about the wheel of life. But if you could go to the very Center you'll find that actually without that central point there is no motion. Meditation is going into that still point. It is not stopping the movement of the wheel. It is not stopping to perform the acts and duties but becoming aware of the still central point and at the same time guiding the movement of the wheel. That is the Art of Living and therefore the Art of Dying.

Swami Veda Bharati

But beware! At the beginning the experience of that Void of fullness, that Presence, in the background of the mind is so subtle that doubt will be your worst adversary. Is that subtle touch of infinity real or just an imagining? But you will soon find that It comes and goes according to Its own purposes and that you cannot force It or control It. Your memory of It is not the same as the experience of It. When we asked Swami Rama what That was inside he answered that It was the Lord, as though it was the most ordinary thing in the world.

This is what is meant by the art of unceasing worship, which at this stage of the path is implied by *ishvara pranidhana* and the practice of Bhakti Yoga. Since it is also a state of deep meditation it can also be considered meditation in action for the Yogi, for whom the process eventually becomes continuous in every day activity.

The *Bhakti Sutras* (Prakash, 1998) express it thus:

35. "Spiritual devotion is developed by relinquishing objects and relinquishing attachments."

36. "By unceasing worship."

Sutra 35 describes nonattachment (*vairagya*). Sutra 36 describes practice (*abhyasa*) as we define it here. The two together describe the two wheels of the chariot of *sadhana*.

The corresponding *sutra* in the *Yoga-Sutra* is:

YS I.12: "By practice and detachment these (mental activities) can be stopped."

Recall that practice (*abhyasa*) is the effort to acquire a tranquil state of mind devoid of spontaneous and random interfering mental activity.

YS I.13 "Exertion to acquire *sthiti* or a tranquil state of mind devoid of fluctuations is called practice."

Aranya, 1981

Such a mind has achieved at the very least, a state of concentration (*dharana*) (the one-pointed state of *ekagra*) where interrupting fluctuations (*vrittis*) only seldomly appear. And ultimately it achieves the arrested state (*niruddha*) which is meditation (*dhyana*) in which the effort of concentration becomes an effortless and natural one-pointed flow of the mind towards its object with no interruption by other fluctuations. Held continuously over a long period this state of *dhyana* will flow into the stages of absorption (*samadhi*) into the Centre of Consciousness to consummate the full identity shift.

To put it differently, what is the content of that tranquil mind that has been achieved by *abhyasa*? Is it a blank, as some would say? Not at all! It is filled with the continuous and growing effulgence of the Centre of Consciousness. It begins as a concentrated mind and becomes a meditative mind, but the object of its flow is the Presence rather than ordinary mental content (*vrittis*). There are no ripples in the surface of the pond to distract and obscure the view of its depths. This is the Still Point, the origin of the *mantra* into which it returns and dissolves in the depth of meditation.

This is not an all or none process. To use the metaphor of the hurricane again, it is a gradual movement of the centre of self identity from the whirling periphery to the still centre. In daily life (meditation in action – holding this state of *abhyasa* in daily life) the periphery is still there. But it falls away as muted and one is centered in the relative prominence of the Still Point rather than in the peripheral chaos itself. Background and foreground have inverted. The Presence and Silence are now foreground and the chaos of ordinary mental-emotional-perceptual (sensory) activity fades into the background where it can be attended to from this new vantage point as one chooses for practical purposes. And when that mental activity is no longer needed it subsides into the Silence. The mind and its functioning are now under control, but all of its functions (*manas*, *chitta*, *buddhi* and *ahamkara*) are intact and can be used as required. The mind has not been destroyed but controlled. Please refer back to the discussion on *niroddha* as control in Part One.

Returning to the *Bhakti Sutras* (Prakash, 1998):

> 49. "Renouncing even the scriptures, a complete, unceasing, intense longing for God is obtained."

In this process of practicing the presence of God, one is to strive for a state of intense, unceasing awareness of that internal Presence. This process results in a relationship with Spirit that is direct and spontaneous. Communication with Its expression as the Inner Teacher can then provide immediate guidance and direction in life. The word *japa* means "repetition." Through long association with *mantra* the word usually is taken to refer to *mantra* repetition. But one can practice *japa* of anything by repeating the remembrance of a thought or idea. Practicing the Presence of God is *japa* on God. ". . . one can continuously remember the Lord or contemplate on the idea that one is in the supreme conscious state, experiencing [that illumination and Light or] the *anahad nada*, which is the sound of the soul, or the *atma* of all *mantras*." (Satyasangananda Saraswati, 2003, p 407).

In this unceasing awareness, some are led by light and some by sound. These spontaneous unstruck subtle sounds of the *anahata nada* emanating from the heart *chakra* which are heard in the right ear form the basis of Nada Yoga. They may have to be distinguished from physiological sounds in the ear that come from blood flow and other sources.

The relationship with the Centre is not mediated; it is direct. All convention, ritual and religion fall away. No rules are needed for the aspirant at this stage on how to live life. One becomes internally rather than externally referenced, following the whisperings of Spirit from within without hesitation. The aspirant may upset some others by not meeting their expectations with conventional behavior. The *sadhaka* may be misunderstood by his or her contemporaries who may criticize. One need only glance at the history books to see what has been done to persecute sages over the centuries. In the Christian Bible Jesus warns his followers to practice in secret. The priests and clerics of orthodox religion may be particularly unhappy with someone who does not need them as an intermediary to reach God. They may feel threatened and disempowered, and lash out. This is a path only for the courageous.

A young man in an audience once entreated Sri Swami Rama to let him renounce and go to a cave to practice under his guidance. Swamiji refused. He instructed the young man to go into the world and accomplish (which in Swamiji's terms usually meant get married, have children and get a PhD!), and then come back to him when he had something to renounce. Swamiji then turned to the rest of the audience and in a commanding voice said that this path was one of conquest. This path is only for the strong and courageous who can first succeed in the world.

As one offers that unceasing awareness to the Presence, it soon begins to flow as devotion and love. After a time the Centre of Consciousness begins to answer both with a flow of intense bliss (and actual force which can be quite hard on the body), and with a sensation of pulling or of attraction. One experiences a drawing of the awareness into It in absorption. But there is no loss of awareness – just the experience in various combinations of force, light, Bliss, sounds in the right ear, stillness, Silence, and the pure knowing of intuition. Sometimes the experience is of an expansion, and at other times of a point. The Centre of Consciousness is both point and expansion and may be represented symbolically by a circle with a dot (*bindu*) at the centre. Its circumference represents the expansion while the dot at the centre represents the infinite point or *bindu*. The word "*samadhi*" is given many translations, but it is most often translated as "absorption."

In his extensive commentary on Yoga and Christianity, Paramahamsa Yogananda (2004, Vol I, p 496) discusses the importance of acquiring the concentrated attention and devotion that make devotional prayer effective. The practice of Bhakti Yoga as devotional prayer will not be effective if the background of the mind is occupied by the distractions of worldly thoughts and desires. God does not manifest so long as other desires have precedence in the devotee's heart and mind. "Thou shalt not take the name of the Lord thy God in vain" (Exodus 20:7). Yogananda points to Jesus' teaching to "pray without ceasing" (1 Thessalonians 5:17).

> Unceasing prayer involves repetition – not vain or mechanical, but spiritualized with ever-increasing, thoughtful, heartfelt devotion. That devotee is sure to find divine contact who continuously keeps the mind on God, intensifying the thoughts of his

prayer, unceasingly reining in the attention regardless of how many times it wanders away. The *Gita* similarly teaches: "On Me fix thy mind, be thou My devotee, with ceaseless worship bow reverently before Me. Having thus united thyself to Me as thy Highest Goal, thou shalt be Mine own" (*Bhagavad Gita* IX: 34). . . . To utter "God" with devotion, and increase the concentration and devotion with each repetition of His name, is to plunge the mind deeper and deeper in the ocean of His presence until one reaches fathomless depths of divine peace and ecstatic joy, the sure proof that one's prayers have touched God. . . . But it takes a long time for prayer to be effective when the mind is outwardly roaming. . . . If one enters the inner temple of silence and worships before the alter of God with prayer and invocation of His presence, He comes quickly. When the consciousness is withdrawn from the sensory surface of the body and its surroundings and centralized in the cerebrospinal shrines of soul perception, that is the most effective time to pray.

Ishvara Pranidhana

What we have just described can also be understood as the practice of *ishvara pranidhana*. In his *Yoga-Sutra* the sage Patanjali is clear that the result of this one-pointed practice of *ishvara pranidhana* is *samadhi*.

> YS I.29 "From that (*ishvara pranidhana*) comes realization of the individual self and the obstacles are resolved."
>
> Aranya, 1981

This idea of unceasing worship is developed further in YS.23–29 which deals with *Ishvara* (Veda Bharati, 1986, pp 277–323).

> YS I.23: *Ishvara-pranidhanad va.*
> "Or, (*samadhi* can be attained quickly through) practicing the presence of God."
>
> Veda Bharati, 1986, p 277

This is not the *ishvara pranidhana* described as part of the *niyamas* in YS II.1. Rather here it means practicing the presence of God, the essence of Bhakti. It refers to the practice of the sequence of *dharana* (concentration), *dhyana* (meditation) and *samadhi* (absorption) – called *samyama* when done together – with the Centre of Consciousness as its eventual object, but in the beginning using the practice of YS I.28 as elaborated below to give *samadhi* as described in YS I.29. When invoked by a true devotee in this manner the grace of God leads to *samadhi*.

This practice of the presence of God requires as support the five *upayas* (methods) described in YS I.20; namely, faith, strength, intentness, mental harmony and discrimination. Added to these is great intensity and momentum of practice (YS I.21, 22). When all of these together reach peak intensity, then the aspirant can drop all other practices, since at this last state God's grace alone suffices to reach the final *samadhi* (*asamprajnata*). When done with high intensity this process of practicing the presence of God becomes a shortcut with the five methods (*upayas*) providing secondary support.

Ishvara in this context is the Supreme Self (*parama-atman*) or *Brahman*. *Ishvara* is non-qualified pure Consciousness, what we refer to here as the Centre of Consciousness, from which consciousness flows in various degrees and grades (deep sleep, dreaming and wakefulness as described in the *Mandukya Upanishad*). Patanjali describes *Ishvara* as a special *purusha* who as pure Consciousness is a form of qualified (*saguna*) Brahman (the Centre of Consciousness as *sat*, *chit*, *ananda* as elaborated in Part One). Beyond that His nature is of no concern! Patanjali takes the position that the concern of the *Yoga-Sutra* is to move the practitioner out of ignorance and suffering into *kaivalya* (liberation) at which point the aspirant will find out for him/herself what *Ishvara* actually is. If the aspirant does not believe in God or in surrender, he or she then does the path of the five methods (*upayas*).

Ishvara pranidhana means to place oneself down in humility and egolessness in the proximity of God. It is to place the mind within, and dwell very near and close to the Centre of Consciousness. One surrenders and places oneself at the disposal of God even if one does not know what God is until one reaches the state of *asamprajnata*. The process is total (mental, vocal and physical), and is described as the secret and easy path.

The term *pranidhana* (to place the mind within) is really a process of *bhavana*: impressing the object of concentration repeatedly on the mind in meditation and in daily life. This is the process of crystallizing the Presence as described by Aziz (Kristof, 2000) in chapter four. *Bhavana* is cultivated concentration, a process of cultivating and absorbing a meaning. It is an internal process of impressing the object of concentration (*bhavya*) repeatedly onto the mind. It is *japa* of the Centre of Consciousness. One rejects all other worldly desires and offers actions to Him as Supreme *Guru*. Actions are not just surrendered after they are performed, but before and during the acts as well. This process of *bhavana* is practiced in daily acts throughout one's entire life as well as in meditation.

In meditation the object of concentration is cultivated. One concentrates on Him (the Centre of Consciousness or Presence) in the heart *chakra*, filling oneself with love as one invokes His Presence, and offering one's entire self to Him without concern or worry (*abhi-dhyana*: will and thought directed towards Him). One thinks lovingly of God constantly. This is meditation in action with the Presence fully manifest behind the mind. Kristoff's model described in Part One develops the sequence of Presence (felt in the head) dropping into Being (experienced lower in the body) and then into Bliss (*ananda*) with the opening of the heart centre.

This process of *abhi-dhyana* is reciprocal. God responds with grace, often in the form of the *guru*, that brings liberation. The practitioner directs thought towards God who then responds with grace whereby he or she attains *samadhi*. This is a process of winning God's favor through devotion. Surrender to the physical *guru* connects one to the Supreme *Guru* (Centre of Consciousness as the expression of the Inner Teacher), for in consciousness they are one and the same. If one cannot mentally surrender to God, then one should surrender to the physical *guru* who in turn connects one to the Supreme *Guru* (YS I.26). Thus practicing the *bhavana* of *ishvara pranidhana* either on the incarnate *guru* or God leads to *samprajnata* and then to *asamprajnata samadhi* in the presence of the Supreme Being whose grace gives liberation (*moksha*).

Who, then, is *Ishvara*? *Sutras* 24 through 26 address this question.

> YS I.24: *Klesha-karma-vipakashayair a-para-mrishtah purusha-vishesha ishvarah.*
>   "A special *purusha* not smeared by afflictions, actions, their fruitions and the domains of their accumulated propensities (is) God."
> YS I.25: *Tatra nir-atishayam sarvajna-bijam.*
>   "In Him the seed of the omniscient (is) unexcelled (and ultimate)."
> YS I.26: *Purvesham api guruh kalena an-avachchhedat.*
>   "(He is) the *guru* even of the very first, the ancient and the former (teachers) (because in Him there is) no delimitation by time."
>   Veda Bharati, 1986

What we are referring to here as the Centre of Consciousness is *Ishvara*. Yoga-Vedanta presents God on three levels of reality (Veda Bharati, 1979a). The highest or most abstract is *Brahman*, the transcendental, absolute, transpersonal Being. The Buddhist and Christian analogs are *Dharmakaya* and God the Father or Logos respectively. Next is God as the imminent spirit of the universe. This is *Ishvara*, the Lord or personal God, also called *Hiranyagarbha* (the Golden Womb – the first *guru* or first wise one, the universal being or teaching spirit of the universe, the original teacher of Yoga also known as *Prajapati* (the Progenitor) or *Brahma*). The first human being is said to have been an incarnation of *Hiranyagarbha* and all revelation comes from the grace that flows from this Golden Womb (Veda Bharati, 1986, p 456). The Buddhist equivalent is *Sambhogakaya* and the Christian term is God the Holy Ghost or Spirit, or teaching spirit in the universe – hence the term Inner *Guru* or Inner Teacher in Yoga. Finally there is the level of *avatara* as a being incarnate and manifest in history such as Jesus, Krishna or Buddha. The Buddhist term is *Nirmanakaya* and Christians refer to God the Son, or God in history. Thus all three traditions have the equivalent of the expression of God as a Holy Trinity.

More specifically, *Ishvara* is the Lord or the Personal God, the Divine with form (*saguna-brahman*). In Advaita Vedanta *Ishvara* is *brahman* as conditioned by *maya* (ensouls the universe; wears the universe as Its body). Although the Absolute has no distinctions, in relation to the world the God-head as *Ishvara* becomes its source and ground, its creator, both the material and efficient cause of the world. The *saguna-brahman* is said to be omnipotent, omniscient, and omnipresent. He manifests in five forms as transcendent (*para*), as various emanations (*vyuha*) and incarnations (*vibhava*), as the indweller (inner teacher or *guru*) (*antaryamin*), and as sacred icons (*arca*). As *para* he possesses six divine qualities: knowledge (*jnana*), strength (*bala*), lordship (*aishvarya*), potency (*shakti*), virility (*virya*), and splendor (*tejas*). He is all-merciful and individual souls attain liberation by His grace. He of course transcends gender and the use of masculine pronouns as designators is only a traditional linguistic convenience. *Ishvara* comes from the verb root *ish* meaning "to have power or control over; to be able to [create, control, direct]; to govern; to impart grace." (Veda Bharati, 1986, p 457). Hence the meaning of "Lord" or "Lordship." In the *Yoga-Sutra* he is neither *prakriti* nor *purusha*, but a special *purusha*, a Conscious Being unstained by the afflictions (*kleshas*) or by *karma* (actions and their fruits).

Thus in *sutra* 24, which is the definition *sutra* (*lakshana-sutra*) that defines *Ishvara*, He is "a special *purusha* not smeared by afflictions, actions, their fruitions and the domains of their accumulated propensities." (Veda Bharati, 1986, p 282). *Samkhya* philosophy stops at giving insight into the nature of suffering (bondage, pain and ignorance) by defining its causes and then explaining the relationship between *purusha* and *prakriti*. This is sufficient for the *Yoga-Sutra* which is a *prayoga-shastra*, a text or science that teaches a practical method by which the connection between *purusha* and *prakriti* can be broken so that *purusha* can dwell in its own nature and a qualified aspirant can receive God's grace that leads to liberation. Beyond this, discussions of the nature of *brahman* are left to Vedanta. The nature of God is not a topic of further interest to the *Yoga-Sutra*. Reach liberation and then find out for yourself what the real nature of God is. Since the Lord is all powerful, He can be only one (for if there were two, and they disagreed, who would prevail?)

His powers of knowledge and action are used to send compassionate grace through the *sattva* of *prakriti* (primordial nature) to liberate beings (Veda Bharati, 1986, p 292). God reveals true knowledge to aspirants thereby raising them from suffering. These are the intuitive revelations of the Inner Teacher. He does this by extending His powers of knowledge and action. When the mind field (*chitta*) is purified through Yogic practice and freed of *tamas* and *rajas* so that its *sattvic* essence shines forth, he touches that *sattva* with His knowledge and action, but without identifying with it like a *jiva* (individual soul) who makes the error of ignorance, mistaking the self for non-self. Thus *Ishvara* is not subject to ignorance (*avidya*) and bondage. His power of knowledge and action sends grace into the purified (*sattvic*) *chitta* to liberate beings. This is God expressing as the Inner *Guru* through intuitive revelation. He accomplishes this by way of the cosmic mind (*chitta*) and thence to the individual *chitta* of the *jiva*. Thus the cosmic *chitta* becomes the instrument of grace flowing from the Lord. This process occurs in perpetual cycles forever: He takes hold of the *sattva* of *prakriti*, the universe is created, and in touch with that *sattva-chitta* He expresses His knowledge and action. When He takes hold of the *tamas* of *prakriti*, the universe is dissolved and He rests in *yoga nidra*.

In *sutra* 25 the essence of a Tradition is explained (Veda Bharati, 1968, p 303). The *sutra* implies that in all beings the essence of *Ishvara's* omniscience exists as a seed from which only a little knowledge manifests in a limited being. That knowledge progressively increases by a decrease of *tamas* (which veils the *buddhi*, determining one's capacity for greater or lesser knowledge – awareness), and by an increase of *sattva* (which increases one's capacity for that knowledge). The knowledge of each delimited being has with it this seed of the omniscient which grows until it reaches the expanse of *Ishvara*. It keeps enlarging and expanding until one reaches an infinite limit of excellence which is *atman* or *Ishvara*.

The Origin of a Spiritual Tradition

The Lord acts from compassion to deliver transmigrating *purushas* by continuously giving them knowledge and virtue through both scriptural revelation and discriminative wisdom. Revealed scriptural knowledge is available to all. But discriminating wisdom (*viveka-khyati*) comes from the practice of *dhyana* and *samadhi* which need the Lord's grace. Knowledge is revealed to the minds of the great sages at the beginning of each cycle of creation and repeatedly to the *rishis* in *samadhi* throughout.

A tradition is a lineage of produced minds (*nirmana-chitta*) called mental offsprings (*manasa-putra*), that imparts knowledge by initiation via a *guru*-disciple lineage through the generations beginning with *Hiranyagarbha*. It is said that Kapila was the first *rishi* to whom Samkhya-Yoga was revealed. He, in turn, initiated a produced mind to teach the tradition and subsequent steps formed the lineage. This is an initiatory process by which the sage as *guru* sends a spark of his *asmita* (I-am-ness) into the prepared disciple's mind thereby transferring the reality and experience of the object of teaching into the disciple's mind. The disciple is then called the teacher's mental offspring. A tradition, then, is a lineage of produced minds or mental offsprings that imparts knowledge through the generations by initiation from *guru* to disciple. The Himalayan Tradition is one such lineage. One can study scriptural knowledge all one wants, but true and full experiential knowledge is transmitted by direct initiation. One must have a *sad-guru* for this. Sri Swami Rama would say to certain disciples, "You I will teach in silence!"

Sutra 26 points out that God, dwelling outside of time, is the *Guru* of all *gurus* past, present and future. He performs this function as the indweller (*antar-yamin*) Who gives them the eye of knowledge. God is the *atman* (the ruling power or Self) of souls, pervading them as their indweller and father. In Vedanta the idea of fatherhood means that souls are to God as sons or daughters are to a father. An alternative metaphor is that souls are to God as sparks to a fire. When God creates or draws forth the universe He multiplies the soul sparks to whom knowledge is revealed and through whom it is transmitted in the *guru* lineage.

Thus by practicing the presence of that one God and surrendering all mental, vocal and physical acts to His will, one receives ever-flowing grace, enters *samadhi*, and is liberated. There are two aspects to the process: constant remembrance which is practicing the Presence as the Centre of Consciousness, and surrender, which is following Spirit without hesitation – with all action, will and desire flowing from the Centre of Consciousness (the essence of Karma Yoga). Killing (not following) the conscience (another name for the Centre of Consciousness) is the only sin in the Tradition. All agendas of the personal ego must be surrendered; it is all or nothing since it is an identity shift of self to true Self. Here both constant remembrance and surrender merge into continuous awareness of the inner Reality: hence, Swami Rama's oft repeated motto – love, serve and remember.

Pranidhana, Bhavana and *Prajna*

Now *pranidhana* is explained (Veda Bharati, 1986).

YS I.27: *Tasya vachakah pranavah.*
   "The word OM is his significator (name)."
YS I.28: *Taj-japas tad-artha-bhavanam.*
   "The *japa* of that name, and cultivating and absorbing its meaning (is called *ishvara-pranidhana*, the practice of the presence of God)."

To reorient ourselves, the structure of *sutras* 23–28 flows as follows. YS I.23 states that *samadhi* can be obtained by practicing the presence of God (*ishvara pranidhana*). Then *sutras* 24–26 explain *Ishvara*. *Sutra* 27 prepares then for *sutra* 28 which explains *pranidhana*.

In *sutra* 27 we are told that the name of God is OM. Certain *mantras* are given special names in *mantra* science. OM is called *pranava*. Swami Veda Bharati (1986, p 310) gives several derivations of this word. The one that is most relevant here is: "From prefixes *pra* and *ni* and verb *dha*, as in *pranidhana*: 'whereby He is placed close, brought close, by those who practice His presence (*pra-ni-dhatrs*).' Or 'whereby one places God in the mind,' for it is by a word or a name that one bears those in mind who are absent or intangible." The other two meanings refer to the devotees who practice His presence and to Him who protects from *samsara* (transmigration).

If one has not yet realized God directly one can only practice His presence using His name, which is OM. Tangible objects do not need a word since they can be experienced directly by the cognitive senses as percepts. But intangible objects cannot be directly experienced by the senses. They are concepts, nominalizations or abstract nouns that can only be symbolized with a word with its inherent meaning. God is one of these, intangible to the senses, and cannot be directly experienced by the unrealized. He can only be signified by His name which is OM, and only in this way can *pranidhana*, His presence, be practiced.

Ordinarily we understand that the link between a word and its meaning is established by convention and usage alone. But this is not the case with OM. The commentators write that the relationship between God and OM is permanent and given by revelation through the Vedas from one creation to the next. The knowledge (meaning) is eternal and one with His self-nature. It is not His possession like an object separate from Him. Thus God = OM; the relationship of name and meaning is one of identity; the two are identical, inseparable.

This being so then OM also carries the inherent power (*shakti*) of God. OM is a power word and eternal. Since OM is the origin of all authentic *mantras*, then *mantras*, too, carry power. This is the origin of *mantra shakti*. These eternal names are to be found in the revealed texts (*agama*) which are the textual authority and tradition of the lineage. Both the lineage and its authority come from revelation, the perception of intuitive knowledge in consciousness. The *mantra* science goes deeply into this process of intuitive revelation with its levels of subtlety from *vaikari* through *madhyama* and *pashyanti* to *paravak* which we will elaborate in Part Five (Tigunait, 1996). Thus the meaning and knowledge that is OM is eternally one with God and uses the sound and word OM as His vehicle. The sound is a modification of *prakriti* (nature) which is subject to creation and dissolution, but the meaning is eternal and one with God.

OM (AUM) is traditionally described as composing the three syllables A (*Brahma*), U (*Vishnu*) and M (*Shiva*) followed by silence. The letters signify the forces of creation, sustaining and dissolution operative in manifest nature (*prakriti*). They are the physical sound of the word which appears and disappears with creation and dissolution of *prakriti*. The silence that follows is the knowledge part of the word which is eternal, absolute, immutable and never modified. It is the silence of *samadhi*.

Thus the three sounds are the vehicles or sonar bodies while the silent knowledge behind them is God's own self as knowledge. OM as eternal, immutable knowledge packaged in a sonar body is not a separate name of God but the same as God (*Mandukya Upanishad*: Nikhilananda, 1987b). As the origin and end of all *mantras*, OM gives to the devotee the fruit of the practice of all other *mantras*.

Now having established the special nature and power of the name as OM, Patanjali goes on to explain the nature of *pranidhana* in *sutra* 28 (Veda Bharati, 1986, p 315). Since one cannot practice the presence of God without the experience of God in *samadhi*, one starts with the symbol OM which YS I.27 has indicated is the same thing. The sonic parts A U M are the objects of concentration, but the silent half (*mora*) that follows AUM is experienced only beyond the mind. Only when the practitioner understands both the nature of the symbol (OM) and what it symbolizes (God) can the actual *pranidhana* which is the *japa*, begin.

Note that a student who has received a proper *guru mantra* by initiation from a qualified initiator (either the master him or herself or a disciple whom he or she empowers to give *mantra* initiation) would use that *guru mantra* for *japa*, for OM is the source of all authentic *mantras*. A *mantra* received through proper initiation carries the *mantra shakti*. *Sutra* 28 then says that *japa* of that name, that *mantra*, as well as cultivating and absorbing its meaning, is what is meant by *ishvara pranidhana* – practicing the presence of God. *Pranidhana*, then, is *bhavana* (contemplation) of the meaning of the word (*mantra*) signifying God. Its real meaning is cultivated and absorbed in meditation. *Mantra japa* begins with the word symbol and ends with the experience of its meaning (not just an intellectual understanding) which is *prajna* (intuition), the realization of the true nature of the object of concentration. You began at your level of capacity, moving through verbal recitation and ultimately into silent mental contemplation. This is not just mechanical *japa* (recitation of the word) but includes *bhavana* of its meaning which is God. The *mantra* signifies God and is one with It. *Japa* must be accompanied with meditation (*dhyana*) on *Brahman*, the Supreme Self, with faith and devotion.

At this stage of the Path what is meant here by God is the Presence aspect of the Centre of Consciousness which is beginning to open as a direct experience in the background of the mind field as we described in detail in Part One. This is the *cit* aspect of the *sat cit ananda* of the Vedantic *saguna brahman*. The object of concentration is the *mantra* pulsing in the silence of that background Awareness or Presence. The *mantra* is the signifier and the Presence is its meaning.

This *bhavana* or contemplation of *Brahman* uses Patanjali's process of *samyama*, going through *dharana*, *dhyana* and *samadhi*. *Bhavana* is a cultivated concentration. It involves impressing the object of concentration (*bhavya*) again and again onto the mind field by preventing any other object from entering the mind. The Chariot of *Sadhana* now takes on a very subtle meaning. *Abhyasa* (practice) becomes a gentle process of returning the mind over and over without strain, conflict or stress to the object of concentration. At the same time through the process of witnessing, *vairagya* (nonattachment) releases over and over any reactivity, emotional or conditioned, that appears in the mind field through a process of surrender and release done from the witnessing stance which as we noted previously, breaks the emotional connection. And so in this process the wheels of the Chariot turn together with *vairagya* releasing each mental fluctuation to subtler and subtler levels, and *abhyasa* returning the awareness over and over to the object of concentration. Releasing and returning; letting go and returning; surrendering and returning. Through this process of *bhavana* the form and nature of the object of meditation is completely realized (*prajna*), leaving no residue of doubt or possibility of misinterpretation (*viparyaya*: false cognition or perception).

By *prajna* is meant the intuitive realization of the true nature of the object of meditation, the process of awakening of wisdom and the wisdom itself. This concentration should remain constant and be continuously maintained. By this cultivation the process of *bhavana* causes the object (the sense or experience of its perception) and the mind eventually to become one. This process is called *vitarka*, which is gross thought, or thought about the names of the particular objects of concentration, which here are the *mantra* word used for *japa* and its meaning which is God. *Vitarka samadhi* occurs when the nature of the object with all of its aspects is finally realized all at once intuitively, and this whole realization is maintained without a break.

And so there are two processes. First there is *japa* of the word (*mantra*), which by its association reminds one of God it signifies. Then the mind comes to dwell on its meaning (God and His attributes – the Presence aspect of the Centre of Consciousness) as *bhavana*.

Notice that the instructions for advanced meditation involve taking the *mantra* to the Silence. Rather than a deliberate forced process, this is allowed to evolve naturally by prolonged observation of the *mantra* alone without the breath. The *mantra* will evolve into increasing and deeper subtlety as a pulsing vibrational energy form which leads the meditator's awareness towards its Source. At this point it will dissolve naturally into the Silence of the Presence in which the meditator's awareness rests one-pointedly. Then with prolonged practice absorption of one's awareness into that Presence leads to its deepening into the levels of Being, the awakening of Heart, Bliss or *Ananda*, and eventually the full integrated experience of the *saguna Brahman* in *samprajnata samadhi*. At this point meditation is actually on the Centre of Consciousness and not the *mantra*. Background becomes foreground. Thus *japa* cannot be done without dis-association of word and its meaning. Practicing the Presence as *pranidhana* is actually this process of *bhavana*, and so it becomes practicing the presence of God truly as the Centre of Consciousness.

Pranidhana, which is *bhavana*, is experienced on two levels (Veda Bharati, 1986, p 315). First the effect and the cause, the parts of the whole, are unified. One contemplates and then one experiences one's self permeated by and unified with *Brahman* like heat permeates an iron ball. Then one discriminates between *prakriti* (symbolized by the iron ball) and *purusha* (symbolized by the heat) and one knows "I am That, I am *Brahman*." This is a Vedantic version of *bhavana*.

As this process proceeds the mind field becomes one-pointed. During the phase when *japa* is recitation, articulate or mental, the mind is in the *vikshipta* state, distracted by other thoughts. But then as the process deepens the meaning of the *mantra*, which is the very Presence of God, becomes the primary experience, and the first stages of *samadhi* ensue. This phase of *samadhi* is *sa-vitarka*, with thought, where the relationship of the word with its meaning is maintained. Later the *samadhi* becomes *nir-vitarka*, *samadhi* without *vitarkas* or thoughts, where there is separation of the word and its meaning and their relationship collapses into unified Presence.

With this entry into *samadhi* the mind field moves from *vikshipta* (distracted) to *ekagra*, becoming one-pointed. The same process happens with the components AUM of OM, however they may be used for meditation (meditations on *Brahma*, *Vishnu* or *Shiva*; the use of the personal *mantra* which evolves from OM; or meditation on the syllables AUM of the OM *mantra*). The concentration is still on the divine consciousness that pervades these objects of meditation. One comes to rest in the Supreme Self, and one becomes filled with that Supreme Self.

Sutra 27 described the power (*shakti*) of a word (*mantra*) as well at its meaning. The power (*shakti*) is *vachaka*, that which enunciates or signifies. The meaning is *vachya*, that which is enunciated or signified. As the *japa* refines itself *vachaka* progressively reduces until only *vachya* remains. The *mantra* as word ceases leaving behind only its meaning as the Presence or Silence shining and totally occupying the mind until the mind takes the form of that object of concentration (YS I.43; III.3), and the mind then seems to become absent.

YS II.1 discusses *svadhyaya* as both *japa* of the purificatories like OM as well as study of the scriptures that lead to liberation. This idea derives from the word *adhyaya* which means study in the sense of formal study of the Vedas. Traditionally this involves precise recitation aloud from memory. This is not *japa* as described here. When the recitation is to oneself only it becomes *sva-adhyaya* (self-study), and then as a mental act it is called *japa*. Note that in this *sutra* 28 under discussion, the word *yoga* means *samadhi* as in YS I.1. As *japa* progresses the mind becomes stilled, and thereby the posture becomes steady. Swami Veda Bharati (1986, p 318) quotes the sage Parashara in the *Vishnu-purana* III.6.2:

"With the aid of silent recitation (*svadhyaya*) let one establish the posture, sitting in yoga. Through yoga too they sit for silent recitation. By perfecting silent recitation and yoga together the Supreme Self shines forth."

As *bhavana* of the meaning of the *mantra* becomes firm, the Presence of God is experienced and *samadhi* ensues. Repeated experience of deep meditation firms up this practice of *japa*. *Svadhyaya* (*japa*) and Yoga (*samadhi*) cannot be simultaneous. This is about taking the *mantra* into the Silence during meditation. One begins meditation with *japa* of the *mantra* which then leads to *samadhi*. One then emerges from *samadhi* back into *japa*. This describes the beginner in *samadhi*. Gradually perfection of *japa* and *samadhi* leads to illumination of the Supreme Self. This is where the process of *pranidhana/bhavana* reaches the silent *mora* beyond the articulate syllables AUM or OM. This is where *japa* becomes one with *samadhi* and is no longer even a mental endeavor.

How then might we summarize the essence of this process of *pranidhana* and *bhavana* on *Ishvara* (the Centre of Consciousness in its aspect as Presence)? Swami Veda Bharati (1986) does it thus:

- One engages in *japa* and *bhavana* (practicing the presence of God) (YS I.28) of OM (or one's *guru mantra*), for a long time, without interruption, with deep faith and with commitment (YS I.14).
  - The articulate form of the word ceases and the repetition becomes mental.
  - By association of word (*mantra*) with its meaning *japa* reminds one of God it (the *mantra*) signifies (meaning). *Japa* refines itself until only that meaning remains. This is taking the *mantra* to the Silence in meditation. This is not a forced process but evolves naturally over a long time.
  - Practicing the presence of God or *bhavana* involves the mind dwelling on this meaning (God and Its attributes), impressing the object of concentration again and again on to the mind field while preventing any other object from entering the mind. This is the Chariot of *Sadhana* in its subtlest form: returning (*abhyasa*) and surrendering (*vairagya*) over and over; remembering the Presence (*abhyasa*) and releasing all other content in the mind field (*vairagya*).
- The word (*mantra*) is replaced by its meaning (the Presence). The power (*shakti*) of the word (that which enunciates, *vachaka*) is extinguished by that which is enunciated (*vachya* – the meaning or God). *Bhavana* on that meaning moves through the stages of *dharana*, *dhyana* to *samadhi*.
  - Concentration is on the divine consciousness that pervades the object of concentration, on the Presence that fills the background of mental space that holds the pulsing *mantra*.
  - One comes to rest in the Supreme Self, filled with It.
- The mind field moves from *vikshipta* (distracted) to *ekagrata* (one-pointed). The mind field becomes harmonized (*samahita*) and flows in a calm, pacific, smooth stream.
- As the *bhavana* of the meaning of the *mantra* becomes firm, the Presence of God is experienced and *samadhi* ensues. This is *prajna*, the intuitive realization of the true nature of the object of meditation.
  - One contemplates and then experiences oneself permeated by and then unified in *Brahman*.
  - One gains the discrimination between *prakriti* and *purusha* and comes to know I am *Brahman*.
- The self now dwells in the Self.
  - All external objects of concentration have been abandoned.
  - No further *samskaras* are gathered.
  - Only the past *samskaras* (*prarabdha karma*) maintain the momentum of the body.
  - The self now dwells in the Self. The identity shift is complete.

Finally, *Sutra* 29 explains the fruit of *ishvara pranidhana*.

YS I.29: *Tatah pratyak-chetanadhigamo'py antarayabhavash cha.*
  "(Through the practice of the presence of God) (accrues) the attainment of inward consciousness (and) the realization of the inwardly conscious self; also the impediments are removed, made absent."
  (Veda Bharati, 1986)

By practicing the presence of God impediments like illness are resolved. One realizes one's true nature as the seer dwelling in its own nature (YS I.3). *Japa* and other practices attract the grace of God which reverses the outward flow of awareness, drawing it inwards until it reaches the ultimate Self-realization. Along the way the obstacles and impediments are removed (YS I.30), some by the practice itself, and some from the grace that clears the paths and channels. This inward flow of consciousness and the removal of obstacles happen together. In Vedantic terms the realization is of the unity of the individual self with the Supreme Self. Through practicing the presence of God one is led to Self-Realization in which one sees the similarity of the natures of the small self and *Ishvara*. Realization of the greater *Purusha* (*Ishvara*) brings the realization of the little *purusha* since they are similar: the Vedantic "That thou art."

We have spent a great deal of time discussing *ishvara pranidhana* which may seem to be laboring a minor point. But this presentation of fine points could be considered the focus of this whole book – once the Centre of Consciousness opens into experience, then what do you do with it? How do you work with it in meditation? The instruction to meditate on It seems very obvious and simple, until one actually tries to do it. This simple instruction is one of the hardest things that the distracted mind can be asked to do. The new disciple will receive an intuition that this experience of the Presence is to be stabilized, to be crystallized, to be made a permanent state of Awareness. But the link to that Centre is still very new and in the process of forming. It is easy to doubt that intuition, much less wonder exactly what the process is for carrying it out. It is very reassuring to find textual evidence for that inner teaching, that inner intuition as well as guidance regarding the exact method. This whole process of *bhavana* forms the essence of meditation at this stage of the path which we will deal with in more detail in Part Five.

Here is the same idea expressed in the *Bhagavad Gita*.

> BG 18.65. "Be aware of me always, adore Me, make every act an offering to Me, and you shall come to Me; this I promise."

> 66. "Abandon all supports and look to Me for protection. I shall purify you from the sins of the past; do not grieve."
>
> Easwaran (1984)

Easwaran (1984) points out that to "abandon all supports" is a terrifying prospect for us. We cannot completely hold on just to the Self; we want to reach out to grab anything, something external for support. Easwaran provides an apt metaphor: " . . . it is only human nature to prefer diversified investments. We want a balanced portfolio of props in life, just in case one or two fall through."

23
The Inward Arc 2

The Reverential Attitudes (The Five *Bhavas*)

In his translation of and commentary on the *Bhakti Sutras*, Prakash (1998) points out that there are five attitudes toward God that an aspirant may adopt in the Indian traditions of Bhakti Yoga: the attitude of a servant, a friend, a parent, a philosopher, or a spouse. In order to develop a personal relationship with a form of God that he or she can best appreciate and understand, the devotee assumes one of these attitudes that corresponds to specific individual temperament so that the vibrations or energy level of his or her personality harmonizes with that chosen form of God.

Bhavas are mental-emotional attitudes used as techniques to cultivate spiritual devotion. Traditionalists consider the list as hierarchical, but what really matters is not the particular *bhava* chosen, but the love and devotion that grows in the devotee's heart.

Prakash (1998) points out the paradox that God plays the roles of both worshiper and worshiped. In his Ramayana, Tulsi Dass has Baba Hanuman say, "From the viewpoint of the body, I am Thy servant; from the viewpoint of the ego, I am a portion of Thee; from the viewpoint of the Self, I am Thyself."

Ramacharitamanas says that the servant of Rama, the servant of God, is greater than God Himself. The greatest of the five *bhavas* is the first – the attitude of a servant. "I am Thy servant. I shall carry out all Thy wishes." This is Karma Yoga, following Spirit without hesitation (Satyananda Saraswati, 1997, pp 92–94).

Ego, Surrender and the Centre of Consciousness

Sri Swami Rama describes the ego as having a higher and a lower side. The ego that helps one go beyond is the higher ego. But the lower ego is limiting. It creates a boundary that separates one from the whole and prevents one from being exposed to higher levels of Consciousness. One is still a Master, but now the mastery is of limitation! This is the small-mindedness that disempowers.

If the mind cannot provide a solution to a problem then the remedy is to go beyond the intellect. But to do this one must accomplish the difficult task of surrendering the ego, something that one never does before another human being. Proper surrender of the ego requires not only faith but some experience of the Reality. The ego is surrendered to the unknown, to the Reality, to the Centre of Consciousness, to that Presence, that Centre of Truth and Awareness within. "I belong to Thee. Let me serve Thee with all my might, with mind, action, and speech, without any selfishness." (Rama, 2002d, p 135). Surrendering does not involve renouncing the ego. It means accepting that higher Reality or Awareness. "Surrendering the ego means becoming constantly aware of the Reality that is within." (Rama, 2002d, p 135). Thus the ego can separate one from the whole, but it can also connect one to the whole if it is properly trained and if it becomes aware of that Reality within. One learns to expand the individual ego to a higher Consciousness where it becomes an instrument that makes one aware of the Reality that lies outside one's boundaries. Then it functions as a higher ego. "I am Thine and Thou art mine. I acknowledge that my existence is because of You." (Rama, 2002d, p 135).

Practice Means to Awaken the Conscience

The only sin in the Tradition is to kill the conscience. Sri Swami Rama points out that the Inner Teacher can also be called the conscience (Rama, 2002d, pp 179–181). It functions like an alarm in your system. It silently says *no* whenever you want to do something that should not be done. It lies beyond mind as the Inner Teacher and whispers guidance to the mind. But habit patterns are so strong that the voice of silence which is the voice of the conscience is not heard. External guidance is not required to tell one what not to do. All of us have a moral sense and we know that we should not hurt, lie or steal. And yet we do so. Once the mind begins to listen to the secret whispers from the Inner Teacher then one is introduced to that real Teacher within which is your own conscience. All yogic teachings are meant for the day when one starts listening to that inner guidance, to that conscience.

Your teacher is trying to make you aware that there is something within you, a teacher within, who is a great friend. No matter who you are, your conscience is always there. If you learn to listen to the voice of the conscience, you can transform your whole personality. That conscience knows everything. No book can teach you; no teacher can teach you. Conscience knows and knows that it knows. Even when you go to a teacher to ask something, you draw your own conclusions and follow your conscience.

But you do not always listen to the teachings of your conscience. In fact, you are constantly killing your conscience. According to the great books of wisdom, the greatest sin of all is to kill your conscience. After some time your conscience stops talking to you because you do not listen to it. You have ignored your conscience so much that it has become silent. It continues to witness your actions but does not say anything. Learn to listen to your conscience.

Sri Swami Rama (2002d, p 179).

But do not be fooled by your mind which can pretend to be your conscience. The mind is different from the conscience. Instructions from the conscience are always for improvement and unfolding the inner being. The mind can lead you astray and try to persuade you not to practice. But you will have to practice for a long time. "Practice (*abhyasa*) means repetition of the same thing again and again to form a strong habit. Habits are motivation in life. If you do not have determination to attain that which should be attained, if you are not constantly aware of the Reality, how can you practice? You will feel lazy and you will not be able to sit in meditation." (Rama, 2002d, p 179).

Relating to the Centre: From Conversation to Absorption

This whole process of dialogue with the Presence evolves over time in a dance from action or "doing" to being, and from duality to non-duality. It begins in the subject-object consciousness of duality as a "conversation" between the individual self and the Centre of Consciousness in its expression as the Inner Teacher. The process is at first hesitant, but as trust builds over a long time a solid relationship begins to form based in trust and faith and evolving through praise to gratitude and then to love. Paradoxically one learns to take that relationship in daily life for granted as the trust builds that one can count on it. And yet one never takes it for granted for the relationship builds on devotion and reverence. With time this devotion flows through praise to gratitude and into love and the conversation becomes a true friendship. The love grows into intimacy as one begins to know the Self within as the nearest, the dearest and closest core of one's essence and friendship becomes a true communion that is constant in all things and events. At the end, intimacy melts into true union with the absorption of *samadhi;* the locus of personal identity shifts from individual self to Self in the nonduality of consciousness-without-an-object. The question, "Who am I?" has finally been answered in a state where all questions are answered because no questions arise.

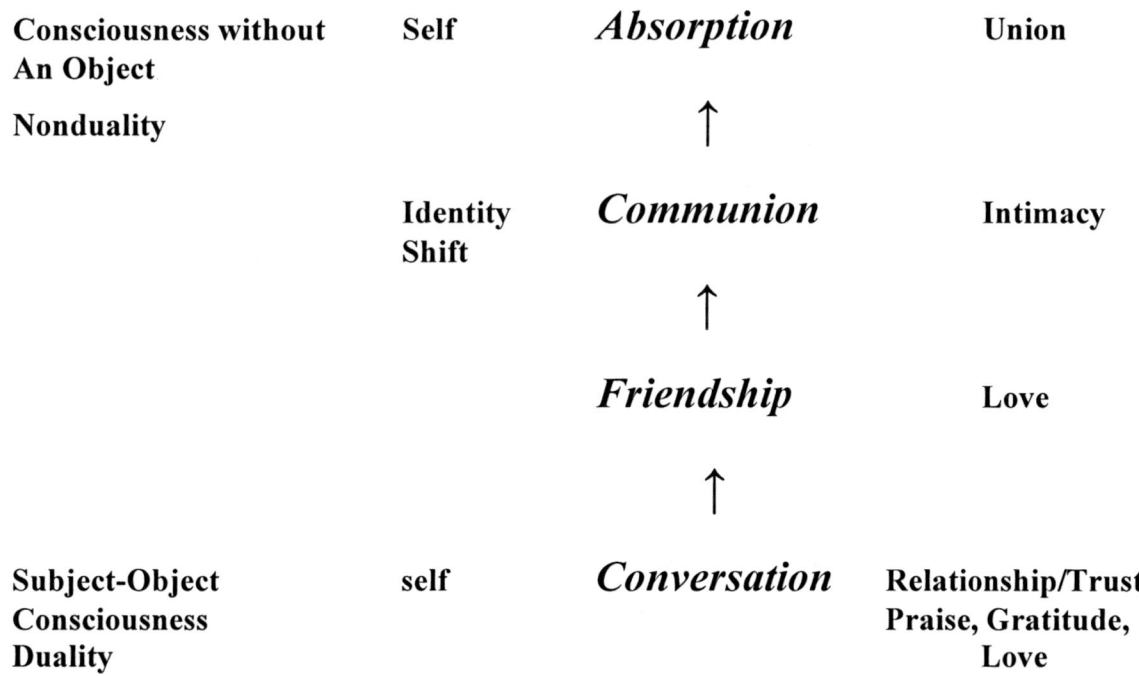

Figure 23.1 The Evolving Dialogue with the Presence
From Duality to Non-duality
From Doing to Being

Consciousness without An Object	**Self**	***Absorption***	**Union**
Nonduality		↑	
	Identity Shift	***Communion***	**Intimacy**
		↑	
		Friendship	**Love**
		↑	
Subject-Object Consciousness Duality	**self**	***Conversation***	**Relationship/Trust Praise, Gratitude, Love**

Integration of the Yogas of Life

Yogas are variously classified by different teachers. In the Himalayan Tradition they are thought of as the Yogas of life and the Yogas of discipline. The former comprise the well-known triad of Karma, Bhakti and Jnana Yogas. The latter make up the royal path of Raja Yoga which has many subdivisions including Mantra, Hatha, Laya, and Kundalini Yogas. Before the opening of the Centre of Consciousness, aspirants consider the three Yogas of life as separate paths to the divine, chosen to suit the character and personality of the student (Rama, 1982a).

But *Brahman,* in addition to being the essence of *sat, cit* and *ananda,* also expresses other energies. Kashmir Shaivism, for example, describes five energies of Lord Shiva as *cit shakti,* the energy of consciousness; *ananda shakti,* the energy of bliss; *iccha shakti,* the energy of will; *jnana shakti,* the energy of knowledge; and *kriya shakti,* the energy of action (Lakshmanjoo, 2000). These expressions embrace the Yogas of life which become integrated within the experience of the Centre of Consciousness. Metaphorically, the Centre, even though essentially a unity, is experienced like a multi-faceted jewel or crystal, now reflecting a flash of green light, now red, now yellow, now blue. These energies are like parts of the spectrum of the white light of consciousness and flow forth as intention, action, knowledge, and bliss all on a ground of Awareness and Being. It is as though one experiences the unity of the *saguna Brahman* at the same time as It projects various energies or functions. One of those is the Centre of Consciousness in its expression as the Inner Teacher which is our focus throughout this book. However, the two are in essence One.

This integration of the Yogas of life proceeds in steps: *jnana → karma → dharma → bhakti* (Niranjanananda, 1995, p 178). The term *jnana* means knowledge, wisdom or comprehension (Grimes, 1989). Here it is used not as mere information as we often employ it in the West, nor even intellectual or intuitive knowledge. Rather it is knowledge in the sense of direct awareness of the Centre of Consciousness, the Presence, and its expression as the Inner *Guru* or Teacher. In Advaita this is the Witness consciousness (*sakshi-chaitanya*), the Awareness that underlies and supports all the states of consciousness, pervading the waking, dreaming and deep sleep states. It is not a state like one of these, but the omnipresent *turiya* or fourth that runs through them all. This is what we are calling here the Presence or Centre of Consciousness.

The aspirant discovers It can provide guidance in daily life. In this sense, Swami Rama used to refer to It as the conscience. Indeed, the only sin is to systematically kill the conscience, meaning not to listen to and follow its guidance. The term *vijnana* refers to the intellect or cognition (Grimes, 1989), but it is sometimes used in the sense of applied knowledge. Live your knowledge is another way to not kill the conscience. If the student is not qualified (*adhikara*) in the sense of prepared, the practice may not "take." The Tradition has many stories to illustrate this: the master filling a student's cup with tea then overflowing it; trying to hold the ocean in a cup; pouring water into sieve, and the like. It is analogous to planting seeds in fallow ground where the means for their growth is absent.

Behold, a sower went forth to sow; and when he sowed, some seeds fell by the wayside, and the fowls came and devoured them up; some fell upon stony places, where they had not much earth; and forthwith they sprung up, because they had no deepness of earth; and when the sun was up, they were scorched; and because they had no root, they withered away. And some fell among thorns; and the thorns sprung up, and choked them; but other fell into good ground, and brought forth fruit, some a hundredfold, some sixtyfold, some thirtyfold. Who hath ears to hear, let him hear.

Matthew 13: 3–9.

With the opening of the Centre of Consciousness the means to right action is now available through inner guidance in daily affairs. But one must remember that this process takes time to mature in proportion to the strengthening of that inner connection. The flow of guidance is filtered through the beliefs, values and attitudes that constitute one's model of the world located in the other than conscious mind, how one pictures reality. These filters can distort the intuitive flow initially and mistakes in action can occur. The uncertainty can make one hesitant, but the solution is to forge ahead and act from and trust the inner guidance as it clarifies. It is like learning to walk, or skate, or ski or ride a bicycle: one gets to fall down a lot until one masters the coordination and the process. One must push ahead by trial and error until one gets it right.

One begins to put that inner guidance into daily action and to express it in behavior. This leads to *karma*, the second step in the process. Living in the world as we do, we are all active, in every moment. As we grow in knowledge our state of Being expands and that reflects in our behavior. In this state action must be understood as a state of co-creativity. To use a metaphor, the Centre of Consciousness can be thought of as the architect of action, while the ego is the project manager that puts the will into action through the personality as a surrendered and aligned instrument. Thus Karma Yoga is action flowing from the Centre of Consciousness. This is a fully conscious and aware process. Since action is carried out as service to the Centre with all fruits surrendered to that Centre, such an individual no longer needs external rules for guidance in what is right action. Action becomes duty surrendered to the Lord. When we would express thanks and appreciation to Sri Swami Rama his reply was always, "I'm just doing my duty." He was expressing right action flowing from that Centre and this was not a personal issue.

Because one is aligned with the Centre, this aligned action leads to one's behavior, actions, speech, ideas and thoughts all lived according to one's *dharma*. This is the third step of integration. By *dharma* here we do not mean righteousness, ethical or moral issues, life philosophy or mission, or even responsibility and duty as this word is often translated. Rather what we mean is what in modern language is often called being in the flow – flowing with the current of life, living by natural principles which govern the cosmos and personality. This is what it means to be aligned with the Centre: to live in synchronicity. One naturally performs right action for the right people in the right place at the right time and in the right way. One co-creates one's destiny with the Centre and life seems to unfold like a flower, like a divine creation, as the whole universe seems to rearrange itself to accommodate one's pictures of reality with a succession of enabling synchronicities – an unfolding life mission.

In this kind of state one falls in love with the process of life, and then the fourth and final step of integration takes place, which is Bhakti. One falls in love with life, with one's mission and with the co-creative process. One lives like an artist who creates for the joy of creating; the outcome is but a byproduct. One is reminded of God's *lila* or play in creation. Creating one's life and destiny becomes a work of art performed with joy. One moves from being a master of limitation to being a Master of Divine Expression, from creating misery and mess to "manifesting heaven on earth" here and now (Alarius, 1988). Sri Swami Rama was an ultimate Master of Divine Expression.

In this state one begins to appreciate the unity of life as well as its plenitude. The disciple knows the protection of the Tradition, and learns he is called forth in proportion to his or her ability to be aligned with the Centre in thought, speech and action. The watchword becomes service above self. Sri Swami Rama used to say that *sheva* (service) is my *puja* (worship). An attitude of praise becomes one of gratitude that flows into love. One lives in a state of high vibrational positive emotions which help one create what one wants and which keeps one aligned with the Centre of Consciousness, and thereby one learns the many faces of love.

One evokes what we call the three G's: gratitude which evokes generosity leading to grace. This creates a virtuous cycle leading back to *jnana*. Sri Ramakrishna said that the winds of grace always blow. One need only put up one's sail to catch them.

24

The Outward Arc

A person is neither a thing nor a process, but an opening or clearing through which the Absolute can manifest.

Martin Heidegger

When we discussed mastery of divine manifestation above we began to touch on the outward arc of *abhyasa*. The inward arc is all about the internalization of awareness into that Centre. But the outward arc is Its expression into manifestation through the surrendered disciple. Both processes occur together and gather momentum as *sadhana* progresses, until full mastery of divine expression is achieved.

There are several aspects to the outward arc. These also express through the Yogas of life mentioned above. The flow of wisdom from the Centre functioning as the Inner Teacher through the awakening of intuition comes from the *cit* aspect of the Centre, accounting for the transcendental Knowing experienced as guidance from the Inner Teacher in a process that is somewhat analogous to modern channeling. Here the Centre of Consciousness is "channeled" by appropriately aligned energy fields of the personality. This is *Jnana* Yoga. The student will also experience the flow of bliss and even a downward force from the Centre. This Force called Consciousness can be difficult for the unprepared personality to contain. Bliss and related love represent the *Ananda* aspect of the Centre and Bhakti Yoga. Finally there is the expression of Will or intentionality into co-creative action. This is Karma Yoga; the Yoga of selfless action, which in its true form is action flowing from the Centre of Consciousness. Karma can be thought of in terms of action as creativity, in the sense of manifestation (Jerry & Jerry, 2001).

These three paths of Yoga are often thought to be mutually exclusive. But in actual fact at this stage of the spiritual path students practice all three to some extent although there may be specialization in one depending on the student's personality. The Centre is experienced a bit like a jewel with many facets. At various moments there may be intuition, now a moment of bliss, then a sense of Will, in a shifting kaleidoscope.

Another aspect of the outward arc is that it is a co-creative process between the small self and the Centre. Action flowing from the Centre of Consciousness is a continuous co-creative process of manifestation. To repeat the analogy, the Centre acts as architect while the self acts like a project manager. At this stage the ego does not disappear but alters its function. The personality then acts as an instrument.

Finally with the outward arc, there is the issue of the attunement and alignment of all parts and energy fields of the personality with the Centre of Consciousness analogous to tuning a radio receiver.

Wisdom and the Opening of Intuition

With the opening of the Centre of Consciousness the expansion of awareness leads to intuition. We discussed intuition at the end of chapter 20.

One needs a good model of how the mind works to see how it takes sensory input and builds it into a model of the world or pictures of reality. These are structured in systems of values, beliefs and attitudes, which are then expressed in feelings and language, and then stored as structured memory in the unconscious mind (Jerry & Jerry, 2001). Neuro-Linguistic Programming provides very practical models for understanding these processes (Grinder & Bandler, 1976).

To understand how a model of the world works one need only put on a pair of sunglasses. The world that one sees promptly turns the brown or green color of the glasses. The color of the glasses is projected, so to speak, onto the world. If one did not know that one was wearing sunglasses than one would assume from experience the green or brown color to be the true color of the world. Belief systems that make up models of the world lie hidden in the unconscious mind. They filter our awareness and project those beliefs onto the world unconsciously so that we experience those beliefs as true, as properties of the world itself.

A small experiment will allow the reader to understand this idea of belief projection. Imagine walking into a room full of people who are staring at you as you find your seat. There is something that you have come into that room to find that you desperately need. Look around the room at all of those people and realize that every one is there to prevent you from getting what you so desperately need. How does that feel? Now take a break for a moment to let those feelings dissipate. Now repeat this visualization in your imagination. But this time as you look around the room at all those people imagine that each one is there to help you find what you so desperately need. This is quite a different feeling and experience, is it not? The difference comes from the projected belief system. All of our experience is filtered by the belief systems in our model of the world. What is more, we are unaware of these belief systems because they are in the unconscious and so we accept the projections as reality, not recognizing how they are caused. We do not experience the world as it actually is.

Intuition can be thought of as perception by the Soul or Self. It is a direct perception of truth that uses the mind as a sixth sense. Intuition is to the Self as light is to the sun, directly illuminating and exposing the reality of all that it falls on. There is a distinction between pure intuition as direct perception and intuition that is filtered through the other-than-conscious mind. The latter is the usual experience of intuition and the resulting distortions by one's belief systems can lead to error. But with the opening of the Centre of Consciousness the flow of intuition is more direct. A purer interaction with the Inner Teacher can now begin. Thus communication with the Centre of Consciousness is about awakening intuition. Perhaps the mystery of intuition as we mean it here is captured best in the idea of a hologram as in the following quotation:

> The Holy Ones are an Intelligence within your intellect.
> Give your profoundest contemplation to this.
>
> Jelaluddin Rumi

How to Work with the Inner Teacher

The process for communing with the Centre of Consciousness is actually quite straightforward. But it takes considerable and persistent practice to perfect, depending on how pure (focused) and undistracted the mind field. The method can be summarized as follows:

- Act "as if" the Centre is open and accessible at least to some degree.
- Relax, quiet the mind, and attune with the Centre by meditation for about ten minutes.
- "Ask" the question – nonverbally will do.
- "Translate" the response.
- Check its veracity with a Yes/No signal until you are skilled enough not to need this.
- Write it down in a journal.
- Act as appropriate on the guidance received.
- This is a skill: practice, practice, practice!
- When the awareness of the Centre becomes stable, the process will become an ongoing "dialogue" without the formality of technique.

This is one of those things like walking that is incredibly easy to do but very difficult to describe! You begin the work by acting as if the Centre is accessible, as though you were talking to someone through a barrier like a door, or over a telephone to someone you cannot see. As the Centre becomes a conscious Awareness that sense of barrier will disappear. A quiet mind is essential for effective communication as well as unwavering focus. This is a bit like tuning a radio or TV receiver to the right frequency to catch the transmission. Here one is tuning subtle energy. The processes of meditation and of practicing the presence of God in daily life are how one gradually attains alignment with the Centre of Consciousness, and that alignment produces the necessary attunement for communication. Communication is also enhanced by emotional purification, and by the reframing of beliefs that constitute one's model of the world. Again, using tuning of a radio as a metaphor, this process of cognitive and emotional purification also removes static that can interfere with energetic communication at any level of vibration. Thus the formula is: purification (emotions + beliefs), + tuning (attunement; alignment), + removing static, and finally + practice, for it is a skill. When asked why questions were not answered internally, Sri Swami Rama replied, "Check the receiver, the transmitter is OK." Like Ramakrishna's comparison of grace to the blowing winds, teaching and transmissions are always flowing from the Inner Teacher. One need only put up one's sail to catch them.

Asking the question is no more than a nonverbal feeling of asking without content – just a kind of nonverbal question mark directed internally to the Centre. The Centre knows the content even before the question is asked. There are many legendary stories where Swami Rama would write something on a piece of paper and then ask a student for questions. After the questions were asked he would show the paper to the student who was astonished to find the questions written on it. Much of the thinking process is preverbal and based in very subtle flows of feeling. It is simply not true that one needs internal dialogue to think. Thought is much faster than that. The response is often instantaneous and comes as an intuitive gestalt, occasionally with the key word or two, which the recipient then must translate into language. Often the energetic gestalt is much richer than can be put into ordinary language, and may unpack into more than one idea or concept. It is important to write the transmissions down as soon as they are received, because they quickly evaporate from memory. Keep a journal of these communications which can be reviewed at intervals over time to gauge the concerns of subject matters that were addressed. This way one can see the progress in one's skills. Add notations about the method used, the process, experiences, etc. so that learning can be documented.

It is also important to act on any advice that is given. If someone seeks good advice from you but repeatedly fails to act on it, and as a result repeatedly gets into trouble, eventually you will stop providing that advice and let that adverse experience be the teacher. This is true also of the Centre. Transmission also means the expression of intuitive wisdom into action, which is the basis of Karma Yoga. If the advice is repeatedly not acted upon that flow is blocked and interrupted and eventually the Centre becomes quiet and stops communicating. We can all be stubborn to some degree at our core, especially when good advice would prompt some major change in our personality. This resistance to guidance has to be overcome. It can be a long struggle.

We now must address one more step – using a Yes/No signal to determine whether the transmissions have been correctly received. One way is to quiet the mind in meditation and then mentally ask for a "yes" signal, noting anything that happens in the way of sensation, sound, images, etc., and record the result. Do the same by asking for a "no" signal. Two or three trials will bring a consistent result. But we recommend the process of muscle testing from kinesiology for something a little more objective. One does not use it to assess the correctness of the advice given. Rather it is used to ask whether the advice has been properly received and understood. This is a critical distinction. The correctness of the advice is determined through the correct action that ensues. A description of kinesiological testing can be found at (http://www.ascending-star.com/kinesiol.htm). When some skill in communication is achieved, then this process can be dropped as unnecessary. One will sense the characteristic communication easily internally.

The Impediments to Yoga

Yoga is union with the Centre of Consciousness, and communication from the Inner Teacher is an aspect of that communion. Hence it is worth visiting Patanjali's discussion of the nine impediments to Yoga in the *Yoga-Sutra* (YS I.30) and their consequences (YS I.31) since they will also impair working with the Centre of Consciousness (Veda Bharati, 1986). *Sutra* 30 lists the impediments as:

- Illness (*vyadhi*)
- Procrastination (*styana*)
- Doubt (*samshaya*)
- Negligence (*pramada*)
- Sloth (*alasya*)
- Non-abstention (*a-virati*)
- Confused philosophies (*bhranti-darshana*)
- Failure to gain ground (*a-labdha-bhumikatva*)
- Instability (*anavasthitatva*)

These distractions (*vikshepas*) of the mind field are the nine impediments or obstacles (*antarayas*) to *yoga* (union) with the Centre. They are impurities or adversaries of that union. They throw the mind off from the path of Yoga, causing it to fall from that union. The aspirant becomes a *yoga-brahshta*: one who has fallen from the path of Yoga. These distractions appear with the growth of *rajas* and *tamas*. They prevent the accomplishment of one-pointedness – the *ekagra* state, the fourth of the five grounds (*bhumis*) of the mind field described in YS I.1, because these distractions (*vikshepas*) consist of a variety of *vrittis*. They must be mastered before the mind field can progress to *ekagra*.

Illness in the Ayurvedic system results from an imbalance of bodily constituents (*dhatus*), fluid essences (*rasas*), and active and cognitive senses plus the mind (*karanas*). They are impediments because the mind reacts to illness with fear and because a sick body disturbs meditation through pain and discomfort. The remedy is through *japa* of the *guru mantra* which allows the mind to stop reacting emotionally to physical illness with depression, and so on. Additionally, use of the *mrityunjaya* mantra is often prescribed in the presence of illness. Proper diet, regulation of lifestyle and habits, and practice of Hatha Yoga purify the body and restore balance so that discomfort ceases to distract the mind.

Procrastination includes the mind's tendency to idleness and mental laziness. The mind has a habit of restlessness and fickleness and will not settle down so that it can be applied in a consistent manner to practice. The individual procrastinates, postpones and finds excuses, and his or her mind cannot be fixed on anything for long. The result is a limited capacity to concentrate. The mind is distracted and will not work for the *sadhaka's* purpose even without an external disturbance.

Doubts about the efficacy of Yoga, the tradition, the texts, one's *guru*, or about one's own capacity and success can be a formidable adversary. The mind oscillates between what is correct and incorrect, what applies and what does not apply: it could be this, it could be that. It is said that along with *viparaya* (perversive cognition; false beliefs and misunderstanding about the tradition and the path), doubt can be the most difficult obstacle to producing the state of mental *nirodha* (control) of the *vrittis* (thoughts).

Negligence refers to not cultivating (*bhavana*) the means to *samadhi*. There is a failure to practice constantly impressing an experience on the mind through repeated observance (*bhavana*), as well as a failure to pay attention to the observance itself and remaining disinterested. One fails to practice the limbs (*anga*) of Yoga such as the *yamas* and *niyamas*. One also neglects to gather the sixfold wealth or six treasures (*shat-sampat*) of Vedanta: *shama* (quietude), *dama* (withdrawal from worldly interests), *titiksha* (forbearance), *shraddha* (faith, humility and surrender), and *samadhana* (freedom from conflicts).

Sloth is a lack of initiative, and perseverance because of the heaviness of the body and of the mind (*tamas*), while non-abstention is a craving for sense objects, a failure to turn away from the world and the attractions of the senses. It is the opposite of *uparati* which is the first stage of *vairagya* discussed in Part Three. One feels a strong pull of the senses (such as the four fountains: sex, sleep, food and self-preservation) that prevents one from concentrating on the path. One experiences lust and sensuality from proximity and contact with sense objects.

Confusion of philosophies refers to *viparaya*: false knowledge, cognition or perception which includes also the afflictions (*kleshas*). One sees facts as non-facts, what is not there in entities, decides against the *guru*'s teachings, and so on. There is no mental oscillation as in doubt. Rather the mind decides in error and takes the incorrect side of an issue. There is total rejection of alternatives. Don't confuse me with facts, my mind's made up! At least with doubt there is oscillation of the mind and the possibility that the fact is really a fact. As noted above, *viparaya* along with doubt are the biggest obstacles to calming the mind field.

By failure to gain ground is meant not reaching the ground of *samadhi*. Despite lots of practice one fails to reach a plateau of achievement of a state of consciousness. There are two reasons. The first is that one has not met the conditions of *sutra* I.14: practicing assiduously for a long time, without interruption, and with complete observance. These must be cultivated with ascetic observance (*tapas*), celibacy (*brahmacharya*), knowledge (*vidya*) and devotion (*shraddha*); in other words, with a positive and devout attitude. The other reason is that the practitioner has little momentum and lower capacity (YS I.21–22).

Finally, by instability is meant the mind field's failure to be sustained in the ground that has been attained. One gains a higher ground, but one falls from it and keeps slipping from it. The prior ground has to be firm or the new ground will be weak. One should not be satisfied with the taste of *samadhi* just a few times. One must practice until *asamprajnata* becomes one's normal state and one no longer falls from this highest ground. Note that all these obstacles are to be considered within the context of *ishvara pranidhana*. Through practicing the presence of God in *japa* all these obstacles are gradually overcome by God's grace.

The effects of these distractions are four (YS I.31):

- Pain (*duhkha*)
- Ill-mindedness (*daur-manasya*)
- Unsteadiness of limbs (*angam-ejayatva*)
- Involuntary inhalation (*shvasa*) and exhalation (*pra-shvasa*).

Duhkha refers to any pain, grief, sorrow or suffering in general, which all beings seek to avoid. It is the realization of the general unsatisfactoriness of life. This is the first of Buddha's fourfold noble truths. It is also a big concern of Samkhya philosophy. Swami Veda Bharati (1986, p 330) quotes the *Karika* as, "Because one intends to prevent the three kinds of pain, there arises inquiry as to the means of that prevention." The second *pada* of the *Yoga-Sutra* deals with the totality of the universal problem of pain (YS II.16, 15–26). It discusses the understanding of pain, the causes of pain, the removal of pain, and the means of removing that pain. Again this is analogous to the Buddhist presentation. The present *sutra* deals more with the personal experience of pain.

Pain can be both universal and personal. It is of three kinds and arises from three sources. Although it is experienced mentally it is attributed to external sources and forces. *Adhyatmika* refers to pain within one's self from physical illness or from mental sources such as passions and desires. *Adhibhautika* refers to pain caused by other beings such as beasts of prey or one's enemies. *Adhidaivika* refers to pain caused by either deities or by natural forces (e.g., heat and cold) and planetary influences.

All pain comes from the movement of *rajasic vrittis*, and it impedes the practice of Yoga. It arises from the nine obstacles discussed above and the movement of mental *vrittis* (thoughts). It is possible to control it mentally so that one suffers it less and one prevents its being a barrier on the path of Yoga. If the mind in daily life is filled with the pain of desire, then the mind in meditation is disturbed (*vikshipta*) and then *sattva* cannot overcome *rajas*.

Ill-mindedness (*daur-manasya*) can also be translated as bad-mindedness (*dur* = bad + *manas* = mind) (Veda Bharati, 1986, p 331). It is the antonym of *saumanasya* or good-mindedness (*su* = good, happy, harmonized + *manas* = mind). The mental pain of desire leads to frustration, anguish, despair and bad moods with emotional disturbance and instability – in other words, psychopathology. The mind in daily life is filled with this negativity and meditation is disturbed.

By unsteadiness is meant shaking of the body and twitching of the limbs in meditation. *Rajasic* tendencies create restlessness and listlessness in daily life. The cause is emotional instability. Mental stability is required for stabilization of the body in meditation. The influence of *sattva* settles the meditation down so that one can sit still and the posture can be steady and comfortable (YS II.46).

Finally, involuntary inhalation and exhalation are symptoms of emotional and mental disturbance. They are the opposite of the total control designated by the word *pranayama*. Thus *shvasa* is the opposite of controlled inhalation (*puraka*), and *prashvasa* is the opposite of controlled exhalation (*rechaka*). Without this control the natural *pranayamas* described in YS II.50–51 cannot be done. In daily life this unnatural state results in gasping and sighing. During meditation the breath flows unevenly with jerks and pauses because desire (*duhkha*) and frustrations (*daur-manasya*) are both present. Hence the importance of regulated "sine wave" breathing patterns in meditation.

All these disturbances are correlates of the nine obstacles (*antarayas*) described in the previous *sutra*. These five are all aspects of a single condition which is the personality disturbed in life and meditation. They must be cured together so that the disturbed state of *vikshipta* can go on to *ekagra*. These are all symptoms of the distracted (*vikshipta*) mind field and do not occur when the mind is harmonized in *samadhi*.

Finally, *sutra* I.32:

> *Tat-pratishedhartham eka-tattvabhyasah.*
> "To prevent and negate those impediments, the distractions and their correlates,
> the practice of a single reality, one principal, is enjoined, prescribed."
> Veda Bharati, 1986, p 333

The distractions are brought under control by the practice of *abhyasa* and *vairagya*. *Ishvara pranidhana* or practicing the Presence (of God) is especially efficacious because it precludes the arising of mental distractions. It is the practice of a single reality, of the mind field's resorting to a single reality or one principle alone (Veda Bharati, 1986, p 335). God or *Ishvara* is that one reality or principle whose presence is practiced, and if successful, the distractions (*vikshepas*) do not arise. Distractions do not arise in a mind harmonized in *samadhi*.

But most of us cannot do this kind of practicing the Presence fully and all of the time. We need the aid of other practices. We start with concentration on gross objects in *savitarka samadhi* and work our way up to *ishvara pranidhana* which employs a continuous directing of the mind towards God until one can maintain oneself with stability in that Presence. The mind must be withdrawn from even thoughts about God (beliefs, notions, attributes, etc.). One must maintain only the awareness of that single Reality. Thoughts and feelings about that Reality are not the same as experience of that One Reality. God is not as He is thought to be. *Abhyasa* and *vairagya* always go together. Both are a precondition for all realizations.

In the Himalayan Tradition Sri Swami Rama described seven basic emotions arising from the four primitive fountains, which we refer to here as the "4–7 model." (Rama, 2002d). In more modern language the model describes the links between emotion and instincts. We mention it here because of the importance of emotional purification in the Himalayan Tradition, and because of the power of emotionality associated with attachment (*raga*) and aversion (*dvesha*) as an obstacle to spiritual practice. The model provides a simple way to conceptualize the interactions of emotions and instincts in this context (Figure 24.1).

From Swamiji's perspective desire is the root cause of all emotions. Desires arise in relation to two of the afflictions (*kleshas*), attraction (*raga*) and aversion (*dvesha*). The latter can be thought of as the inverse of desire. Desires produce emotions which in turn, give rise to thoughts and to motivations toward speech and action. Desires and then emotions can arise from external stimuli which are both stored as *samskaras* and *vasanas* in the unconscious mind, and which trigger the expression of these corresponding stored entities into thought, speech and action as described by the theory of *karma*. Desires and emotions may also arise internally from the instinctual activities of the four primitive fountains: food, sex, sleep and self-preservation (Rama, 2002d). Anger and related emotions arise when desire is blocked or frustrated. I may become jealous of what others have that I lack. The issue is not that anger is bad and that one should never be angry. There are times when anger is appropriate, but it should never be uncontrolled; it should never disturb the inner calm of the Centre. If desire is fulfilled then greed can arise which leads to attachment with clinging from fear of loss. Also pride and egotism can arise with the sense of ownership and what I have achieved or gained that allows me to feel superior. This Yogic model is a very different way to conceptualize emotions than the models currently in use in neuroscience.

Emotions and the Four Primitive Fountains

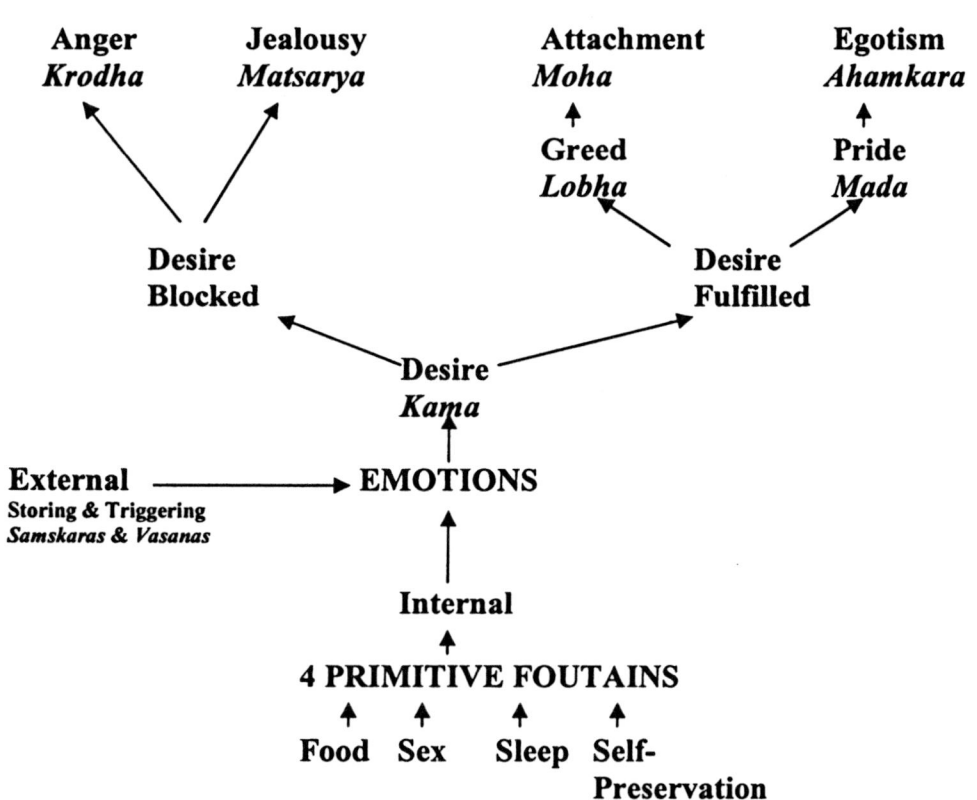

Figure 24.1. The Relationship between Emotions and Instincts (The Four Primitive Fountains)

Surrender and Detachment

Eknath Easwaran's commentary on verses 6 and 7 of chapter 12 of the *Bhagavad Gita* (1979, pp 345–350) encapsulate the idea of the chariot of *sadhana* beautifully.

> 12.6–7 "But they for whom I am the supreme goal, who do all work renouncing self for Me and meditate on Me with single-hearted devotion – these will I swiftly rescue from the fragment's cycle of birth and death to fullness of eternal life in Me."
>
> Easwaran, 1979, p 345.

We have all heard the story of what to do when confronted with a child holding a sharp knife in the hand by its blade. To directly take the knife would injure the child. Instead the child is presented with his favorite sweet. He takes it with the free hand. Now both hands are full, one with the knife and one with the candy. Again he is presented with his favorite sweet. The child reaches for it, dropping the knife safely as he does so.

Here Easwaran presents us with a similar dilemma. Krishna (representing the Centre of Consciousness) offers us the gift of immortality, asking us to reach out and take it. But our hands are full of sweet mangoes. He asks us to let go, to free our hands to receive his gift. But we want our cake (or mangoes!) and eat it too. Why not just give us your present first, we say, and then we'll throw away the mangoes! In this essential conflict we are split between our higher and lower natures, the selfless and the selfish. Part of us wants to reach for the highest, but the other part cannot relinquish personal desire. But the only goal is that Centre, the Lord. Everything is for the sake of the indwelling Self and not just to please yourself or others.

If a part of the illusion is real then it is all real. The transition to the unchanging Real has to be total. Eventually everything must go: no exceptions. "Thou shalt love the Lord thy God with all thine heart, and with all thy soul, and with all thy might." (Deuteronomy 6:5). To do this one must go deep below the surface level of consciousness using meditation, but everything personal must be released to open the doors to deeper awareness.

Easwaran notes that this struggle between ego consciousness and Awareness is described vividly by Augustine in his Confessions, a struggle that raged within him for over twelve years. "I was bound . . . by my own iron self-will . . . For a will that is bent awry becomes selfish desire, desire yielded to becomes habit, and habit not resisted becomes compulsion." This brings to mind the cycles of action and reaction, of *karmas* and *samskaras* and *vasanas* that characterize the conditioned individual mind. Augustine goes on to write that "The new will being born in me . . . was not yet strong enough to overcome the old will that had been strengthened by so much use. Thus two wills warred against each other within me – one old, one new; one physical, the other spiritual – and in their conflict they wasted my spirit." (Easwaran, 1979, p 347). Augustine then provides the clue to victory: "I was in both camps, but there was a little more of me on the side I approved than on the side I disapproved. . . . It was I who willed and I who was unwilling; . . . Therefore I strove with myself and was distracted by myself. . . ." This describes what we call the hill of *sadhana* discussed above.

Easwaran (1979, p 347) points out that this is not two selves in conflict, but a single self alternating from one side of an issue to the other. Nor is this mental oscillation the obstacle of doubt as described in the nine obstacles above in YS I.30. It is deeper and more fundamental than this for it lies in the process of the identity shift from individual self or ego consciousness to Self or Transcendent Awareness of the *Atman* which is the essence of the path. To succeed you increasingly put more of yourself into the higher side of light.

Sri Swami Rama repeatedly emphasized the importance of developing *sankalpa shakti* or will power: I have to do it, I must do it, I WILL do it. With each failure (and there will be many as your strength grows) you get up and try again with the attitude that you will never give up no matter how many lifetimes it takes. And here the role of *shraddha* or faith in the *guru*, the practice and the teachings is key to sustaining that drive to enlightenment (*mumukshutva*) – the fifth of the basic instincts or fountains we all possess.

Easwaran (1979, p 347) writes: "In the latter stages of spiritual development, even the greatest mystics have cried out from the depths of their heart when they see how far off the goal is and how frail their strength, how limited their capacity. As Augustine says, it is like trying to wake up out of the seductive torpor of a dream – knowing it is time to wake up, longing to see but unwilling to open our eyes. If we could watch our dreams, we would see that there is no freedom in the unconscious; our dream actions are all compulsive. And Augustine says, it is the same in waking life: our will is not our own." Intellectually you want to give yourself to the grace of the Inner Teacher but you continue to be ruled and bound by your individual wishes and desires of the personality.

If I am truly an omnipotent Self and I know intellectually that I am immersed in this dream, why can I not just wake up by willing it? But knowing is not enough. In my unconscious my will is fast asleep and I want to go on dreaming. I need something more than just that knowledge; I need what St. John called a "burning fervor" that can create the total commitment that lets me leave some personal desire behind without so much as looking back. The Sufis say, "When the heart grieves over what it has lost, the spirit rejoices over what it has found."

This is a long process. The inner experience of the Centre comes and goes over a very long time. Paramahansa Yogananda advised taking the role of the naughty child. When the child cries the mother comes. She will try to distract it with another toy for a little longer. One should play the inconsolable child and not be content with anything other than the mother herself.

Finally in the struggle one comes to the point where one is done with the world. In the final stages of meditation one needs dedication and total trust to let go so that the identity shift can proceed; so that one can cross the chasm of separateness into the unitive state. This requires developing an all-consuming devotion and love for that Centre, for the Lord and Inner Guide. This is not blind, but an unshakable faith in the Real, in That which never changes.

Easwaran (1979, p 349) further points out that this process leads one to the theme of death and immortality. Hang on to passing physical pleasures and be assured that in the course of time you cannot avoid the suffering that overtakes the physical sheath. We have a built in margin for error in the first half of life. The body and personality have tremendous reserve and can absorb a great deal of punishment with little complaint. But with aging that reserve gradually disappears. Easwaran writes, "But as we grow older, if we fail to assess wisely, life is not going to ask us if we are ready to give up our attachments. It is going to take them from us, and in the taking is most of the suffering of old age and death." As we walk the path, we let go of selfish attachments within our capacity bit by bit, voluntarily, and not under duress, until finally we no longer need to hold on to anything else for support. Although difficult at first, ultimately it is the way to be free. This is the great promise; when consciousness becomes completely unified one transcends beyond change and death into eternity. It is time to awaken from the dream.

Kindling this burning desire for the Centre, for the Lord, is the role of *abhyasa* as we interpret it here. It lets you to be done with the world, which is *vairagya*. The two wheels of the chariot of *sadhana* turn together.

All of this discussion seems to be dualistic in its presentation. It is very much rooted in Bhakti Yoga. Great philosophical debates have raged over the centuries about the relative merits of dualistic (*dvaita*) versus non-dualistic (*advaita*) conceptions of reality, with the latter considered to be the highest state as in Vedanta. We do not see these as opposing opposites. Rather we see them as evolving stages of consciousness as it proceeds through the identity shift.

Initially when the Centre first opens, appearing and reappearing for the longest time as the subtlest and dimmest Presence behind the mind, the aspirant's locus of consciousness is predominantly within the mind field and the personality as an individual ego, and mostly body-identified. In this state the Presence is experienced as "other," as an object. If the Self is ultimately our true nature, how it can experience Itself as an object in subject-object consciousness is a great mystery. Perhaps It recognizes Itself as a reflection in the inner surface of *buddhi* which has been sufficiently purified by prior Yogic practice and by the grace of the *guru* and initiation. When the chasm of separateness has been crossed into the unitive state, which is the identity shift, then there is Yoga, union, when individuality and subject-object consciousness dissolve and one knows "I am That."

The role of the sage in the Himalayan Tradition of Yoga is to awaken within the student the divine flame, that spark of divinity that all human beings carry within them, and which Sri Swami Rama called the Teacher within or Inner *Guru*. This happens by higher initiation through the bestowal of *shakipata* at some level of intensity commensurate with the student's capacity to receive at that point in time. It is the descent of divine grace through the competent physical *guru*. Once that divine flame is lit one truly becomes a disciple. Once that divine spark is ignited the final struggle is engaged and there is no turning back. The life of the new disciple is changed forever and can never be the same again. This is the essence of our message in this book.

We conclude this section with the following quotation from Paul Brunton's *Secret Path* (1935, pp 32–33):

A Sophist approached one of the Wise Men of ancient Greece, and thought to puzzle him with the most perplexing questions.

But the Sage of Miletus was equal to the test for he replied to them all, without the least hesitation yet with the utmost exactitude.

1. What is the oldest of all things?
   "*God*, because He has always existed."
2. What is the most beautiful of all things?
   "*The Universe*, because it is the work of God."
3. What is the greatest of all things?
   "*Space*, because it contains all that has been created."
4. What is the most constant of all things?
   "*Hope*, because it still remains with man, after he has lost everything else."
5. What is the best of all things?
   "*Virtue*, because without it there is nothing good."
6. What is the quickest of all things?
   "*Thought*, because in less than a minute it can fly to the end of the universe."
7. What is the strongest of all things?
   "*Necessity*, which makes man face all the dangers of life."
8. What is the easiest of all things?
   "*To give advice*."

But when it came to the ninth question our sage pronounced a paradox.

He gave an answer which I am certain his worldly wise querent never understood, and which to most people will give only the most superficial meaning.

The question was:

What is the most difficult of all things?

And the Miletian sage replied:

"*To know Thyself!*"

This was the bidding to ignorant man from the ancient sages, this shall be the bidding yet.

Thyself, of course, is the Centre of Consciousness.

25
Practicing ABHYASA

Now let us look at the methodologies for *abhyasa* or practice. Here the situation is a little more intricate. With *vairagya* one is releasing what blocks access to the Centre of Consciousness. But with *abhyasa* one is looking directly at that communication.

Recall that this communication or communion is two-way. The inward arc involves progressive absorption into Being, while the outward arc brings manifestation into activity or doing. The latter includes both intentionality and the function of the Centre of Consciousness as the Inner Teacher.

With *abhyasa* we are concerned with the inward arc which has three aspects. One is the *sat* aspect which refers to an experience of profound Existence or Being – the experience of total Rest or Silence and the quality of *Shantih*, known as the Peace that passes all understanding. Associated with this is the second aspect, *bhakti*, which manifests as an experience of devotion and reverence, mixed with praise and gratitude. Finally there is the aspect of the relationship between the student and the Inner Teacher, that begins as a kind of conversational exchange between the two which then the blossoms into a friendship as the relationship forms and then moves to the communion and absorption of *samadhi*.

Now how do some of these practices shown in Table 25.1 work with *abhyasa*? There are two processes at work here. The first is the production of stillness and one-pointedness that are a part of the aspect of deep Rest, Being and Existence. Processes like *Kaya Sthairyam* or surveying the body using progressive relaxation with mindfulness are used to develop stillness and stability of the upright physical body. Then the various *asanas* or postures of Hatha Yoga condition the body so that one can sit absolutely still for long periods of time. The various practices of inner silence (*antar mouna*) and meditation (*dharana* and *dhyana*) also apply here, as do those of *pranayama* and related techniques such as the application of *sushumna*. Special breathing techniques up and down the spine (*sumeru* breathing) during meditation prepare the central channels for the ascent of the *kundalini* and also produce a centering effect. Indeed centering is another way to think of the process of *abhyasa* directed towards the Centre of Consciousness. All of the inner limbs of Raja Yoga including *pratyahara* and *samyama* (the combination of concentration, meditation and *samadhi*), are at work here. The practice of silence, done properly, is a great aid (Veda Bharati, 1999). To be silent means to rest in stillness in the Centre of Consciousness in all things. While not speaking is a step in the right direction, running about passing notes to others is not what it is about.

Table 25.1 Some Methods for Practicing *Abhyasa*
Methods to Produce Stillness and One-Pointedness • *Kaya Sthairyam*, progressive relaxation • Practice of silence • *Antar Mouna* • *Pranayama* • *Pratyahara* • *Dharana* and *Dhyana*
Methods Producing Remembrance, Surrender, Expansion, Absorption and Awareness • *Ishvara pranidhana* (practicing the presence of God) • Bhakti Yoga: devotion, worship, music, chanting • Attitudes of gratitude, generosity, and grace • Meditation • Concentration on the subject aspect of subject-object consciousness • Awakening Awareness through witnessing • Contemplation including journaling   Who am I? of Ramana Maharshi • Releasing techniques (Sedona Method)

The second process is one of constant remembrance in a state of surrender along with expansion of awareness into the Presence of the Centre of Consciousness leading to absorption into Its aspect of Being. This is the essence of Bhakti Yoga with all of its practices of devotion, worship, music, reverence, etc. Essential here is the practice of *ishvara pranidhana* (surrender to God) or practicing the presence of God as a form of constant remembrance of the Centre. The Tradition neatly encapsulates all of this in the phrase "love, serve and remember." There are related attitudes, high energetic vibrational states that facilitate alignment with the Centre. We describe them as the three G's: gratitude, generosity, and grace. An attitude of praise towards the Centre awakens gratitude which, in turn, awakens the love and reverence that evoke grace. Again all of the upper limbs of Raja Yoga apply here including *pratyahara* and the processes of *samyama*. Meditation is the core practice for *abhyasa*. There are particular meditations on space and expansion in the Heart Centre in Vedanta that may be used (Niranjanananda, 1993b). Franklin Merrell-Wolff (1994) found that concentrating on the subjective pole of subject-object consciousness was especially efficacious for awakening transcendental states.

There are also methods for awakening the Presence or Awareness aspect of the Centre of Consciousness from a process of witnessing and directly in meditation. These have been explored in detail by Aziz Kristof (2000). Methods involving contemplation and even journaling can be helpful, including the "Who am I?" contemplation of Ramana Maharshi (1974, 1988). Indeed the passion for Yoga (union) at this stage of the practice can lead to a continuous and ongoing inner contemplation or rumination that keeps the awareness centered on the Centre of Consciousness. Contemplative walking is helpful (Veda Bharati, 2000). One should review Swami Veda Bharati's five pillars of *sadhana*: stillness, silence, fasting, celibacy and conquest of sleep (Veda Bharati, 1997). The release techniques (Sedona method) of Lester Levenson are also very helpful (Dwoskin, 2003). The ultimate result of all this work with *abhyasa* is the shift from subject-object consciousness to Consciousness-Without-an-Object, from small self to Self, the essence of the identity shift that leads to Self Realization.

Part Five

Meditation in the Himalayan Tradition

26

Meditation Unites the Wheels of the Chariot of SADHANA

Meditation (*dhyana*) lies at the core of the Chariot of *Sadhana*. On the one hand its process of sensory-emotional dissociation is key to the development of nonattachment (*vairagya*), and on the other, it is the essential process for one-pointed absorption into the Centre of Consciousness which here is called practice (*abhyasa*). It holds the penultimate position as the seventh rung in Patanjali's Classical or *ashtanga* Yoga which lies at the basis of the Himalayan Tradition. Thus it deserves special consideration in our exploration of the Chariot.

No one can teach you to meditate! What passes for authentic instruction in Yogic meditation is the art of concentration (*dharana*). When one-pointedness of the mind field is mastered it passes spontaneously into meditation and then into the various levels of *samadhi*. The term "meditation" is used variously to describe methods and processes, but actually it is a state of being that dawns within when concentration is mastered. Our purpose here is not to provide an exhaustive dissertation on meditation, which has been done better elsewhere (for example, Jnaneshvara Bharati, 2004; Rama, 1992a; Sovik, 2005; Tigunait, 1996; Veda Bharati, 1974; Veda Bharati, 1981). Rather we wish here to explore how the opening of the Centre of Consciousness as a real experience in the aspirant's inner world alters his or her practice of meditation.

When one sits to practice something new has been added to inner space. That Presence or the internal sounds may come and go, wax and wane, over many years. But It brings an irrevocable and transformational change to one's inner world to which one must adjust. When you meditate, what do you do with that Presence, with those sounds? Stick to the breath and the *mantra* and ignore It? Focus on It instead? But when you do sometimes It seems so elusive and subtle, like noticing something in peripheral vision that seems to vanish when you look at It directly. At times It is hard to find, and at other times It dominates, draws and absorbs the attention fearfully. How do you work with It, knowing intuitively that the task is to crystallize its Presence as a stable Awareness at all times? Because meditation means so many different things to so many different people we begin our exploration by defining what we mean by it here in this context.

What Do We Mean Here by Meditation?

The Tradition of the Himalayan Masters is a continuous master-disciple lineage and oral tradition that can be traced back 5,000 years as recorded in the cave monasteries in the Himalayas. It is said to be one of the most ancient of Traditions and includes all of the known meditation methods. Many of these methods have subsequently become specialized, for example, mindfulness and insight meditations in Buddhism which are currently popular in the West.

In Raja Yoga the Sanskrit word for meditation is *dhyana*. By tracing this word through its linguistic evolution it can be shown that Zen and Buddhism evolved from Indian Yoga (Austin 1999, 2006; Swami Veda Bharati, personal communication). In 520 B.C.E. the Indian monk, Bodhidharma, traveled to China to teach. There the word *dhyana* became Ch'an-Na and later Ch'an. The Ch'an school of meditation became part of Mahayana Buddhism. Then the Buddhist monks transplanted Ch'an meditation to Japan where it was pronounced as Zen. Thus Zen became a school of Buddhism that emphasizes meditation and evolved from the spread of the art of meditation from India to China and then to Japan. Zazen is its system of meditation.

Meditation and Yoga are inextricably linked. If Yoga is defined as the science of spirituality, then meditation is its principal tool for exploring inner space. Our position is echoed by the Dali Lama (2005, pp 134–7) who recently has made the case for the use of meditation as a first-person method for the scientific study of consciousness to supplement the usual objective third-person approaches of traditional modern science. We have described the typology of the various common forms of Yoga elsewhere (Jerry & Jerry, 2001, p 169). Meditation occupies the central position in all Yogas. *Dhyana* is the final common pathway for all the Yogas of life and discipline preparatory to unlocking transcendental awareness. So when we talk about meditation, we are also talking about Yoga. All of the six prior limbs of Patanjali's Classical Yoga build the foundation on which meditation and the full capacity for it can flourish.

Meditation has been applied clinically in the West. But in the clinical setting we are not talking about the primary purpose of meditation, but about its byproducts. Swami Veda Bharati, Georg Feuerstein and many others in the authentic Yoga community have expressed concern about this Western tendency to redirect the primary purpose of Yoga practices. The essential role of meditation is as the primary tool for inner exploration on the spiritual path. In particular be on the lookout for the peculiarly Western adaptation that might be called "New Age Yoga." This is Yoga that has been altered and diluted for commercialism and personal copyright. If one is going to make the commitment to study Yoga and meditation be sure to get authentic teaching by knowledgeable and properly trained teachers.

Then what do we mean here by meditation? It is very hard to define since it is an internal state. One can begin with what it is not: sitting still, worrying, daydreaming, sleeping, fantasizing, contemplating, thinking or doing guided visualizations, listening to New Age music, or any number of things that people call meditation and are not. When someone says he'll meditate on a problem he really means he'll think about it, contemplate it. In some parts of rural Canada, to meditate means to sit on the commode!

A current rage is the use of auditory binaural beats to create a whole brain alpha rhythm state. To assume that alpha or any other rhythm recorded from a meditator always indicates a state of meditation is naïve. But to then assume the reverse, that creating an artificial alpha state is equivalent to a natural alpha state, and that this is the same as meditation is unwarranted. Anecdotal reports using this approach describe strong emotional catharsis which is interpreted as therapeutic, but one can also interpret it as a method that produces adverse side effects in almost everyone who tries it!

Beginning with two dictionary definitions, here are several Western definitions of meditation.

SOME WESTERN DEFINITIONS OF MEDITATION

Because meditation has many forms and there is yet no coherent theory of meditation, there is no unified definition of meditation in the West.

> "The action or practice of profound spiritual or religious reflection or mental contemplation."
> > (*The New Shorter Oxford English Dictionary*, 1993, p 1731)

> "A deep, serious thought; reflection on a religious subject as a spiritual exercise."
> > (*The New Lexicon Webster's Dictionary*, 1987, p 621)

Neither of these dictionary definitions correctly describes meditation. Rather they describe contemplation. Meditation is the antithesis of active thinking.

Definition by Its Effects:
The relaxation response. (Benson, 1975)

Definition by Its Goals:
A state of complete concentration devoid of any extraneous thoughts; a state of choiceless awareness. (Shapiro, 1980)

> "An internal regulation of attention from moment to moment." (Kutz, Borysenko & Benson, 1985; Goleman, 1977)

> "A family of techniques, which have in common a conscious attempt to focus attention in a non-analytical way, and an attempt not to dwell on discursive, ruminating thought." (Shapiro, 1980)

> "An exercise which usually involves the individual in turning attention or awareness to dwell upon a single object, sound, concept or experience." (West, 1979)

Benson's definition by its physiological effects (the relaxation response) again is not correct. The other definitions above are much better. Here is a definition by Swami Veda Bharati, a *Dhyana* Yogi from the Himalayan Tradition:

> "Meditation is a state of mind in which you experience complete tranquility. Not emptiness of the mind, but tranquility, a peacefulness of the mind in which the conflicting forces of thought stop, and the mind then flows along a single stream of consciousness."

The technical definition of meditation also requires an understanding of *dharana* or concentration. Here are the two terms as defined in Patanjali's *Yoga-Sutra* (Aranya, 1981), the core text for Raja Yoga:

A Technical Definition of Meditation
Dharana
(Concentration, fixity)

- Fixing the mind on a particular point in space – defined as the object for concentration.
- Active, requiring will.
- The thought process is intermittent like a succession of similar drops of water.
- A still one-pointed mind.

Dhyana
(Meditation)

- The continuous, uninterrupted flow of the mind towards its object of concentration.
- Effortless, arising spontaneously.
- The flow of knowing is continuous like the flow of oil and not interrupted by any other knowing or thought.
- With continuous knowing it appears as though there is a single idea present in the mind.

Patanjali's *Yoga-Sutra* III: 1, 2

Epstein distinguishes two distinct attentional strategies (Goleman, 1977): concentration on a single object, and moment-to-moment awareness of changing objects of perception (mindfulness). The latter encourages the development of an observing self and also initially promotes the emergence of unconscious material. He claims that concentration stabilizes the mind so it can practice mindfulness (Delmonte, 1990).

We emphasize again that actually no one can teach you to meditate! The processes we usually call meditation are actually concentration (*dharana*). If one succeeds in making the mind one-pointed and still, then concentration moves spontaneously into meditation. *Dhyana* is an inner state in which the one-pointedness is burst through and the awareness explodes into expansion and then into *samadhi*, of which there are many levels. Enlightenment is gradual and incremental and not just a big "Aha!" So meditation can be defined as a process, referred to as a method of concentration, or as an internal state of awareness. Meditation methods can be considered in two broad categories: concentration meditation (e.g., *mantra* meditation), or mindfulness meditation (moment to moment awareness).

27

The Structure of Himalayan Meditation

Swami Veda Bharati (1998) has summarized the essential components of the Himalayan Tradition of Meditation. It is said to be the first and most comprehensive meditative tradition which has given birth to the other major meditative traditions and continues to nourish them all. It comes to us through a very ancient and unbroken *Guru*–disciple lineage in which knowledge is passed on experientially by transmission of a pulsation of spiritual energy, *shakti*. It is an initiatory path of pure meditation. It combines the wisdom of the Classical Yoga of Patanjali's *Yoga-Sutra* with Vedanta and with the philosophy and practices of Tantra in an integral and unified system that relies on a tradition of oral instruction and initiatory experience.

One of its basic components is the purification of thoughts and emotions through the practice of the *yamas* and *niyamas* of Classical Yoga, the four right attitudes (*brahma-viharas*; YS I.33), the antidotes to disturbing thoughts (YS II.33), and the conquest of the nine obstacles (YS I.30) and their five accompaniments (YS I.31). These lead to a solid foundation of ethical behavior, loosening of *karma*, and mental-emotional clarity and stability that allow the mind field to become one-pointed and then controlled in *samadhi*.

Mindfulness of body, breath and mind has an important place, as does breath awareness in which students are taught a controlled diaphragmatic breathing that is slow, smooth and without jerks or breaks in the flow of the breath that leads to a natural *kevala-kumbhaka* or breath suspension. Breath awareness underlies the process of purification of subtle energy channels through *pranayama*, especially varieties of *nadi shodhana* (alternate nostril breathing to produce autonomic and subtle energetic balance), as well as *pratyahara* in which the sense faculties are calmed by certain breathing practices.

The first step in the Tantric path is *kundalini* breathing or *sumeru* breathing with personal *mantra* (obtained through initiation) and awareness of the subtle energy flow in the spine. *Japa* and *mantra* practice in nine major stages are used to travel through the levels of subtle energy from *vaikhari* (articulate speech) to *madhyama* (mental level) to *pashyanti* (revelation) and into supreme absorption in the *para* (the transcendent), the supreme Silence. Processes are taught for *dharana* (concentration) and *dhyana* (meditation proper). The complex and detailed interior exercises of *yoga nidra* are carried out in *shavasana* to enter the subtle body, master the ability for conscious sleep, for accelerated learning, for healing, to master the art of dying, and to enter *samadhi*. Mastery of all of these steps requires transmission (initiation) by a qualified preceptor in the oral tradition.

Five Steps to Stillness

Mantra meditation from the Himalayan Tradition has a consistent structure that gives it its power. That structure remains constant, but it is endlessly elaborated and made more complex as the student advances, like variations on a theme in music. The method is also integral to all of the eight rungs of Raja Yoga. Meditation alone is poorly effective unless it is practiced with all of the eight rungs in an integrated way. This makes for a complete method that addresses all levels of the personality at once as described in the Vedantic model of the *koshas* (sheaths). It is practiced after *hatha* and *pranayama* and integrated with release (relaxation) and breath awareness which contribute to its efficacy. *Pranayama* should include the practice of *nadi shodhana* or alternate nostril breathing in order to balance the subtle energy body to allow the application of *sushumna* with greater ease. A meditation practice assumes observance of the supportive *yamas* and *niyamas* which raise one's life to the level of one's meditation by avoiding the creation of personal problems and dysfunctional relationships which would disturb meditation. We particularly urge the reader to study carefully Swami Veda Bharati's text *The Song of Silence: Subtleties in Sadhana* (2004), pages 73–94 for an exquisite discussion of the finer points of meditation. Here is the basic structure:

THE INTEGRAL STRUCTURE OF HIMALAYAN MEDITATION

(*ASANAS*)
(*PRANAYAMA*, especially *nadi shodhana*)
(*BHUTA SHUDDHI*)

PREPARATION
Posture: Head, neck and trunk straight; the posture steady, comfortable and absolutely still
(Optional: Draw around oneself 3 concentric circles of white light intoned with *bhur, bhuvah, svah*)
Withdrawal from place, space and time

RELAXATION
(*Shavasana* → sitting)
(Progressive relaxation with tension – optional if relaxation is found to be hard to learn)
Progressive muscle relaxation
(Progressive muscle and joint relaxation as a more advanced step)
(Advanced: methods from *yoga nidra*)

BREATH AWARENESS
(Crocodile posture → *Shavasana*)
Diaphragmatic breathing at the navel (exhalation to inhalation: 1:1 → 2:1), regulated like a continuous sine wave
Diaphragmatic breathing at the nostrils
(Optional: Mindfulness with breath awareness)
(Advanced: Application of *sushumna*)

MEDITATION
Meditation with breath at nostrils using *So'ham*: *So* on inhalation, *Ham* on exhalation
(Advanced: personal *guru mantra* with *sumeru* breathing, → *mantra* without breath, →
    refine to the Silence)

CONCLUSION
Gently!
Palm the eyes
Bring the awareness into the room maintaining the inner state

Let us review each of these briefly in turn so that one can see how the integrated structure derives
its efficacy.

1. Preparation. This first step allows one to withdraw from the external into the inner world,
and creates a personal space where one can meditate without distraction. Posture is important. Sit
so that the head, neck and trunk are erect and straight and the body is still, steady and comfortable. There are special *asanas* for meditation (Rama, 1992a; Sovik, 2005), and, indeed, the cultural
asanas have as part of their purpose preparing the body so that it can sit for prolonged periods (3
hours or more) without any movement. Any posture is appropriate that meets these requirements,
including a chair. For seated postures a folded blanket slipped under the edge of the buttocks can
relieve the tendency to slouch. The posture must be absolutely still and refined to avoid swaying,
swirling, slumping, twitching and other movements. Then comes the process of withdrawing the
awareness from place, space and time to create an inner space of solitude and security.

2. Relaxation. Usually a standard progressive relaxation is used. This may surprise the reader
who associates it with Western psychology and stress management. But it is not often realized that
progressive relaxation comes from Yoga. Jacobson brought the method from India in early 1900s
(Jacobson, 1929). Indeed, it is surprising how much of modern stress management is Yoga, even
the physical exercises (Winter, 1983).

Relaxation is learned in the posture called *shavasana*, the "corpse posture." The student lies on
the back with the body aligned, the feet shoulder width apart, the arms alongside the body and
slightly apart from the body with the palms turned upward. The head and neck can be supported
by a thin pillow and optionally the eyes covered. The posture is aptly named since meditation along
with sleep are the two models used in Yoga for the process of dying (Veda Bharati, 1979b; Jerry &
Jerry, 2001). One uses this posture for the relaxation for four to eight weeks until it is learned. Then
the relaxation can be done in the sitting posture. This may seem paradoxical, but the metaphor of
clothes (the limbs) hanging limply from an upright coat tree (the erect spine) is apt. This is a skill
that improves with long practice until complete relaxation can be done with a single exhalation.
For the beginner most of the time in the process is spent with the relaxation and much less with
the meditation itself. With practice relaxation can be done quickly and then proportionately more
time is spent with meditation.

During the process one moves slowly through the body beginning with the scalp and progressing in sequence to the forehead, eyebrows and eyes, corners of the mouth, neck (pause for three breaths), shoulders, upper arms, forearms, hands and fingers (pause for three breaths as though the breath were flowing through the arms to the fingertips). Then move back up from fingertips to the hands, forearms, upper arms, shoulders to the chest and heart centre (pause for three breaths as though through the heart centre). Then move to the upper and middle back, stomach, abdomen, lower back, pelvis, hips, thighs, calves, feet and toes, and let the whole body breathe from toe to top and top to toe for at least three breaths. Finally repeat the same sequence in reverse order, releasing any remaining muscle tension. A more advanced method adds relaxation of the major joints to the sequence (shoulder joints, elbows, wrists, hips, knees and ankles). For the experienced student Swami Veda Bharati (2004, p 77) recommends the sequence forehead (for the mind), joints of the jaw and throat centre (for speech and subvocalization), shoulders (for manual activity), heart center (for emotions), navel region (for desires and smooth flow of the *prana*), and thigh joints (for locomotion). Complete by relaxing all these points in reverse.

Some individuals find relaxation difficult. They can be taught progressive relaxation with muscle tension. The muscles are tensed and relaxed in sequence so that the student can learn to distinguish the sensations of contraction from relaxation. The usual method is directive. But nondirective or suggestive language can also be used. One relaxes or releases the mind in the muscle and the muscle then relaxes automatically. This is a mental letting go, a process of dissociating consciousness from its identification with the physical body. There is nothing that you do physically with the muscle itself. The sequence goes down the body from head to toe to release tension from the major muscle groups and then refines the process to release any residual tension on the way back up. There is emphasis on the shoulders and the arms where we hold most tension. Pauses at the throat, the fingertips, and the heart centre are for duration of three breaths each. Some students find a relaxation with eyes closed to be frightening. Let the eyes be open until confidence is achieved, and the methods of energy psychology can be used to relieve any feelings of anxiety.

As the practice progresses relaxation can be deepened either by adding relaxation of the joints as well as the muscles, or by adding some of the exercises like *shithali karana* from *yoga nidra*. The latter is a set of progressive relaxation exercises that lead to conscious sleep. Note that there are many Western modifications of the basic progressive relaxation exercise. Payne's text (1995) describes over 20 variants of physical and mental relaxation for clinical use; his text should be consulted for details. But the Yoga science takes the process far beyond this.

Is this hypnosis? Yes! A surprising answer given the loud protestations to the contrary that one usually hears from teachers of Yoga who almost universally criticize hypnosis as something evil and who generally know nothing about it or have any experience of it. But in saying "Yes!" we are not saying that meditation is hypnosis. This is just a preliminary state of relaxation and meditation takes one far beyond it. Hypnosis, like all internal states, is difficult to define. By hypnosis here, we refer to Ericksonian hypnosis which deals with light trance-like states that all of us experience in varying degrees daily. Indeed as the nasal ultradian rhythm shifts between *ida* and *pingala* through *sushumna* every ninety minutes, one passes through a transient Ericksonian trance. Erickson used this natural phenomenon as the basis for his naturalistic approach to inducing trance in his clients. Rossi (1991) has evolved the phenomenon into a formal therapeutic process he calls the "20 minute break." Progressive relaxation is a standard way to induce a light trance by self-hypnosis. The EEG will show alpha rhythm with the eyes closed, and the appearance of alpha is commonly (and incorrectly) taken as synonymous with the state of trance. But the word "hypnosis" often is carefully avoided because of popular discomfort with the idea.

We once led a workshop group through a full Himalayan meditation at an international conference on Neuro-Linguistic Programming, which included extensive material on Ericksonian hypnosis in addition to many other topics. One member of the audience was Erickson's daughter, who is an internationally recognized Ericksonian hypnotherapist. If anyone knew what hypnosis was about, she certainly did! Afterwards she came up to us and congratulated us on the outstanding process we had used for inducing trance in the group!

3. Breath Awareness. Initially breath awareness is taught by rolling the body over into the crocodile posture. The student lies prone with the forehead on the crossed forearms and the legs shoulder-width apart, toes pointing out or in as is comfortable. In this position the chest muscles are fixed so that the student breathes predominantly with the diaphragm. One concentrates on the sensation of the stomach muscles pushing against the floor on inhalation and relaxing back on exhalation. Since the lower ribs rotate a bit like a bucket handle eventually the student learns to sense this motion at the sides and the back of the lower rib cage as well. In this way the student learns diaphragmatic breathing correctly. This kind of breathing is natural for an infant, but our process of education and socialization changes us into chest breathers with all of the tension that comes with it from sympathetic nervous overstimulation. Diaphragmatic breathing is critical to the correct use of the breath in meditation. One practices in this posture for four to eight weeks so that proper diaphragmatic breathing becomes a habit. Then both the relaxation and breath awareness can be done in the sitting posture.

In the sitting posture diaphragmatic breathing is done with the attention on the gentle rise and fall of the stomach muscles in the region of the navel with lateral movement of the sides of the lower ribs with inhalation and exhalation. Initially it is done in a 1:1 ratio of inhalation to exhalation. Later exhalation can be prolonged to twice the length of inhalation. This 2:1 diaphragmatic breath is more relaxing even than progressive relaxation itself. It can be done any time where there is stress, such as in traffic, during a meeting, etc. Once diaphragmatic breathing is established at the navel (the epigastrium or upper abdomen), the attention is then switched to the flow of the breath at the nostrils, with attention to the sensation of airflow, of moisture or dryness, and of warmth or coolness.

The physiology of breath awareness is important. Diaphragmatic breathing improves the flow of air to the bases of the lungs. Normally the distribution of blood in the lungs favors the bases. During chest breathing the chest wall expands and pulls the lungs outward to create a partial vacuum which draws in the air. But in chest breathing the airflow is predominantly into the upper and middle parts of the lungs which have the least blood distribution. With diaphragmatic breathing, the diaphragm contracts and flattens downwards creating a more complete vacuum that not only pulls in more air, but also pulls it down into the lowest lobes where the blood supply is the greatest so that gas exchange is optimized. In exhalation the diaphragm relaxes back into its dome shape forcing air out of the lungs. This movement up and down of the diaphragm is transmitted through the abdominal organs to the wall of the upper abdomen around the navel and epigastrium as well as the sides of the lower ribs where it is felt as a rising and falling or expanding sensation. Thus diaphragmatic breathing means improved airflow to the bases of the lungs with optimized gas exchange.

The reader will be familiar with the division of the autonomic nervous system into sympathetic and parasympathetic branches. Both act on glands, the pupils of the eyes, the lungs, blood vessels and internal organs. The sympathetic system creates arousal and activation, while the parasympathetic system mediates rest and inhibition. Sympathetic dominance has characteristic physiological effects. There are increased cardiac rate, blood pressure, sweat secretion, pupillary dilation, and inhibition of gastrointestinal motor and secretory functions. One sees desynchrony of the EEG, with increased skeletal muscle tone, and elevation of certain hormones such as adrenaline, noradrenalin, adrenocortical steroids and thyroxin. The resulting behavioral effects include arousal, alertness, heightened activity and emotional responsiveness. In contrast, parasympathetic dominance is associated with reduction in cardiac rate, blood pressure and sweat secretion, with pupillary constriction and increased gastrointestinal motor and secretory functions. There is synchrony of the EEG, loss of skeletal muscle tone, blocking of the shivering response and increased secretion of insulin. The behavioral effects include inactivity, digestion, relaxation, drowsiness and sleep.

The breath is closely linked to autonomic balance. Inhalation reflects and stimulates sympathetic input with its tendency to arousal and fight or flight, while exhalation reflects and stimulates parasympathetic input with its tendency to inhibition and the possum response. These alternating inputs affect the nerve supply of the diaphragm and respiratory muscles. Usually breathing is somewhat irregular. Inhalation is often prolonged compared to exhalation and there are often pauses at the end of each. This irregularity produces an imbalance of nervous input into the autonomic nervous system with sympathetic dominance. Pauses in the breath in some individuals can adversely affect heart rhythm. This changing sympathetic and parasympathetic input is reflected in the sinus arrhythmia seen in the electrocardiogram, with heart rate speeding slightly with inhalation and slowing with exhalation. It is also seen in the fine, continuous variation in heart rate from beat to beat which can be measured as heart rate variability.

For breath awareness the instructions are that the breath should be gentle and easy, deep but refined, within the comfortable capacity of the student, with the breath flowing smoothly without jerkiness or sound, the breath even with inhalation and exhalation equal in length, and with no pauses within or between breaths. The breath should flow like oil in a continuous, uninterrupted stream. This is the definition of a sine wave. With "sine wave breathing" both sympathetic and parasympathetic inputs are equal and so the result is equalization of autonomic nervous system input and hence a balancing of the whole psychoneuroimmune (PNI) host resistance mechanism. Indeed, the Yogis have always known that the secret to control of the psychoneuroimmune system which integrates the autonomic nervous, immune and endocrine systems is through control of the breath.

This sine wave breathing is established first at the navel while observing the rise and fall of the upper abdomen. Then the attention is transferred to the touch of the breath in the nostrils and the same pattern established there. Optionally one can remember one's *mantra* merged with the flow of the breath. At this point one can choose to move on to the next step in the process, or choose to do prolonged breath awareness meditation or mindfulness as the principal practice. It can also be used to quiet a restless mind.

Pratyahara (sensory withdrawal) is the next step in Patanjali's Classical system after *pranayama*. This is done by applying *sushumna*. One observes the touch of the breath in the open or active nostril (3, 7, 11 or more breaths), and then in the opposite, closed or passive nostril while intending it to open. The final step is awareness of the breath at the point (*nasagra*) where the bridge of the nose joins the upper lip until the breath flows equally in both nostrils together as though in a single stream. It will feel as though the two sides have merged into one and that a single unified breath flows through a central channel. Optionally the *mantra* can be added throughout. The mind interiorizes, and becomes quiet and pleasant. True meditation can only occur when the application of *sushumna* has been mastered. It represents at the subtle level a shift of the flow of life energy from *ida* and *pingala* (which produce the unequal air flow in the nostrils via the parasympathetic and sympathetic nervous systems respectively) into the *sushumna* channel in the centre of the spine (associated with the flow of the breath equally in the two nostrils). The cerebral hemispheres are balanced and the mind field becomes unified and balanced.

Observe how the breath, *mantra* and mind flow together in a single stream, then how the whole mind and consciousness become a smoothly flowing stream. Eventually when the mind stream itself can be observed independently of the flow of the breath, true meditation begins (Veda Bharati, 2004, p 79). The breath will not flow smoothly unless the body is relaxed, the breathing is diaphragmatic, the emotions are calmed and the state of the breath is observed continuously. Learn to relax the involuntary tensing that occurs with inhalation. Finally, the pause between breaths must be mastered and eliminated by counting the inhalations and exhalations of the breaths (one through five and five through one, extending to one through ten and ten through one) to prolong the time that the mind flows easily, and by observing the transition to the next breath. The pause at the end of inhalation is easier to eliminate, but the pause at the end of exhalation is a challenge. A slight tension of the upper abdominal muscles during exhalation can make it easier to learn. The practice produces a spontaneous refinement and attenuation of the breath until it stops in a natural *kevala kumbhaka*. "The mind becomes a chamber of silence, and an unprecedented control over autonomic processes ensues, finally leading to the first stages of . . . *Samadhi*." "One who masters the pause between the breaths becomes a death-conqueror." (Veda Bharati, 2004, p 83). Death is considered as the long pause between two breaths: the last breath of the present body and the first breath of the next. Conquest of the pause leads to the ability to set the time and place for dropping the body (Veda Bharati, 1979b).

4. Meditation. Only now in the practice do we reach the actual meditation process. The preparation up to this point is what makes this kind of meditation so powerful a method. The student is initially taught meditation with a *mantra* along with breath awareness at the nostrils. This is a concentrative type of meditation that uses the sound of the *mantra* as the object of concentration. Mantra Yoga is one of the "chapters" of the "book" of Raja Yoga. The word "*mantra*" comes from the Sanskrit verb *man*, "to think" (the source of the English "man" – the one who thinks, the meditating one), and *tra*, to protect, guide, lead. *Mantra* is a thought that protects guides and leads.

Lots of objects can be used for concentration, but some are easier than others. A *mantra* and the breath are some of the easiest and most commonly used. Some people advocate counting, as in Benson's relaxation response. Lord Tennyson used his own name. One can choose any *mantra* but it should come naturally to you and be conducive to continuous awareness in union with the breath. In the Himalayan Tradition the mantra *so'ham* is used.

So'ham is the sound the breath naturally makes: "*so*" on inhalation, "*ham*" (pronounced "hum") on exhalation. The *mantra* should synchronize with the breath, and *so'ham* does this easily. Indeed, with experience one can spontaneously hear these sounds which the breath makes all the time. The Tradition says that for this reason one is in spontaneous meditation all the time: *so'ham* with each breath, repeating itself 21,600 times a day at 15 respirations per minute or 900 per hour (although with relaxation the breathing rate can drop to 2–3 per minute). To the Western mind *so'ham* is a meaningless sound which is an advantage. It is not necessary to associate meaning to get results. The continuous remembrance with attentiveness is what brings results.

But *so'ham* does have a meaning. It means "I am That."

THE *SO'HAM* MANTRA

sah aham becomes *so'ham* with Sanskrit *sandhi* (euphony)
sah means "he, she, it, that"; *aham* means "I"
so'ham is a nominal sentence (two nouns) with the verb "to be" implied

That (am) I or I (am) That;
I (am) He/She (Divinity);
I (am) Shiva;
I (am) Consciousness (Divinity, Spirit)

All authentic *mantras* have their origins in the Vedic texts. Here are examples for *so'ham*.

The breath comes out with the sound Ha (Ham) and is taken in with the sound Sa (So). Thus each individual continuously repeats the mantra Hamsa . . . Hamsa . . . Hamsa (Soham . . . Soham . . . Soham). Therefore, this mantra is repeated throughout the day. This is called ajapa gayatri and can bring liberation to yogis.

Yoga Chudamani *Upanishad* (v. 31, 32, 33)

The more you repeat this mantra (Soham), the greater the fruits, both temporal and spiritual. Therefore with intense effort, in all conditions, at all times, you should repeat the mantra.

Kularnava Tantra (Chapter 3)

Yo'sav-aditye purushah so'sav-aham
   The person who shines in the sun
   That One I am.

Yajur Veda XL, 17

By going out he utters "sa," by coming in he utters "ha." In this way he recites the mantra hamsa, repeating so'ham, so'ham, so'ham day and night. This sacred recitation is always existing for him.

Vijnanabhairava Tantra 155

He recites this mantra with breath twenty-one thousand six hundred times in a day and a night. This recitation, which is of that supreme energy of God consciousness, is very easy for those who are aware and very difficult for those who are not.

Vijnanabhairava Tantra 156

Having said that the English translation is not essential, one can remember the meaning continuously as a method of affirmation for people who have had deep transcendental experience and who want to maintain that state of Awareness. It is a way to intensify identification with the Centre. Some take the task of remembering it twenty-four hours a day until it becomes a spontaneous pulsation in the mind field, when talking, reading, writing, walking, sleeping, etc. Everything is done with this sound pulsation in the background. Consciously remembering a *mantra* is called *japa*. Eventually it pulses spontaneously by itself, even in sleep. Then it is called *ajapa-japa*. This perpetual process is very powerful for transforming the mind and unlocking its potential. Going to sleep in the *mantra* is also very powerful since there is a point where there is access to the unconscious mind. The *mantra* drops in with time and fills the sleeping state as well.

In many traditions, including the Himalayan Tradition, eventually *so'ham* is replaced by initiation into a personal *mantra* which is individualized to one's personality and is even more powerful since it brings an internal link to the Tradition itself (Veda Bharati, 1981; Tigunait, 1996). Everything written above then applies to the personal *mantra*.

Any number of other words can be used: Shalom, biblical verses, etc. depending on one's religion.

So'ham is also called the *hamsa* or *hamsah* mantra, because the two words appear in a long sequence of repetitions depending on how the syllables are parsed. This is a natural *mantra* that emanates spontaneously from within as the natural sound of the breath. Thus it has been called the *mantra* of the Self. It is highly regarded in the Vedas, the Tantra Shastras, and the Siddhas sing of it in their poetry. One text that reveals its science is the Vijnana Bhairava Tantra, a supreme scripture of Kashmir Shaivism. It is described in *sutra* 24 which is the first *upaya* (practice) or practical method of *dharana* that is revealed in the text. It is also discussed in *sutras* 155 and 156. The text is a dialogue between master and disciple, husband and wife, the supreme Lord and His beloved. The *Guru* is *Bhairava* or *Shiva* (Consciousness) and the disciple is *Bhairavi* (*Shakti* or *Shiva's* creative energy – the mother of the world). *Bhairavi* listens to *Bhairava* describe the state of the formless supreme Reality, and then asks him to reveal a simple means for knowing It. He responds with 112 methods for knowing Truth, of which the first and the most sublime is the awareness of the *hamsa* which all of us have within ourselves. *Dharana* usually is rendered as concentration in Patanjali's Classical Yoga. Here in Kashmir Shaivism it has a special twist. A *dharana* "is an awareness through which you hold God within." (Muktananda, 1992, p 29). The Vijnana Bhairava contains 112 of these *dharanas* (Osho, 1974; Satyasangananda Saraswati, 2003; Singh, 2003).

The sound of the breath coming in and going out is the repetition of the *so'ham mantra*: *so* on the in breath and *ham* (pronounced hum) on the out breath. It is a natural *japa*, a natural *mantra* repetition that always goes on in all living, breathing creatures. Kabir said that God Himself was repeating his *mantra* while he relaxed and listened to it. This is *ajapa-japa* or unrepeated or spontaneous *mantra* repetition. Niranjanananda (1993b, pp 68–154) provides a detailed description of *ajapa dharana* with *so'ham*. Swami Muktananda (1992) writes a very deep commentary on this *sutra* 24 of the Vijnana Bhairava Tantra elaborating the deeper nature of *Hamsa vidya*, the science of *Hamsa* from the perspective of Kashmir Shaivism. In her extensive commentary of the Vijnana Bhairava Tantra, Swami Satyasangananda Saraswati (2003, p 148) discusses *sutra* 24 as a *dharana* on the two points of generation of *prana* and *apana*.

The role of the breath in meditation is very important. Meditation here takes the definition from the *Yoga-Sutra*, *Bhagavad Gita* and *Brahma-Sutras* as "the continuous flow of one and the same cognition not interrupted by an external cognition." (Veda Bharati, 2004, p 84). For this the mind needs a support, an object of meditation. Swami Veda Bharati (2004) points out that this support or *alambana* is something for the mind to "hang on to" internally so the attention can flow continuously without interruption as the thought repeats itself in an identical sequence like a series of points forming a line. The breath is the easiest experience of flow and the mind takes the shape of what is presented to it. "Present to the mind something flowing like a stream; the mind will begin to flow like a stream." (Veda Bharati, 2004, p 84). "Thus breath awareness in itself does not constitute meditation. Breath awareness is used to trick the mind into flowing into a state of meditation." One observes how the breath, mind and *mantra* flow together as a single stream. One becomes absorbed in this observation of the *mantra* and of the flow of the mind on that *mantra*. Eventually one can drop the breath flow and observe only the flow of the mind as an even-flowing stream (Veda Bharati, 2004, p 86).

We noted above that people divide meditation into two types: mindfulness and concentration. But is the distinction so clear-cut? What is mindfulness? *Vipassana* (insight) meditation introduced by the Buddha some twenty-five centuries ago uses mental activities designed to experience a state of uninterrupted mindfulness. It is a state of pure awareness, bare attention, nonjudgmental and nonconceptual witnessing, present moment awareness and alertness in the here and now that is devoid of ego or self-reference. It is a pure perception of the passing flow of experience as it really is.

It is not an intellectual process of thinking, but rather just pure awareness. Gunaratana (2002, p 141) calls it "participatory observation" because the meditator is both participant and observer at the same time. One feels and experiences one's thoughts, emotions and physical sensations and at the same time one watches oneself doing so. It is a state of deep observation with total nonattachment. Indeed, it is the essence of *vairagya* as we discussed in Part Three.

Mindfulness (*sati* in Pali) is the essence of insight (*vipassana*) meditation which uses breath awareness at the nostrils (*anapana-sati* in Pali or *pranapana-smrti* in Sanskrit (Veda Bharati, 2001, p 793)). In meditation the attention is placed on one object. If the mind wanders from this focus, it is mindfulness that reminds you that your mind has wandered and brings it back to the object of meditation.

> Mindfulness is at one and the same time both bare attention itself and the function of reminding us to pay bare attention if we have ceased to do so. Bare attention is noticing. It reestablishes itself simply by noticing that it has not been present. As soon as you are noticing that you have not been noticing, then by definition you are noticing and then you are back again to paying bare attention.
>
> Gunaratana, 2002, p 143.

Now the distinction between mindfulness and concentration in meditation is not so black and white as it may seem. Gunaratana (2002, 149) points out that although concentration and mindfulness are different processes they each play a role and work together in meditation in a balanced fashion. Concentration is one-pointedness of mind: a single, active, uninterrupted, pointed focus on one object using the force of will. It provides the power to keep the attention focused on one object. "Mindfulness picks the objects of attention, and notices when the attention has gone astray. Concentration does the actual work of holding the attention steady on that chosen object. If either of these partners is weak, your meditation goes astray." (Gunaratana, 2002, p 149). Mindfulness guides the practitioner's development in meditation because it has the ability to be aware of itself, and to let the aspirant know how s/he is doing.

> Concentration and mindfulness go hand in hand in the job of meditation. Mindfulness directs the power of concentration. Mindfulness is the manager of the operation. Concentration furnishes the power by which mindfulness can penetrate into the deepest level of mind. Their cooperation results in insight and understanding. These must be cultivated together in a balanced manner. Just a bit more emphasis is given to mindfulness, because mindfulness is the center of meditation.
>
> Gunaratana, 2002, p 154.

5. Concluding Meditation. In coming out of meditation the important thing is to do it gently. Palming the eyes while the awareness begins to exteriorize is an effective way to do this. As one brings the awareness into the room, one tries to hold the sound of the *mantra* and the inner stillness as long as possible into one's subsequent daily activities. With prolonged practice that inner centeredness will start to pervade the daily round more and more completely.

For students in the Himalayan Tradition there are many sources of information and help to learn meditation. Swami Rama's text on Meditation is the main source. Swami Veda's (premonastic name Usharbudh Arya) *Superconscious Meditation* and *Mantra and Meditation* are highly recommended as is Pandit Rajmani Tigunait's book *Mantra and Initiation,* and *Moving Inward: The Journey to Meditation* by Rolf Sovik. Practice audiotapes by Swami Rama and Swami Veda are also available. Swami Veda has several tape courses on beginning and advanced aspects of meditation. Swami Jnaneshwar's web site www.swamij.com also has extensive material on meditation in the Himalayan Tradition.

Additional Resources for Meditation

For the Himalayan Tradition (Himalayan Institute Press at http://www.himalayaninstitute.org):

Swami Rama's *Meditation and Its Practice.*
Pandit Rajmani's *The Power of Mantra and Mystery of Initiation.*
Sandra Anderson & Rolf Sovik's *Yoga: Mastering the Basics.*
Rolf Sovik's *Moving Inward: The Journey to Meditation.*
Swami Veda's *Superconscious Meditation, Mantra and Meditation, Meditation and the Art of Dying, The Song of Silence: Subtleties in Sadhana,* and *The Himalayan Tradition of Yoga Meditation* available at http://www.swamiveda.org/yoga_books.htm or http://themeditationcenter.org .
Swami Jnaneshwar's website at http://swamij.com .
(Swami Rama and Swami Veda have many lecture and practice tapes available.)

From the Bihar School of Yoga:

Swami Satyananda Saraswati's *Sure Ways to Self Realization: Meditations from the Tantras, Yoga and Kriya.*
Swami Niranjanananda's *Dharana Darshan.*

Additional resources include:

Alper H (Ed) (1991). *Understanding Mantras.* Motilal Banarsidass, Delhi.
Brother Lawrence's *The Practice of the Presence of God.*
Coward H & Goa D (1991) *Mantra: Hearing the Divine in India.* Anima Books, Chambersburg, PA.
Humphreys C (1987). *Concentration and Meditation.* Element, Rockport, Mass.
Michael Murphy & Steven Donovan (1999). *The Physical and Psychological Effects of Meditation.* Institute for Noetic Sciences, Sausalito CA.
Swami Vishnu Devananda (1978). *Meditation and Mantras.* OM Lotus Publication Co., New York.

The Vijnanabhairava Tantra is a collection of 112 meditation methods. The following are excellent translations:

Osho (1974). *The Book of Secrets: 112 Keys to the Mystery Within.* St. Martin's Griffin, New York.

Jaideva Singh (2003). *Vijnanabhairava or Divine Consciousness: A Treasury of 112 Types of Yoga.* Motilal Banarsidass Publishers Private Limited, Delhi. Reprint.

Swami Satyasangananda Saraswati (2003). *Sri Vijnana Bhairava Tantra: The Ascent.* Yoga Publications Trust, Munger, Bihar, India.

Swami Muktananda (1992). *I Am That: The Science of HAMSA from the Vijnana Bhairava.* SYDA Foundation, South Fallsburg, New York.

The practice of mindfulness is a foundation in all meditative systems. In the Himalayan Tradition and the Yoga-Sutra of Patanjali it is called smrty-upasthana.

Thich Nhat Hanh (1990). *Transformation and Healing: Sutra on the Four Establishments of Mindfulness (Satipatthana Sutta).* Parallax Press, Berkeley, CA.

Thich Nhat Hanh (1990). *Our Appointment with Life: Discourse on Living Happily in the Present Moment.* Parallax Press, Berkeley, CA.

Thich Nhat Hanh (1996). *Breathe! You Are Alive: Sutra on the Full Awareness of Breath (Anapanasati Sutta).* Parallax Press, Berkeley, CA.

Thich Nhat Hanh (1987). *The Miracle of Mindfulness: A Manual on Meditation.* Beacon Press, Boston.

Bhikkhu Nanamoli (1991). *Visuddhimagga: The Path of Purification.* PBS Pariyatti Editions Seattle (BPE), Seattle, WA. (This is the commentary by Bhadantacariya Buddhaghosa.)

Bhante Henepola Gunaratana (2002). *Mindfulness in Plain English.* Wisdom Publications, Boston.

Tape courses include:

Sharon Salzberg & Joseph Goldstein (2001). *Insight Meditation.* Sounds True, Boulder, Colorado

Jon Kabat-Zinn (2005). *Guided Mindfulness Meditation.* Sounds True, Boulder, Colorado

28
Learning Meditation

Sri Swami Rama (Rama, 2002a) constantly praised the virtues of meditation and taught it very systematically as a science which has been practiced and studied for thousands of years by aspirants who sought to make their lives more serene, creative, and fulfilling. He would say that meditation would improve one's health, relationships, and the skillfulness of all one's actions. He was fond of pointing out that this is because meditation can give one something that no other technique can accomplish. It can introduce you to yourself on all levels, and then finally lead you to the Centre of Consciousness within, from where consciousness flows in various degrees and grades. He described meditation as self-effort, a probe into one's inner life that would eventually reveal all secrets.

He described meditation as an inward method for understanding all the levels of the mind, especially the unconscious mind. One meditates with the desire to meet God who is within. He saw meditation as something very concrete and definite that can help free the mind from disturbances and obstacles. Not only is it a way of calming the mind, but it is also a method of self-training. It is not a passive process nor is it something negative that creates hallucinations. He would say that meditation makes you aware; it acts like a mirror in which you can see yourself. In meditation you consciously control your mind and allow it to expand. He defined meditation as the mind flowing spontaneously towards its object, while concentration means making the mind one-pointed. Once concentration is mastered it flows spontaneously into meditation which then expands that one-pointed mind into universality. During concentration on an object the mind flits here and there and comes back. But in meditation it flows without any interruption. Concentration is a narrowing down; meditation is expansion which leads eventually to the eternal in *samadhi*.

For Swamiji, **preparation for meditation** was almost more important than meditation itself. First one must build one's determination. He would say that one decides with firm conviction and full strength: "*I will do it. Today I* HAVE *to meditate. At such and such time I will meditate, no matter what happens.*" He pointed out that prayer is another way to build determination: "*Oh Lord, help me obtain the goal I have set. Help me attain meditation.*" He taught that this is *sankalpa shakti*, the power of will. One achieves this by learning to train the attention, by giving full attention to whatever one does from morning until evening. He provided an important clue: interest is the key to attention. Interest absorbs the mind in its object of attention. Without interest in one's duties or one's meditation, mere repetition of a *mantra* will be mechanical and boring, and will not be helpful. Mindfulness is important. One trains attention by paying attention, and the more one pays attention, the more one becomes aware. This practice strengthens the mind and slowly makes it one-pointed and inwards. Then the student does not have to fight and struggle to meditate.

Stillness is the next step and Swamiji advised that one should take one or two months for stilling the posture. Working with the body first helps to make the mind inward and one-pointed. From the very beginning use a meditative posture that is comfortable, and that produces steadiness so that the body is without tension. A good meditative posture keeps the head, neck and trunk erect in a straight line, and arranges the limbs so that they are not a disturbance. Choose one posture, do not change it, and practice that same still posture every day all by itself. While this is done the mind will disturb with thoughts so it must be kept pleasantly busy. Let the mind survey the whole body from head to feet and then from feet to head two or three times. One can also use progressive relaxation or do *kaya sthairyam*.

In a few days the subtle physical sensations such as twitching, jerking, feelings of warmth and perspiration cease. Sri Swamiji would point out that foolish teachers call these sensations *kundalini* experiences. Rather they are experiences that arise from the subtle body that resents being disciplined. Swamiji would say that one quarter of the battle has been won when one has quieted the body. "Meditation means stillness." He would say, "One should learn to be still." He would advise one to observe a lake to see what happens when one becomes still. When waves agitate the surface one cannot see through to the bottom. When the lake of the mind is stilled then the Reality which is hidden at the bottom will be seen. Swamiji would quote the Bible, "*Be still and know that I am God.*" "You have not to search for God." he would say, "Just learn to be still and God will reveal himself to you, for Truth alone has power of revelation."

Sitting for meditation means that for a long time without any break one should practice every day at the same time. Experiment for a week by meditating at exactly the same time for not more than 15 or 20 minutes. Do not sit for a long time in the beginning because the body is not accustomed to being in one posture for a long time and the posture will become distorted. Swamiji recommended that a student go slowly and steadily and watch his or her progress. Expecting too much creates feelings of guilt. Do not meditate when you are very tired to avoid falling asleep, or when you have eaten too much and you will be disturbed by indigestion and burping. Also you cannot meditate when you are anxious or tense. Meditation time is not meant for thinking or worrying.

Students ask, "How many hours or minutes shall I do meditation?" It depends on the capacity of your mind. Swamiji would say that you waste time and energy if you sit for two hours and worry or sleep. Learn to know the capacity of your mind and then sit down quietly. If you sleep or the mind is uncontrollably dissipated then get up. At the next session try again at your capacity to relax and watch the breath. It is a skill that takes time to master. "Do not fight with your mind." he would say.

Breath awareness is the next step. One needs an object, focus or support (*alambana*) to train the mind, and the easiest and closest is the breath. Swamiji taught that mind and breath are inextricably linked. One takes one or two month's time to train the breath to be very serene, without jerks, noise, or pauses. Swamiji would advise avoiding a long pause, for "pause means death," he would say. Having made the body still, watch the breath to make it calm and serene, and do nothing else. Let the mind watch the breath; nothing else, inhaling and exhaling without any pause. The eyes will remain slightly open. The mind will become very calm and not jump. Swami Rama would say that sixty percent of the distraction of the mind is created by bad breathing habits. This exercise is enough, and after a few days the mind will see the stream of energy that is flowing.

Now comes *sushumna* **application**. To meditate successfully one must establish tranquility. This is done by applying or awakening *sushumna*, a simple method of breath awareness. Focus the mind on the space between the two nostrils where the bridge of the nose meets the space above the upper lip. Focus the mind on the breath as it flows past this point. The goal in learning to apply *sushumna* is to change the flow of the breath in the nostrils mentally. This is done by creating a relaxed focus on the right or left nostril. If a nostril is blocked, then focusing the mind on it will open that nostril and it will become active. When you have learned to mentally change the flow of the breath in the nostrils then a time comes when both nostrils begin to flow evenly. Depending on your capacity and the strength of your desire this may take some months or perhaps a year. When both nostrils flow freely this state is called *sandhya*, the wedding of the sun and moon, or *ida* and *pingala*. Swamiji taught that once this experience can be maintained for five minutes the aspirant has crossed a great barrier. The mind has attained some degree of one-pointedness and has become focused inward. This is a form of *pratyahara*. When the nostrils flow evenly the mind cannot worry because it is disconnected from the senses. The mind becomes calm and pleasant and attains a state of joy that is conducive to deep meditation.

Mantra is the object used for meditation. Swamiji taught that the word means that which dispels the darkness of ignorance, removing agony and pain from the mind. *Mantra* is sound, a syllable or a set of words that is prescribed by a competent teacher who knows you well. Swamiji taught that once you have a *mantra*, you do not need any guidance, for *mantra* will guide itself. *Mantra* helps the mind to become one-pointed and that is its only function here. He advised one not to try to find out the various literal meanings, translation and applications of a *mantra*. He would say that when you practice something like mental repetition of a *mantra* for a long time it becomes your habit and then you start to enjoy it. Do not repeat it mechanically, he would advise, but concentrate and remember the *mantra*, what *mantra* is, the meaning of the *mantra*, and it can help you to attain the highest state. "*Mantra* will lead you to meditative silence where the great Lord, the inner dweller, dwells in perfect silence."

Swamiji taught that **letting go** is important to learn. When you sit to meditate do not allow any external stimuli like sensations or sounds to disturb you. In the early stages of meditation thought patterns will come and go through the mental space; learn not to allow these thought patterns to disturb you. To do this, Swamiji advised one to learn to let go. Releasing and allowing all thought processes to go away will calm the conscious mind. Say to yourself, "*No, not this,*" and allow all the thought forms to go away. Strengthen your will, he would say, by making a determination that no matter what thoughts come they will not affect you. He taught that "They are not you; they are only thoughts, so do not identify with thoughts and emotions that arise from the mind. No thoughts or emotions should affect you; release and allow all the thought forms, both pleasant and unpleasant, to go away. Just let them go. Remain a witness to them and do not associate into or engage them." He said that this will expand the capacity of your conscious mind and eventually you will discover that the conscious and unconscious minds are one and the same. Then with systematic practice you will be able to access the entire store of knowledge that is hidden within the unconscious mind and attain a superconscious state.

Witnessing and inspecting are very important. He would say, "First learn to let go, and then learn to witness anything that goes through the mind without being affected by it. Do not be influenced by thought patterns; do not identify with any thought patterns. Remain detached and avoid associating emotionally with mental contents. Learn how to be detached and how not to be identified." He also pointed out that again the power of will, *sankalpa shakti*, comes to the fore. "Be very strong from within. When you decide or want to do something, do it. Nothing should be able to influence, impress, or affect you." As the logo on the T-shirt says, *Just do it*! But be sure to distinguish this from stubbornness or an inability to take advice. Finally, he would say, "Learn the art of inspecting. Say to yourself, *I have the power not to be distracted. I am a seer; I am drishta. I can inspect.* Witnessing means only watching; in witnessing you do not inspect. Inspecting is an advanced stage of witnessing. Sharpen the faculty of introspection so that you understand which thought patterns should be allowed and which should not." He taught that some thought patterns are helpful, some are not helpful and create obstacles, and some are neither. Then understand, he would say, which to accept and which to reject. Nourish the thought patterns and feelings which are helpful and reject those which are not helpful.

The order is important. First develop the power to let go, then to witness, and then finally to inspect. Swami Rama would advise taking three months to learn these three steps, and to allow two months to develop breath awareness, and one month to still the body. Then he would say that in the seventh month you will be in *samadhi*!

Meditation in Silence. The final step of meditation is to remain in the Silence. This is the Centre of Consciousness which is indescribable and inexplicable. This Silence awakens intuitive knowledge, and then the past, present, and future are revealed to the student.

This Silence lies beyond body, breath, and mind; it emanates peace, happiness and bliss. This Silence becomes the meditator's personal abode, and is the final goal of meditation.

Meditation in action. Both meditation in action and meditation in Silence are important. Swamiji would say that for learning to be perfect in the world while functioning in it, you have to learn to meditate in Silence. He also said that when you learn to be gentle to yourself, to still your body, to make your breath serene, and to calm your mind, that which is hidden behind will come forward.

Meditation in Silence leads to meditation in action. Swamiji would say that "you do not need liberation or God after death; you need Him here and now in this world." In meditation in action you remain aware of the Reality (the Centre of Consciousness) all the time, wherever you go, whatever you do. "You do your duties without identifying with the work. You understand the purpose of your life. You are free."

29

Some Considerations about Meditation

Christian Meditation

There is a meditative tradition in Christianity that is not widely known. Original Christianity is, in fact, a Yoga tradition – a mix of Bhakti and Karma Yoga (devotion and selfless service) with an initiatory (baptism) master-disciple relationship. Yogis consider that Christ was a very advanced Yogic adept, and many say the lost years were spent in Kashmir and the Himalayas among other places, where he mastered Yoga.

The Christian meditative tradition has descended from the early Christian monks, the Desert Fathers, as a simple tradition of silent, contemplative prayer. Father John Main has reintroduced it to the West in recent times. His method is summarized below and clearly resembles the *mantra* meditation we have just been discussing.

CHRISTIAN MEDITATION

Sit down. Sit still. Close your eyes lightly. Sit relaxed but alert. Silently, interiorly begin to say a single word. We recommend the prayer-phrase, "*Maranatha*." Recite it as four syllables of equal length. Listen to it as you say it, gently but continuously. Do not think or imagine anything – spiritual or otherwise. If thoughts and images come, these are distractions at the time of meditation, so keep returning to the simple work of saying the word. Meditate each morning and evening for between 20 and 30 minutes.

Father John Main (Willoughby, 2000)

Here the *mantra* is *maranatha* which is a word in the Aramaic language spoken by Jesus which is taken to mean *Come Lord, Come Lord Jesus* or *the Lord comes*. It is pronounced with a long "a" sound (as in "car" or "far") as a balanced rhythmic word that harmonizes with the breath. It is one of the oldest Christian prayers. It has been used for a very long time by the early monks. The word *Maranatha* is the final instruction of St. Paul's teachings to the Corinthians, and the final instruction of St. John's Book of Revelations. It is also the last word, the final teaching of the whole Christian Bible. As a non-English word with no associations it does not encourage thinking or images. It has a threefold purpose: a point of focus and absorption allowing distractions to be ignored; it leads to a condition of simplicity; and saying it is an expression of Christian faith in the Christ who lives in human hearts – in other words, it is a form of continuous prayer. Other *mantras* can be chosen such as Abba, the name of Jesus, the Jesus prayer or any part of it, or any short phrase of Christian scripture.

The Himalayan Tradition uses a diversity of *mantras* for meditation. It encourages students to follow the teachings, traditions and *mantras* of their own religion. Indeed the lineage may prescribe a *mantra* during initiation that comes from and is practiced in accordance with one's religious affiliation. In Christian meditation John Cassian recommended, "Oh God, come to my aid; Oh Lord, make haste to help me." Whatever is used, the choice of the *mantra* is important for it is an expression of the meditator's Christian faith. In the Christian tradition one can choose one's own *mantra*, but ideally a teacher gives a *mantra* to a student. The Holy Spirit is recognized as the Inner Teacher and could inspire a self-chosen *mantra*. The method of meditation including frequency, length of time, etc. is the same as in the Himalayan Tradition, and it uses the still, steady posture with an erect spine in a suitable Yogic sitting *asana*. But its essence is continuous inner prayer and remembrance in the Bhakti fashion. What makes it Christian? The World Community for Christian Meditation says that meditation is Christian because of the Christian faith of the person meditating.

As in the Himalayan Tradition, the *mantra* is used with the breath. One breathes naturally with the attention on the *mantra* which is said continually, but it is allowed to integrate itself quite naturally with the breath. For some people it coordinates with other bodily rhythms like the pulse, but most people say the *mantra* with the breath. Breathing in one says the *mantra*; breathing out one is silent. Or breathing in one repeats "Mar-ra" and breathing out one repeats "na-tha." It can also be done as "Ma" with inhalation; "ra" with exhalation; "na" with inhalation; "tha" with exhalation. Breathing should be diaphragmatic, associated with good posture and be an important aid to relaxation. Father John Main did not stress breathing in the interests of keeping the method simple and not allowing the discipline to be turned into a technique. Focusing on a technique can let one forget the purpose of the practice.

The mind's focus of attention can rest either in the heart centre, in the space of the spiritual heart or cave of the still, silent heart, feeling the coming and going of the *mantra*. Or it can be done in the space between the eyebrows, the *ajna chakra*, in the field of the mind. The attention rests in that space as the *mantra* comes and goes. One chooses the centre either on the instruction of the preceptor or based on how one might feel one's attention drawn. One can use a set of 108 *mala* beads as a counter and timer for one's practice time of twenty to thirty minutes. Repetition should not be mechanical, but should be accompanied by feeling, calmness and awareness of the meaning. It can also be used with a *purashcharana* to develop stability and capacity for practice.

Also parallel to the Himalayan Tradition Father John Main noted that after many years the *mantra* would lead one into complete silence, even for very brief moments. This experience should not be anticipated or desired. If you note in your mind that "I am silent" or a similar sentiment, then you are thinking and this is not complete silence.

In the Himalayan Tradition the *mantra* changes over time. It will be repeated with effort mentally but felt in the mouth in the beginning. As it goes deeper it goes more into the mind and after a while is no longer felt in the mouth. Effortable thinking of the *mantra* by the mind becomes progressively the *mantra* repeating itself more and more spontaneously in the mind. Having to start the *mantra* willfully becomes the *mantra* arising spontaneously by itself. The *mantra* refines itself from recognizable words and phrases gradually into a pulsation that progressively simplifies its complex wave form and leads the practitioner deeper and deeper into the mind field which, in turn, settles down and becomes progressively still. Eventually the pulsation leads one to the silence, and it may dissolve into the silence, leaving absolute stillness to be enjoyed. The process moves to subtler and subtler levels through saying into thinking and then into listening. Father John Main describes the same progression with the *Maranatha mantra* through four stages. Over weeks, months and years it requires less effort and force to say it; he describes it as becoming more gentle and faithful. The *mantra* is first said with effort in the head, then with greater ease and acceptance of distractions in the heart, and finally one listens to it with full attention; thinking becomes listening. Eventually it leads to the silence which cannot be anticipated.

The *mantra* may also have significance in the Yoga tradition.

> Maranatha is also a Sanskrit word: "Mara" is Kama Deva, the primordial master of Sri Vidya, one of the most esoteric schools of Yoga; "Natha" means "Lord." In Sanskrit literature, especially the literature that originated in the northwestern region of the Himalayas, the words "Mara Natha," "Sri Natha," and "Mina Natha" are used to refer to the supreme form of God. Thus it is likely that maranatha was revered as a mantra by the sages who lived and practiced in the Kashmir Himalayas, a place where some say Jesus himself lived and practiced during the years not recorded in the New Testament. In fact the shrine where Christ is said to have lived is called Amaranatha.
>
> Pandit Rajamani Tigunait (Willoughby, 2000)

The World Community for Christian Meditation (2004) provides an extensive discussion of Christian meditation and Swami Jnaneshvara Bharati discusses it in the context of the Himalayan Tradition (2004).

Meditation and Non-Attachment

Meditation has been likened to "washing the mind." When the mind is quieted the lid comes off the unconscious and all of the "stuff" (technical term!) starts to come up. There are three sources of disturbance:

- The environment – input from the five senses, with sounds as especially disturbing;
- The body and its discomforts; and
- The mind's restlessness as the unconscious contents start to surface.

Disturbances originating from body are dealt with by other practices like Hatha Yoga, diet, breathing and learning to sit still. Focusing on bodily sensations until the restless mind gets bored and moves away exploits the mind's restlessness by allowing it to move beyond bodily sensations.

Disturbances originating from both the five senses and from mental restlessness are dealt with in the same way – by mindfulness – by observing the intrusion of either the external sounds or the extraneous thoughts and feelings, acknowledging and observing their presence (thereby detaching from them because of the observer or witness position), and then bringing the awareness back to the sound of *so'ham* or the personal *mantra* flowing with the breath at the nostrils.

The state of witnessing, of detachment, of being the observer, is key here. The disturbances are simply allowed, witnessed, observed with complete disinterest and detachment, and then allowed to release like so many "clouds" of energy floating through the mind's "sky." If one associates into the thoughts or feelings and loses the detached observer position, one will have to restart the process: re-establish the upright posture which will have slumped, re-establish the relaxation, and bring the mind back to the flow of the sound with the breath at the nostrils.

In other words, we propose that meditation works like visual-kinesthetic dissociation (V-KD) in Neuro-Linguistic Programming (NLP) to break the links between emotion and internal image to produce detachment as we discussed in Part Three. Associating into the emotion again just strengthens it for the next time. One sits anchored in the meditation posture, witnessing the mind (i.e., yourself) repeating the *mantra* over and over (watching the *mantra* repeat itself over and over in the mind field). This is a dissociated or even doubly-dissociated internal state. The foreground is the *mantra* flowing with the breath, and extraneous thoughts, feelings or sounds float through the background and release.

This process of detachment through V-K dissociation is the basis for both the relaxation effects of meditation (releasing or letting go), and for its therapeutic effects in cleansing the mind of unconscious inputs and eventually bringing it to silence. *Antar mouna* and other forms of mindfulness work by the same process so that the two become a powerful combination for producing *vairagya* (detachment).

But in the long term meditation does much more than this. It raises the mean (average) vibratory set-point of the subtle energy field that is the mind. A still mind is not a dull and vacant mind. A still mind in the sense meant here is a high-energy mind, a vibrant and aware field of energy. Yet it seems still, like a top that is rotating so rapidly and with such high energy that it appears motionless. Such a mind has lost its tendency to emotional reactivity no matter the provocation. In the far reaches of such a mind the edge of eternity can reflect.

> Aequanimitas
>> Thou must be like a promontory of the sea, against which, though the waves beat continuously, yet it both itself stands, and about it are those swelling waves stilled and quieted.
>
> Marcus Aurelius

So in summary, there are two processes going on here: concentration and mindfulness. The preliminary practices of stillness, diaphragmatic breathing and relaxation are all forms of concentration. The feeling of the touch of the breath in the nostrils is a very refined sensation. It produces *pratyahara* (sensory withdrawal). The activity of the other senses naturally quiets and they withdraw. Then one can concentrate on the mental sound of the *mantra* which is the literal expression of an inner and inward energy that leads the awareness back to the Centre of Consciousness which is its Source.

Raising the vibrational set-point of the mind extends to all the energy fields of the personality. All of the practices of Raja Yoga combine to achieve this total transformation. This step by step process must be coordinated. Periods of progress alternate with periods when nothing seems to be happening. But during these times of apparent stagnation the gains are being integrated into all of the *koshas* of the personality and external behavior before going the next step. If the integration is incomplete, if one or more energy sheath surges ahead, falls behind or comes out of alignment with the others, the basis for illness is established – what the Mother, Sri Aurobindo's partner, called "Yogic illness" (The Mother, 1972).

Obstacles to Meditation

Meditation is not as simple as it looks. In chapter 24 we reviewed the impediments to Yoga (union) as described in Patanjali's *Yoga-Sutra* (I.30) and their adverse consequences (YS I.31). They also become the obstacles to meditation. Johnsen (2000) provides a modern discussion in this context.

In Part Three we discussed at length the issue of emotional and mental purification of the personality in the context of developing non-attachment (*vairagya*). Volatile emotional states and the pressure of restless mental agitation can present a formidable obstacle to the serious meditator until some progress has been made in stabilizing the mind field. Simply sitting and witnessing the mind with mindfulness until the agitation slowly subsides can be a useful strategy.

Swami Sivananda (1986b, pp 240–373) discusses a long list of physical, mental and higher obstacles to meditation, as well as distracting inner experiences, and Christmas Humphreys (1968) provides sound counsel in his excellent text on concentration and meditation from a Zen Buddhist perspective.

Swami Veda Bharati (1974, pp 91–102) describes five stages of thoughts arising in the mind during meditation. In the first stage the random thoughts of the uncontrolled mind sweep the attention away through association, and can even lead to fantasies misinterpreted as messages and directions from the teacher or great masters. Mental agitation leads to physical tension; the erect posture slumps. The corrective is to ignore these random thoughts and fantasies. Do not associate into them and engage them. Observe that they are there, perhaps even with labeling: *thinking, thinking*; reestablish the erect posture, relax the muscles and joints with a slow exhalation, and bring the mind back to the *mantra*. The key is to remain dis-associated as an observer and release the thoughts, let them go. The process then becomes a purification of the mind. If one engages and associates into the train of thoughts, particularly with the associated emotions, they are strengthened and go back down into the subconscious to arise again another day. In the beginning this will have to be done over and over again for a very long time. The other obstacle at this stage is sleep which can sweep away the awareness without the meditator even noticing until s/he awakens with a start. Not meditating when one is tired or sleepy, or after a meal can help. One may have to get up and walk or splash cold water on the face.

In the second stage the random thoughts still arise from the subconscious, but they no longer produce chains of associated thoughts. The witnessing process for dealing with them is still the same. Provided one can maintain the dis-association of the observer stance the momentum of *samskaras* and hidden *karma* is reduced. A student may even feel he or she is getting worse as unknown hidden negativities arise. One should continue to practice the *yamas* and *niyamas* in daily life and remain a witness to these negative thoughts also.

In the third stage arising thoughts become specific. They deal with practical problems that the conscious and subconscious minds are preoccupied with at that time. Their content reflects a meditator's progress or lack thereof as well as the influence of current life conflicts and problems. Swami Veda Bharati recommends that the dichotomy between life and meditation should be resolved by raising one's life to the level of one's meditation. As the mind elevates and the inner personality is transformed, harmony manifests in all of one's actions and interactions in the external world. The environment stops being a source of obstacles with its temptations and resistances.

In the fourth stage problems seldom arise. They are replaced by solutions, inspirations, projects, poetry, music, creative thoughts and guidance for success. Note down the solutions and guidance after the meditation is over and act on them as appropriate. Avoid getting caught in the ego trap of thinking yourself to be a great person because you are favored with these revelations as a chosen Divine instrument.

The fifth stage brings communion with the superconscious. One learns to distinguish its intuitive whisperings from material arising from the subconscious. Guidance for stages four and five is given personally by the master to the disciple.

Conclusion

Is all of this hard to do? The method seems so elegantly simple – just remember and follow spirit without hesitation, and yet an enormous effort seems to be required to rediscover ourselves, to find the answer to "Who am I?" In his commentary on the *Bhagavad Gita for Daily Living*, Eknath Easwaren (1979, p 235) recounts a traditional story that epitomizes the challenge for the householder.

The story concerns the monk Narada who believed that householders are not capable of much progress on the spiritual path. But one day in heaven Krishna, who favored householders, had the opportunity to adjust Narada's position when he asked Krishna why he as the Lord liked them so much when they were not very regular in their practice.

Krishna responded by asking Narada to carry a little oil lamp around the temple three times, but not to let the flame go out. As soon as he left, Krishna called the wind god Marut to ask him to blow for all he was worth.

Marut blew up a hurricane and Narada was hard put to keep the flame from going out. But he held the lamp close to shield it from the wind and made it around the temple three times with the flame still flickering.

On his return Krishna congratulated him for his success, and then asked him how many times he remembered to repeat His, the Lord's name, the *mantram*, as he was going around the temple. Narada hemmed and hawed, made long excuses about the wind, and then finally admitted to the Lord that he didn't remember Him even once.

Sri Krishna then pointed out to Narada that these householders face so many problems. They must contend with television, 9/11, hurricanes, tsunamis, the generation gap, Wall Street, Madison Avenue, and all the rest; in the storms of daily living the wind blows against them all the time. Said Krishna, "If they are able to remember me only a little part of the day, I am very pleased." (Easwaren, 1979).

A student once asked Swami Rama for a new practice. He had been working with his *mantra* for three months, and now he wanted to move on to the next stage. Swamiji eyed him calmly and asked if the *mantra* went by itself without his actively trying to remember it. No. Was it always present in every moment of the day? Well, no. Was it present in his dreams? No. "Then," said Swamiji, "Keep practicing!"

30

Meditation and the Centre of Consciousness

How does meditation change when the Presence aspect of the Centre of Consciousness opens into awareness in the mind? How does one cope with this new awareness in the practice of meditation? What strategies can be used to crystallize this Awareness until it becomes a stable background in the mind? How does one deepen this experience into Being and Bliss? Let us begin by setting the stage with two quotations.

Swami Rama sometimes used the word "desirelessness" for detachment or nonattachment. He spoke of meditation and the Centre of Consciousness thus (Rama, 1999a, p 28):

> Whenever you have time, sit down quietly, compose yourself, and just start remembering that Centre deep down within you beyond the thinking process.

> Desire is the very root of all mysteries. You must become desireless and maintain the here and now [i.e., the awareness of the Centre] by constant awareness. Remember the Centre of Consciousness within you. Constant awareness is the most important thing, and it is possible for you to achieve. . . . you must first become peaceful and tranquil.

> You cannot experience anything of God if your mind remains agitated and dissipated by desires. You must first become calm, peaceful and tranquil. . . . Just for a few seconds ask yourself not to have any desires. What will be the condition of your mind then? Immediately your mind will flow in an ocean of joy and bliss [i.e., be filled with the effulgence of the Centre]. When you are able to lead your mind to the state of desirelessness, then it is considered to be real meditation [i.e., desirelessness implies a quiet mind free of disturbing thoughts]. The purpose of meditation is to lead you to that higher state. . . . if you attain that Centre within with the help of meditation, then you will have peace of mind.

> You should learn to play your part while having constant awareness of the Reality that is within you [i.e., this is meditation in action]. You should allow all desires to be swallowed up by the one desire for attaining the higher purpose of life [i.e., this is a one-pointed mind focused on the Centre of Consciousness]. . . . When the desire to know God is strengthened, it swallows all other desires. Finally this desire is fulfilled by attaining a height beyond itself called desirelessness [i.e., a silent mind field].

This and the next quotation emphasize the interplay between nonattachment and the practice of the Centre of Consciousness which lies at the core of the Chariot of *Sadhana*: *vairagya* and *abhyasa*.

> Meditation is not a technique. The technique alone will not do. The State of Meditation is a condition of Being in which you don't do anything. In this state, you rest within Totality becoming absorbed into the Universal Presence. The State of Meditation is the state of surrender. This profound surrender unites you with the Beyond.
>
> Kristof, 2000, p 13

Examples of Meditation on the Centre of Consciousness:

1. Here is a shortened meditation from the Himalayan Tradition by Swami Veda Bharati.

Meditation on the Centre of Consciousness in the Himalayan Yoga Tradition

Bring your awareness only to the spot where you are sitting. Be aware only of the space that your body is occupying. In the time stream be aware only of that tiny ripple called this moment and this space, only one ripple at a time, not bringing forth the momentum of the previous ones, not anticipating the next one, only dwelling in the moment.

Now observe the fact of your being, without any qualifications attached to that being; no names, no sizes, no boundaries, no genders, no titles, no limitations, no load from past experiences, no identification from the moment before. Only be in the given moment. Be aware of Being – no words for this Being, no thoughts about this Being, only an awareness of Being, Being without associations, without conditions, without titles, without identifications from past events, without anxieties concerning future events – only Being in this moment. Be aware of your Being.

Now be aware only of the fact of Awareness, pure Awareness. Observe the nature of this Awareness. Observe the nature of this Consciousness, pure Consciousness without a title, without an object, without condition, an ever-flowing stream of fullness, Consciousness – conscious of being Consciousness. Be that.

By now in this process of self-awareness all your emotions will have merged into serenity. All *prana* warps will have been smoothed out, straightened out, and your breath will have begun to flow evenly, gently and smoothly. Maintaining the awareness of your Being as a Consciousness, weaving the consciousness stream into your breath, be aware of the flow and the touch of your breath in your nostrils. Exhale and inhale gently. Let there be no break in your stream of consciousness, so there will be no jerks in the breath stream. When the consciousness flows as a single stream there will be no break between your breaths. Remain aware of the Atman, the spiritual Self: pure Consciousness that breathes forth, and into Whom the breath merges back again, and from Whom the breath emerges, and into Whom the breath returns and merges again.

Maintain the flow of consciousness in your breathing. Remaining aware of the flow, gently open your eyes, but let there be no alternation in your consciousness. And God bless you.

© Swami Veda Bharati, 2001

2. A longer example has been published by us elsewhere (Jerry & Jerry, 2001, p 178)

Direct Meditation on the Centre of Consciousness

Sit erect in your meditation posture with the head, neck and trunk straight.
    Let the body become steady, stable and absolutely still.

With a single, long exhalation, travel through body from head to toe and relax any tension in the muscle groups.
    Exhale any tension you find.

Let the breathing become diaphragmatic and connected,
    Quiet, deep, slow, smooth, equal and continuous.
    Let the whole body breath this way from top to toe and toe to top.

Now sense the energy field of the body.
    Feel the body's aliveness.
    This field is a gateway to the Inner Presence.
    Become one with, absorbed in that aliveness, the energy of that aliveness.
When your *guru mantra* appears just let it go, let it pulse continuously in the background as you relax and let it lead you deeper into stillness, into pure Silence.

A Silence that is absolutely still.
A Silence that is a Conscious Presence; a Presence that can only be referred to as THAT.
    As though the whole of infinite inner space is alive, aware.
    As though the space in a room were pure awareness, pure conscious Presence, containing within it all the contents of the room and yet unaffected by their presence.

Similarly the whole of inner space is pure Awareness, pure conscious Presence, containing within It all the contents of the mind and the ego, the small self, and yet remaining unaffected by them.

A Nothingness, a Space, a Void of purest Awareness. Yet a Nothing that is Something.

A Void that is a Plenitude. A Fullness of infinite potential.

Recall the opening words of the *Isha Upanishad*:

"That is full; this is full. This fullness has been projected from that fullness.

When this fullness merges in that fullness, all that remains is fullness."

The power and presence of the eternal NOW.

That Presence may be effulgent with the softest white or golden light.

And if the mind is still enough you may detect a continual whispering.

The whispering of a flow of purest knowing and certainty.

This is the Inner Teacher.

The gentle caress of a downward flow of bliss.

This is the Inner Beloved. Love whispers.

You may even be aware of the subtle sounds in the right ear in the background.

For some are led by sound and some by light.

Thoughts, images or feelings may flow through the inner space of the mind.

Let them go like clouds scudding through the space of the sky.

The Presence becomes foreground; thoughts become only a distant murmuring background that no longer disturbs the Presence.

If there be even the slightest stirring of that silent Void, let it come forth as your *mantra*.

Then refine it back into that Silence.

Move back and forth between the pulsing of the *mantra* and the Silence as needed to stabilize the Presence.

Just be absorbed in THAT, in total Silence, in total Stillness, in total Awareness.

Rest in *Shanti*, in total Peace, in the "Peace that passes all understanding."

Now let your *mantra* reappear.

Lead it gently and slowly towards the surface of the mind.

Join it with the breath, the two flowing together at the nostrils as though from a common point deep in the mind.

Maintaining the stillness and the *mantra* in the mind, gently cup the eyes with the palms of the hands.

Remaining inwardly attuned, gently open the eyes to the palms, lower the hands to the thighs, move the body and be comfortable.

An experienced meditator can drop right into the Presence directly. We maintain the basic meditation structure and sequence in abbreviated format, but the experienced meditator will find it unnecessary to be quite so formal once the State of Presence begins to become established in the mental background in daily life. One can find and return to It back behind the mind at any time.

One simply assumes an erect meditation posture, comes to inner stillness, relaxes the body from head to toe with an exhalation, and drops into the Centre or Presence directly, inhaling and exhaling deeply and slowly, and diaphragmatically, breathing to and from the State of Presence with the *mantra*, and then relaxing into that Presence as it comes to the foreground – holding It steady. After the meditation one brings that Presence into daily life, holding it in background awareness as long as one can in daily activity. This is meditation on the *cit* or consciousness aspect (in the sense of awareness, knowing or knowledge) of the *saccidananda* (existence-consciousness-bliss) which is the very essence of *saguna Brahman* in Advaita Vedanta.

3. Aziz Kristof (2000) describes a complete meditation on Presence, Being and Heart which works with the Centre of Consciousness as the *sat cit ananda* (or in his terminology: Presence, Being and Heart). One is trying to realize the *saccidananda* of *Brahman* as an integrated experience. Awareness, Being and Bliss (to use Aziz's terms), are not three independent things to be realized separately. Each merges into the next in the meditation sequence for a cumulative realization of the *saccidananda* as an integrated experience of Consciousness.

Aziz (Kristof, 2000) describes three pillars of meditation (Presence, Being and Heart) on what we here call the Centre of Consciousness. He calls it the complete meditation. It seeks an inner wholeness, a unity of the I AM (his term for *Atman* or soul and also *Brahman*), the *sat cit ananda*. This reflects our interpretation of his writing, for he himself refuses to link his terminology to traditional nondualistic terminology. He puts forth his teaching as a new dispensation for a new age (personal communication). The three pillars are Awareness, Being and Heart.

The first step in his method is the awakening of Awareness (Intelligence or Knowing) which is the Presence. The process of concentration activates Attention. A continuity of this Attention shifts Awareness to a higher state where the Presence is recognized as the Centre of Awareness in the mind in relation to the *ajna chakra*. The process of accomplishing this involves two steps: awakening and stabilization. There are four methods he uses to awaken the Presence which we discussed in chapter 4. To review, the first is observation of the mind which leads to observing the observer. Another is observation of a thought like a *mantra* and ascertaining who the observer is. Contemplation can also be used where one asks who the thinker is. The fourth way is to go for direct recognition of the Presence in the background behind the mind. In outline, Aziz (Kristof, 2000) describes them this way:

1. Direct recognition:
- "Letting go. The body still and posture erect. Be present to the Now/Centre of Consciousness/Presence.
- Inhale up to the head, retain the breath, recognize and become the Presence, crystallize the Attention, then exhale and relax with this Presence in the head space, and repeat.
- This state of Presence is the Witness, choiceless Awareness, your real Me, pure Subject, the state of Self-Consciousness, the silent background of the mind which does not change in spite of the coming and going of thoughts, perceptions and endless experiences.
- Stay with this Presence in a centered way, but relaxed."

2. By observation of the mind:
- "With curiosity and detachment be aware of arising thoughts, noting their unreal quality without becoming entangled.
- Who is the Observer? Observe the Observer. Recognize the One Who is behind, in the background, the One Who is looking at your mind, the Subject. Gently turn the attention back, feeling the One behind."

3. By observing the mantra:
- "Observe the pulsation of your *mantra*.
- Who is the Observer? Who is the One observing the movement of the *mantra*? Gently turn the attention back and feel the One behind."

4. Through contemplation:
- "Instead of observing the mind, and being fully conscious, repeat in your mind very slowly, contemplatively and with great intensity, a thought, like "Attention in!"
- As you repeat it, watch it, see it, feel the Me behind, the One Who is repeating the thought.
- You are just behind the thought. Feel it. The moment you feel it, stay with it, this feeling of Me, this sense of I Am, just behind the thought
- Take one more breath up to the head, retain the breath, crystallize the attention, become this Presence which is just present without any object.
- And with exhalation, relax with this Presence inside the head."

Once It has been identified It must be stabilized or "crystallized" to use his term. This is done by a long process of holding it and then letting it go (relaxation, surrender) until its presence in the mind is spontaneous. Steps three and four are reminiscent of Ramana Maharshi's sequence (1988): "To whom does this (thought, *mantra*, etc.) arise? To me. Who am I?"

The next step is the awakening of pure Being (pure rest). This involves a gradual maturation of the consciousness-energy system from a predominant focus in individuality towards transcendence. The process centers around surrender. One tries to be fully Now in the experience of the Presence. Through surrender there is a vertical letting go into immersion into Being located at the *hara* in the belly. It involves slow diaphragmatic breathing with complete exhalation.

- "Inhale up to the head. Stop breathing. Centralize your attention in the head space. Then with exhalation gently relax, but from within your Presence. Allow it to expand like a space of Awareness inside your head and around your head, and just abide in this space.
- Moment to moment make sure that the Presence is present, not allowing yourself to lose It or to get caught in the mind.
- Now relax into that Presence, letting go vertically into that Now, by connecting with the breath in the belly, relaxing into Being but from the place of Awareness, from the place of clear Presence within your head.
- Just being, resting within; moment to moment, letting go into that vastness. Presence and letting go, surrender, and profound relaxation of being.
- Rest within in a state of non-doing, and non-activity, passivity which is full of potential."

The final step is awakening of the Heart (sensitivity). There are two levels: energetic activation of the heart centre, and then awakening to subtle sensitivity – the feeling of the Soul. At this point the Soul recognizes the Divine through Intelligence, surrender and utmost sensitivity, and then merges with It. The process involves awakening of intention within which leads to grace. It is of the essence of Bhakti. It uses meditation and breath in the *anahata chakra* facilitated with prayer and music. He describes it as a long and complex journey.

- "The heart is the gateway to the Divine.
- Placing your hand gently on the middle of the chest, feel your heart as you gently breathe into the chest.
- Breathing through the heart center, go deep into the cave of the heart. Feel the love of the One who is dwelling in the depth of your heart. Be present and resting within, feeling and merging with the heart which then opens up like a flower and you enter inside.
- Gently breathing into your heart, feeling your heart, letting go into the heart and into Being, remaining one with your soul, one with Awareness, one with your Heart and resting in Being. Remain like this, just sitting, calmly abiding."

Meditation and Being

In figure 30.1 we present meditation as a state of pure being which has three aspects. They are Presence, Being or Heart/Bliss to use Aziz's terminology, or *cit, sat* and *ananda* in *advaitic* terms, the *saguna brahman*. C of C refers to the Centre of Consciousness as we have been using the term here. The first step in the process awakens the Presence, and this is an active process involving "doing things" in meditation.

The subsequent steps, however, require a total change in strategy. Being and then Bliss are reached by doing nothing, by releasing doing, by surrender and by opening to the descent of grace. It is a calm abiding in the Presence until the states of Being and then Bliss arise in their integrated fullness.

This kind of passive resting in Being is very difficult for us to understand and do because we are used to achieving things by doing. We want to know how something is to be gained, what is the process for it, what practices are we to do. To answer: Nothing – just be, is very hard to accept.

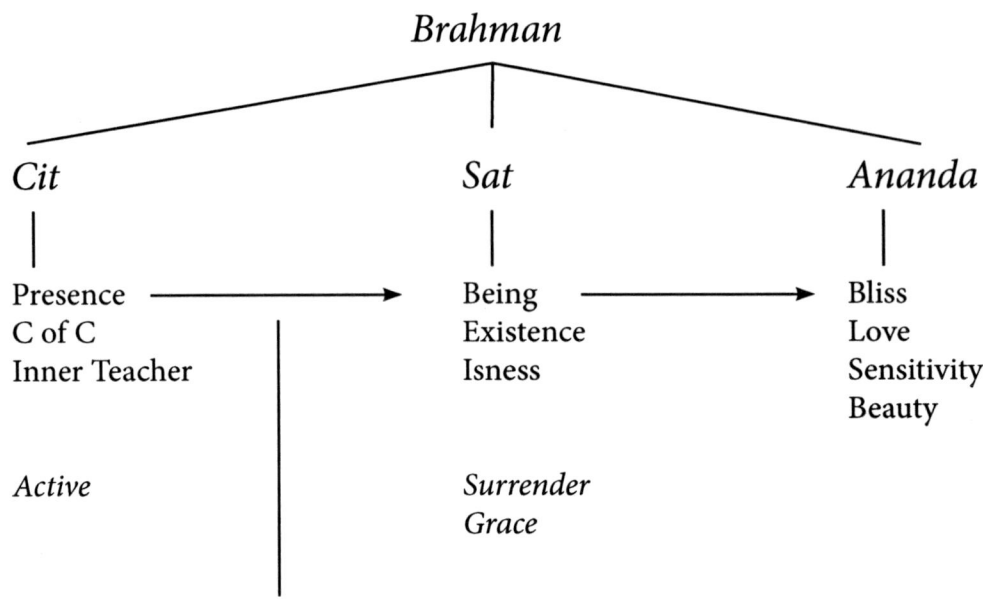

Figure 30.1 The relative roles of action and surrender in meditation

The Importance of Surrender

Osho (1974, pp 22 –26) points out that a method means depending on your self; it requires that you exert your will and do something. But on the path of surrender, surrender itself is the only method. Methods are nonsurrendering, but with surrender there is nothing more to do; surrender has no method. Surrender is reached through love which is sufficient unto itself and needs nothing more. Surrender comes when all efforts, all methods have failed; it happens in total helplessness. Surrender is the most difficult thing in the world for you cannot train yourself to surrender and to ask how to surrender is absurd. It is either there or it is not. Like love, it just happens, and the two are a deep unity. It is a state that is totally open and vulnerable and can bring with it a sense of insecurity and danger. It is the essence of the true *guru*-disciple relationship.

But one can understand what blocks surrender and try to remove that. The key blockage comes from the individuality, the ego. As an individual personality you cannot surrender; surrender happens when you are not. You are identified as an ego and surrender cannot coexist because surrender transcends the individuality. Hence the need to find the answer to the question, "Who am I?" as propounded by Ramana Maharshi (1988).

But here there is a paradox. The purpose of the inquiry is not to find out who I am, but to discover that I am not; to dissolve the small self based in the mind into the identity shift to the Self. There is no answer; the question itself will dissolve. When the small "I" is not, the real "I" shines. That Being is void, the Presence, and now you become surrender itself. There are no techniques.

Ramana Maharshi (1988, p 4) describes the process this way:

" . . . As each thought arises one should inquire with diligence, 'To whom has this thought arisen?' The answer that would emerge would be 'To me.' Thereupon if one inquires 'Who am I?' the mind will go back to its source, and the thought that arose will become quiescent. With repeated practice in this manner, the mind will develop the skill to stay in its source. . . . the 'I' which is the source of all thoughts, will go and the Self which ever exists will shine. Whatever one does, one should do without the egoity 'I'. If one acts in that way, all will appear as of the nature of Shiva."

Osho compares surrender to a valley and the ego to a peak. As an ego one is above everyone and nothing can enter you. But with surrender one becomes a valley; one becomes depth rather than height. The grace of divinity can pour into such a bottomless vacuum and fill one totally. There are minor and major surrenders. Surrendering to a master lets the master's energy flow into you. This is part of the meaning of receiving the master's *darshan*. If you cannot feel that energy flow into you then you have not surrendered in even a minor way. There are many minor surrenders before the final major surrender. The minor ones prepare you for the final death of the total surrender, the identity shift that brings about the death of one's identity as a small self. The master helps you with the minor surrenders until you have the courage for the total surrender. And then with just a touch or a look by the master, it is accomplished – enlightenment dawns.

31
Working with the Centre of Consciousness

The Object of Meditation Is the Centre of Consciousness

When the Centre of Consciousness dawns as the Presence, It gradually becomes the object of meditation directly. Until then all objects used for concentration are symbols, representatives of that Centre. Is there textual evidence for this statement? Shyam Sundar Goswami (1999, pp 59–67) has collected many scriptural references to this idea, some of which we summarize here.

> By controlling the desiring mind, a wise yogi should hold the Divine Spirit in his consciousness in concentration; this is *Dharana.*
>
> *Amritanadopanishad,* 15

> *Dharana* is of three kinds: the holding-concentration on the divine aspect of the self; holding-concentration of the void in the *hrit* (heart) centre; and holding concentration on the five divine forms in the five intra-spinal subtle centres
>
> *Shandilyopanishad,* 1.9.1

> . . . with the purified and spiritualized mind he should concentrate on *Vasudeva* who is the Supreme Spirit. When concentration is so deep that the whole consciousness is moulded into the *Vasudeva* form, then that concentration will lead to liberation.
>
> *Trishikhibrahmanopanishad, Mantra* Section, 145–9.

> Concentration on the universal form of God has been advised.
>
> *Darshanopanishad,* 9.1–2.

> The final stage of *dhyana* is the concentration on Brahman (God) without form.
>
> *Darshanopanishad,* 9.3–5.

> When concentration reaches the phase of "*ekatanata,*" monoformity (of consciousness) of the Divine Being abiding in all, that is *dhyana.*
>
> *Mandalabrahmanopanishad,* 1.1.9.

> The object of the formless concentration is the Supreme Power-Consciousness which is beyond mind and speech, unmanifest, omnipresent, and unknowable.
>
> *Mahanirvanatantra,* 5. 137–140.

Experts in yoga say that *dhyana* is to make the form of Deity held (continuously) in consciousness.

Prapanchasaratantra, 19. 22–23.

Dhyana is the concentration on the Deity of *mantra*.

Kularnava, ch. 17, p 83.

Deep concentration on the conscious form of the Deity of *mantra* in your consciousness is *dhyana*.

Gandharvatantra, ch. 5, p 26.

The mind operating at the sensory level is the root-cause of all the worldly knowledge. If the mind is dissolved, there will be no worldly knowledge. Therefore, keep the consciousness fixed on the Supreme Being in deepest concentration.

Adhyatmopanishad, 26

In superconcentration, God is held by concentration, and consciousness becomes godly.

Shyam Sundar Goswami, 1999, p 63.

When the penetration of the objective world into consciousness is prevented by sensory control, then the Supreme Spirit in its divine form is held in consciousness in concentration. At the beginning, concentration does not go very deep, so it breaks and the one-pointedness of the consciousness is interrupted. But concentration quickly regains its power. This is holding-concentration. When concentration grows deeper, and interruption does not occur, it continues; consciousness is now only in the divine form, which is continually being held. This single-pointedness of consciousness is deep concentration. When the deep concentration becomes deepest, I-ness is lost, the whole world is lost, what remains is only the spiritually illuminated consciousness of divine form, it is the state of superconscious concentration. When the light-like concentrative consciousness is absorbed into Supreme Consciousness in supreme concentration, there remains solely the Supreme Spirit, and nothing else. This is non-mens (mind-transcendent) concentration.

Shyam Sundar Goswami, 1999, p 65.

By yoga (non-mens or mind-transcendent concentration), yoga (superconscious concentration) should be controlled, and the multiformed consciousness by the one-pointed consciousness in which God is held; thus being in Supreme Consciousness, which is beyond all knowledge, the yogi becomes that.

Soubhagyalakshmyupanishad, 2.12.

Consciousness may become free from the *vrittis* by the control of the perceptive, intellective, volitive and affective aspects of the mind, and becomes monoform and single-pointed, in which only the Supreme Being is held in concentration.

Shyam Sundar Goswami, 1999, p 66.

With one-pointed attention, you must feel and perceive that this universe and your body are simultaneously one with God consciousness. Then the rise of that supreme God consciousness takes place.

Vijnana Bhairava Tantra 36.

Or by aiming at the pure element (*shuddha tattva*, the supreme Shiva) of Shiva, he possesses Shiva's unlimited energy.

Shiva Sutra I.16

In the Pratyabhijnahrdayam text of Kashmir Shaivism the Centre is given an interesting link to the *sushumna nadi*. Singh (1987, p 41) describes it thus:

Sutra 17: By the development of the centre is acquisition of the bliss of the spirit. By the development of the centre can the bliss of the spirit be obtained. *Samvit* [universal or supreme consciousness] or the power of consciousness is called the centre, because it is the support or ground of every thing in the world. In the individual, it is symbolized by the central *nadi*, i.e., *sushumna*. When the central consciousness in man develops or when the *sushumna nadi* develops, then is there the bliss of the universal consciousness.

In *sutra* 18 various means for the development of the centre are listed. The main method of Pratyabhijna is *madhya-vikasa* (the development or unfoldment of the centre) where the word *madhya* refers to the Central Consciousness which is *Samvit*, the pure I-consciousness or pure subjectivity. It also refers to the *sushumna* or central *pranic nadi*. This method is *vikalpakshaya*, the dissolution of all *vikalpas* or thoughts. One concentrates on the heart centre, not allowing any thoughts to arise and leading the mind to a thoughtless (*avikalpa*) condition while holding the Self as the real experient in the focus of consciousness. One thereby develops the *madhya* or consciousness of central reality and enters the *turiya* and then the *turiyatita* states.

Other methods are listed, of which *sankoca* and *vikasa* of *shakti* are notable in this context for developing the *madhya* (which also means to develop the *prana-shakti* in the *sushumna*) (Singh, 1987, p 42, p 152). *Sankoca* of *shakti* means to withdraw the consciousness from going outward through the senses, turning it inwards towards the Self, the Centre of Consciousness – in other words, *pratyahara* or sensory withdrawal. Even while the senses are functioning and the mind goes outward through them to external objects, one withdraws the attention from them and turns it inwards to the inner Reality which is the source and background of all activity. *Vikasa* of *shakti* involves holding the consciousness steadily within, concentrating on the inner Reality, even while the senses are open to and perceive their external objects. It is concentration on the inner reality even while the senses are active and open – the practice of *bhairavi mudra*. *Sankoca* is withdrawal of attention from external objects, while *vikasa* is concentration of attention on the inner consciousness, not allowing it to go out at all even when the cognitive senses are open and active. "It means remaining steady within like a gold pillar, even while the senses are directed towards their objects." (Singh, 1987, p 153). The same practices are described in the Spanda Karikas in verse 7 of section three (Singh, 1980, p 139) where he translates the commentary as: ". . . if the yogi gets established in his imperishable Self, viz., the spiritual Consciousness, . . . if he is steadily absorbed in that state, either by withdrawing his sense, etc. within himself (*sankoca*) as a tortoise withdraws its limbs within itself or by the device of the expansion of all-embracing consciousness (*vikasa*), then he acquires omniscience, and omnipotence appropriate to *Shiva* everywhere."

Singh (1987, p 42, p 153) describes another way to achieve *sankoca* and *vikasa* of *shakti* that relates to the *kundalini*. When *prana* and *apana* enter the *sushumna nadi* and the *kundalini* rises the *yogin* leads it to and restrains it at the *ajna chakra* (condition of *urdhva-kundalini*) and then practices *prasara* (*vikasa*) and *vishranti* (*sankoca*). As he emerges from *samadhi* he retains its experience which is practicing *prasara* or *vikasa*, and merging back into *samadhi* and resting in that state is *vishranti* or *sankoca*. For these processes to work, clearly the Centre of Consciousness has to be experienced at least to some degree by the aspirant. Working with these processes will then help to crystallize that experience make the identity shift from self to Self.

The same idea is expressed in Section 1 of the Kashmir Shaivism text Spanda-Karikas (Singh, 1980, p 100). This is a collection of verses (*karika*) on the *spanda* which literally means a "throb." It refers to the creative pulsation or vibration in the motionless Consciousness of Shiva which brings about the manifestation, maintenance and withdrawal of the universe. The route to *Shiva* (Consciousness) is through *Shakti* (Energy). The 21st verse is translated by Singh as: "Therefore, one should be always on the alert for the discernment of the *Spanda* principle. Such a person attains his essential state (as *spanda*) even in the waking condition in short time." Constant awareness of the divine not only in meditation but also during daily life in the waking state results in a transformation of the mind from within that brings the acquisition of Integral Divine Consciousness. The commentator refers to the *Bhagavad Gita* XII, 2: "Those who merging their mind in me, always united with me, wait upon me." Then by ever-present absorption in It the practitioner becomes fully enlightened and liberated while living. Singh quotes Utpalabhatta as to how that discernment should be practiced: "I am only pure Consciousness: this world is only a glorious manifestation of myself."

Hints on Working with the Presence in Meditation

In the final phase of the standard meditation as described above, the *mantra* is refined into the Silence, and the meditator rests in the stillness of that Silence. When the Presence dawns as an actual experience, however subtle or faint, that Silence moves from just stillness into a conscious, still Presence, Awareness or Witness. The pulsation of the *mantra* will be felt in the centre or core of that Presence. Simply rest in the stillness of that Presence with the mind one-pointedly fixed on the pulsation of the *mantra* if it is also present. Additional steps can be tried to enhance or stabilize the experience to see what works best for the individual practitioner. One will be guided by intuition as to what to do. Here are examples to give the practitioner some hints:

- Let go of the *mantra* pulsation and any passing thoughts and let the Presence Itself be the principal focus. Like a figure/ground reversal, bring the background which is the Presence forward, and let all other mental content fade into the periphery. Later with the movement from Presence into Being any remaining mental content will be experienced from and as contained within an encompassing, transcendent space of pure existence, Being or Isness.

- Use a modification of the Sedona releasing method. Welcome the Presence, allow it to be as fully present as you can. Then mentally and gently ask yourself: Could I just allow/accept That? Would I? When? Repeat four or five times and observe what happens.

- If the attention is momentarily carried away by thoughts, emotions, images or other mental content, just note the distraction and then bring the attention back to the Presence. If the distraction is persistent, then try to release it: observe it, welcome it, allow it to be fully present, then ask yourself: Could I just let this go? Would I? When? Alternatively observe the thought and ask: To whom has this thought arisen? To me! Who am I? This approach of Ramana Maharshi (1988) tends to return the mind into the Presence and release the distraction.

"When other thoughts arise, one should not pursue them, but should inquire: 'To whom do they arise?' It does not matter how many thoughts arise. As each thought arises, one should inquire with diligence, 'To whom has this thought arisen?' The answer that would emerge would be 'To me.' Thereupon if one inquires, 'Who am I?' the mind will go back to its source, and the thought that arose will become quiescent." (Ramana Maharshi, 1988, p 4).

- The breath can also be used to stabilize and intensify the experience of the Presence. Simply breathe as thought the breath were flowing through It. Or on inhalation intensify It, as though pulling It into the mind, and on exhalation relax, surrender, let It go and expand. Using *sumeru* breathing up and down the spine, with inhalation lift the energy up the spine as though it were a bucket of water and "pour" it into the Presence, relaxing on exhalation down the spine. Or imagine a wave of energy up the spine on inhalation crashing into the Presence like a wave on a beach, flowing back down the spine on exhalation pulling the Presence with it down the spine into the *chakras* and *sushumna* channel.

- With meditation in action, hold the Presence in background awareness and carry out all actions as if they were flowing from that Centre through you as a surrendered instrument. Give up being the doer of action. Karma Yoga is the experience of action flowing from the Centre of Consciousness. Initially this is most easily practiced with something mechanical like walking or walking meditation.

Practices with the Centre of Consciousness

Other activities by which the aspirant can work to stabilize the Presence can include:

- Walking in nature. One can also do this with one's *Guru mantra* or *mantras* such as *akhanda* or *mrityunjaya.*

- *Chankramanam* or walking meditation, but done in the Presence. It may feel at times as though the mind were still in the Presence and the body walking separately within that Space. For details see Swami Veda Bharati's booklet on *Contemplative Walking* (2000), Swami Satyananda Saraswati's text on Kriya Yoga (1981, p 729), or manuals on Buddhist *Vipassana* or Insight meditation (Salzberg & Goldstein, 2001, p 52).

- Observe a period of silence or take a silence retreat. The trick here is that all activities are carried out immersed in the stillness of the Presence, regardless of whether one actually speaks or not. Keeping silence of speech facilitates that inner absorption. For details please see Swami Veda Bharati's booklets on *Silence* (1999) and *Five Pillars of Sadhana* (1997).

- Keep a spiritual journal (Niranjanananda, 1993c, p 157).

- Practice eating and carrying out routine physical tasks such as doing dishes, cleaning or gardening in Silence. By Silence, again is meant doing the activity immersed in the stillness of the Presence and as though the activity was flowing from the Presence.

- Carry out Yogic practices such as *asana* and *pranayama* immersed in and as though flowing from the Presence. This requires intense bare attention in the Now and full awareness as a Witness to the practice without evaluating, judging or thinking about each movement – just observe. It is mindfulness, but immersed in the Presence. If practices are done mechanically from habit without moment to moment awareness one receives only about 20% of their benefit. Some have even recommended practicing a month on and a month off to avoid practices becoming a habit. We would prefer continual practice, but with mindfulness.

- Consider taking a Yoga retreat in a foreign country with a very different culture. This undoes habitual behavior and breaks psychophysical conditioning so that the Presence can slip into the gap thus created.

- Swami Veda Bharati recommends hourly one minute meditations to turn the mind repeatedly back to the Centre. For a moment be still. Relax the body with an exhalation. And remember the *mantra* flowing with the breath with the mind turned towards the Presence. During a busy day this simple process can be very hard to remember to do. Use a kitchen timer set hourly to remind one to do the practice. Or link each meditation to the beginning or end of transitions between routine daily activities (Veda Bharati, 2004, p 88).

- Increase the length and number of meditation sessions per day. Most students do one or two sessions morning and/or evening for twenty minutes or half an hour each. Lengthen each session to 45 minutes or an hour each. Or increase the number of sessions to three or four daily by adding sessions before lunch and before dinner. Avoid the period between noon and 3PM. But a short and fully aware practice is preferred to a long one that is filled with sleep and daydreaming. When increasing length of time work within your capacity. Quality is always to be preferred over quantity. Increase your capacity for length gradually. The objective is to spend as much time as possible immersed in the silence of the Presence.

- Give your practice an extra stretch with *purashcharanas*, but they should be done in the Presence. Like interval training with exercise, they will increase your capacity for meditation. Participate in the annual *Guru* Purnima celebration which revolves around this kind of extra boost to practice for the 40 days ending on the day of the full moon each July. Completing 125,000 repetitions of the *Guru mantra* during this period, sometimes with some *malas* of *gayatri*, *mrityunjaya* or other special *mantra* that the teacher may assign is a usual type of practice. The teacher may also assign a *purashcharana* of a special *mantra* like *gayatri* as 100,000 times the number of syllables in the *mantra* (2.4 million repetitions). This should only be done under careful supervision by an experienced teacher and can take up to five years to complete depending on how much time can be made available for it daily. All such purifying practices should be done immersed in the Presence as much as possible.

- Practice exercises that enhance the capacity for witnessing. Periods of mindfulness meditation can be done. Count the breath one to five and five to one, then extend to one to ten and ten to one, etc. How many breaths does it take to go from one place to another, such as home from yoga class? Swami Rama advised counting from one to 100 and back or even one to 1000 and back without losing the count. In doing such practices, adopt the musician's rule of five. A passage is played over and over on an instrument until it can be played perfectly five times in a row. If there is any mistake (or the mind loses the count in the case of meditation), even at the fourth repetition, you go back to one and start all over.

- Adopt attitudes that keep you present, like curiosity. Be like a banker and approach all things with interest! The key to meditation is focus and awareness. And the key to focus and concentration on something is to be interested in it.

- Develop a conditioned response linking the *mantra* with the Presence. When the *mantra* is repeated it invokes the Presence automatically. Then keep the *Guru mantra japa* going at all times.

- Repeatedly throughout the day pause and turn inwards mentally and check that the Presence is there in the background, or whether it has really gone and dedicated practice is needed to reestablish It. Initially for a very long time expect that the Presence will come and go, sometimes over long periods, until it is fully stabilized. This is a work of many years. Our habitual conditioning is not so easily altered and this is a radical change to our experience of inner space. Based on modern neuroscience one suspects that rewiring of neural networks (neuroplasticity) could be involved as a physiological basis of support for stabilizing the higher states of consciousness of the Presence, and this is a slow process that comes about with long and persistent practice.

The energy flowing from above with the Presence can at times be intense. The Centre may come and go periodically to give your nervous system a rest while your energy fields readjust to the higher flow. Each step has to be integrated into all of the *koshas* (energetic sheaths) of the personality. If some sheaths surge ahead of others and come out of synchrony illness can result. Do not push the process. Work with patience within your comfortable capacity.

The objective of all of these practices and strategies – and many more you will devise on your own (these are just examples to stimulate your own creativity) – is to make the Presence *sahaja* – spontaneously available as a natural state of awareness at all times and in all situations, twenty-four hours a day. In this way the Presence is stabilized or crystallized, and can be recalled into awareness consistently at any time.

32

Dharana, Pranidhana *and* Bhavana

The Central Role of *Dharana*

In the introduction to her commentary on the *Vijnana Bhairava Tantra* (2003, p 29), Swami Satyasangananda Saraswati of the Bihar School of Yoga develops in detail the importance and central role played by *dharana* in the Tantric meditations described in this text.

Dharana means "to hold" or "to possess." It is a state that is obtained when you can hold or possess something to the exclusion of all else in *chidakasha*, the space of Consciousness. *Dharana* is a total focus on any one object, thought, idea, feeling, memory, person or act. It can be practiced on any object, image or person, on psychic centers, *nadis*, or on thought, idea or feeling. It reveals the hidden power of the chosen symbol and opens up new dimensions of awareness. It is effortful. Correctly done, it leads to *dhyana* (meditation) spontaneously, which is a state of complete and spontaneous or effortless absorption in the object of *dharana*, from which one is led without any effort to *samadhi*.

In the *Yoga-Sutra dharana* is the sixth limb of *ashtanga yoga*. Patanjali says that "Binding the mind to one place is *dharana*." It refers to a one-pointed focus on something, a way to focus the awareness which is normally scattered by external perception. *Dhyana* which follows it is a state of total, unbroken awareness of that something. Total awareness means that only one thing and no other occupies the mind, be it form, or idea, feeling, action or experience. In selecting an object it is important to choose something that can spontaneously and effortlessly as well as totally absorb your attention – body, mind and soul. This total absorption can then lead to *samadhi*.

Awareness rests in the present moment in concentration. Fix the mind on an object and remain focused in the present. Keep bringing the wandering mind back to the object until with practice awareness becomes steady, fixed and focused on the object and on the space it occupies in the present moment or time. Gradually these three (time, space and object) merge into one another and there is an explosive experience at the nucleus or *bindu* of the psychic centre where they meet.

Without perfection of *dharana* no further progress can be made on the spiritual path. It is the gateway to higher states of awareness. Once it is mastered the aspirant need make no further effort towards enlightenment, for *dhyana* and *samadhi* follow as a natural consequence. Once the Centre of Consciousness is realized then effort is used to sustain that experience of inner illumination in day-to-day life. So *dharana* is the point of transition to higher dimensions of awareness.

In *dharana* awareness is completely withdrawn from the senses and crystallized at one point. Concentration trains the awareness to hold onto whatever object has been chosen without fluctuation. It is not a process of thinking. It is a process of inner perception, of inner seeing. The thinking, conceptual mind plays no part. Indeed, if the thinking mind is active then *dharana* cannot occur.

The faculty of awareness (*chetana*), which is subtler than the mind, is active in *dharana*. This awareness illumines the object on which concentration is focused. This occurs naturally when one tries to solve a problem. One quiets the mind and focuses the awareness on the problem. The aspirant trains this awareness to focus inwards and crystallize at one point. Once this is accomplished, the inner path that the aspirant is to traverse and later the destination are gradually revealed. Initially that inner point, that object of concentration, is hazy and may feel unfamiliar. Later it will attract the aspirant's awareness like nothing has attracted him or her before because of the bliss (*anandam*) that is generated from within; awareness becomes Awareness, the Presence within. The meditator is pervaded by feelings of well-being, love, oneness and totality. But until this happens one keeps practicing.

The Dalai Lama reported a conversation with a Tibetan monk who said that learning to concentrate the mind was the hardest thing he had to do in his whole life.

> "*Dharana* is an invaluable accomplishment that surpasses all others; it is the epitome of human achievement. All other achievements pale in comparison."
> Swami Satyasangananda Saraswati (2003), p 33

Previously we have talked about the use of meditation to raise the level of energy or vibration of the mind field. Such a refined mind can then hold higher Consciousness. From studies of neuroplasticity in modern neuroscience one can expect the prolonged practice of *dharana* to be accompanied by a reorganization of synaptic connectivity and the formation of new neuronal connections – a rewiring of the brain itself to become an enhanced physical receiver for higher states of consciousness.

A recent study using MRI imaging as healthy subjects participated in tests of memory and attention has shown that distraction may underlie memory problems with aging (Gazzaley et al, 2005). Focusing on relevant information is not enough. Attention involves both the need to focus on relevant information as well as suppressing irrelevant and distracting information. With aging the ability to focus attention on relevant information is preserved but there is a deficit in suppressing distractions.

To attain this kind of metal receptivity one refines the inner tools of perception that make up the inner instrument or *antahkarana* (*manas, chitta, buddhi* and *ahamkara*) until they vibrate at the frequency of higher Consciousness (*chetana*). *Dharana* is the method for refining the *antahkarana*. It brings the scattered forces of the mind to focus on one thing to the exclusion of all else, thereby generating the one-pointed or *ekagrata* state. Eventually you transcend yourself, cease to exist as an I-thought, leaving only the experience of Consciousness or pure Awareness, and attain a fully controlled state (*nirodha*) that corresponds to *samadhi*.

Experiences in meditation prior to mastery of *dharana* come from the conscious and subconscious minds. When *dharana* merges into *dhyana* inner experiences have their source in the causal or unconscious mind.

> "Spiritual experience begins only when *dharana* has been perfected and the state of *dhyana* dawns."
>
> Swami Satyasangananda Saraswati (2003), p 43

Thus in Classical Yoga *pratyahara, dharana, dhyana* and *samadhi* form a natural progression. *Pratyahara* is perfected so that awareness is withdrawn from the external world into internal perception. *Dharana* is a natural consequence of *pratyahara* where awareness is internalized and fixed on one point for a period of time. Then the consciousness begins to flow freely. When there is no break, obstruction, diversion or distraction the flow of consciousness gains intensity and *dhyana* occurs. Then *dhyana* develops naturally into *samadhi* or inner illumination. All four of these steps progress like a natural process of growth.

To be carried out safely the inner journey has to be grounded. The Centre of Consciousness acts as that ground. *Dharana* is an essential process to train and give direction to the mind and the awareness so that they do not fly out of control. The ordinary mind is directed by and follows the ten senses (*indriyas*) – the five cognitive senses (*jnanendriyas*) the five active senses (*karmendriyas*). The mind follows wherever they lead. *Dharana* is the mental training that frees one from this influence and allows one to focus and direct the awareness as one desires without interference from the senses. Fixing the awareness at one point gives the mind a specific direction in which to travel. The awareness must be trained before it is allowed to roam freely. Until concentration is mastered the mind must not be allowed free flight which can be damaging and even irrevocable. Without a point of reference, a ground, the awareness can wander off for long periods and even get lost in egoism and uncharted dimensions of Consciousness. Without grounding the result can be insanity and the inability to distinguish what is real. Thus it is fortunate indeed that *dharana* guards the gateway to higher Consciousness and must be mastered before it can be entered.

For this reason in Tantra symbols that are used for *dharana* are *mantra, yantra* and *mandala*, or sound, form and light. The object of focus becomes a base for awareness so that it does not get lost when it moves into the unknown. This is why the object of *dharana* is one that the meditator feels strongly and naturally drawn to (like a personal *mantra* received through initiation). If there is a natural attraction for the object of concentration then the mind will stay fixed on it and not be easily distracted but keep returning to it. Then the awareness will not wander off for long periods and get lost. *Dharana* is the bridge that allows for safe passage from external to internal reality.

A witnessing attitude (*sakshi bhava*) or stance is critical for success. Two sources of content fill the mind during meditation. At first the lid is taken off the subconscious mind and its contents erupt into awareness, disturbing the meditation process. Later inner psychic experiences may manifest. It is important not to get caught in either of these phenomena, to become attached to or to engage them so that the awareness is carried off and the symbol which is the object of meditation and the meditation process itself are lost. Whatever comes up one must continue *dharana* on the symbol despite these inner experiences; keep bringing the awareness back to the *mantra* over and over and not get carried away.

This awareness is maintained by a mental stance or attitude of witnessing. Part of you does the practice and another part watches you do the practice and witnesses your experience from a position meta or beyond or "above." When the Centre of Consciousness becomes an inner experience the witnessing moves into that Presence, which is a stage beyond even witnessing. Witnessing is of the mind, but the Presence transcends the mind. Two things result: non-attachment and release of the disturbing mental content with consequent purification of thought and emotion. One is able to continue the inner journey through the subconscious and unconscious mind with *dharana* on the symbol directly to the goal without being diverted, sidetracked or lost.

Swami Satyasangananda Saraswati (2003, p 71) also points out that witnessing leads to the development of dual awareness. Eventually this is critical for crystallizing the experience of the Presence when it dawns. It is a simple practice conceptually but very difficult to attain and to maintain. The awareness expands to include both the inner and the outer worlds and experiences simultaneously. Most of us can hold one or the other with some clarity, but not both together, much less as a unified single witness to both. Eventually Awareness will expand from the waking state through the states of dreaming, deep sleep and into *turiya* as a simultaneous homogeneity. Meditation is not immersing oneself in inner experience alone, but achieving a homogeneous Awareness (the Centre of Consciousness as Presence) that holds full knowledge of both the outer and inner worlds simultaneously with all experience included. In this way *dharana* can penetrate deep into the inner world and still retain the outer awareness of the symbol or *mantra*.

Pranidhana and *Bhavana*

In Part Four we dealt in some detail with *abhyasa*, and particularly with *ishvara pranidhana* or practicing the presence of God, or practicing the Presence (the Awareness aspect of the Centre of Consciousness) in this context. We suggest the reader review this material at this point in comparison with our statement here that the Centre of Consciousness becomes the object of meditation.

In Part Four we pointed out in the context of *mantra* practice that *pranidhana* (the idea of placing the awareness within) means *bhavana*. We wrote that, "*Bhavana* is cultivated concentration. It involves impressing the object of concentration (*bhavya*) again and again onto the mind field by preventing any other object from entering the mind." We hope that now this key devotional practice of *Ishvara pranidhana* as described in the *Yoga-Sutra* is clearer as it relates to the manifestation of the Centre of Consciousness into awareness. It quite literally becomes practicing the Presence (of God, the Centre of Consciousness). This why in Part Four *ishvara pranidhana* was the centerpiece for our discussion.

Paramahamsa Yogananda (2004, p 492) addresses *pranidhana* and *bhavana* from the Bhakti perspective of personal, silent, devotional prayer – "prayer that touches the heart of God."

"Sometimes, no loud or even whispered words can I pray; for when deep feeling for God possesses you, you cannot utter any words. That love is secret within, an inner communion, silently giving its oblations into the Spirit. Like a sacred fire, that love burns the darkness from around the soul, and in that light one beholds the mightiness of Spirit."

Yogananda calls this "the method of divine romanticism in seclusion," by which he means the scientific art of interiorization of the mind by *pratyahara, dharana* and *dhyana* into interiorized silence where true prayer and divine communion are both possible and effective. Shutting off the distraction of sensory inputs is one aspect, but failing also to quiet the tumult and distraction of the mind is like asking a friend to call you on the telephone and then keeping the line occupied with incoming and outgoing calls so your friend can get only a busy signal, and then wondering why your friend failed to answer your request to call. Yogananda writes that "God hears all prayers; but His children do not always hear His response." To succeed one must master the process of conscious interiorization into the inner silence. Saint Teresa of Avila described it as entering the "interior castle" to commune with Christ. "They become markedly conscious that they are gradually retiring within themselves. . . . I think I have read that they are like a hedgehog or a tortoise withdrawing into itself [referring to the *Bhagavad Gita* 11:58]." Yogananda interprets Jesus' teaching: "But thou, when thou prayest, enter into thy closet (withdraw the mind into the silence within), and when thou hast shut thy door (the door of the senses), pray to thy Father which is in secret (in the inner transcendent divine consciousness); and thy Father which seeth in secret shall reward thee openly (shall bless you with the ever new Bliss of His Being)." As the Biblical phrase says: "Be still and know that I AM God." The voice of the Inner Teacher can only be heard communicating through the silence of intuition when mental restlessness ceases. "In the devotee's silence God's silence ceases." Swami Rama (2005) writes of the sequence of purification (silencing mental restlessness) leading to silence and then to union. Yogananda writes: "Silencing the thoughts means tuning them in to God. That is when true prayer begins. . . . He speaks to us in silence, telling us to come Home."

This devotional process leads to a constant holding of the Centre of Consciousness. Yogananda (2004, pp 526–529) describes this in terms of putting God first in one's daily life. "During the busyness of the day, the true God-seeker spiritualizes all actions with the thought of Him. He learns to keep the mind most of the time at the Christ center, the *Kutastha* center [*ajna chakra*] of the *yogi*, and finds the Infinite Christ pouring over his consciousness wave after wave of quiet heavenly joy." This is meditation in action. He then refers to the *Bhagavad Gita* VI: 30: "He who perceives Me everywhere and beholds everything in Me never loses sight of Me, nor do I ever lose sight of him." Yogananda continues: "When the devotee puts his mind on God, he will see that out of the invisible, out of the unseen skies, a perceptible Presence will speak to him. It is possible to talk to God. His voice can be heard in words, as well as through intuitive feeling, if the devotee loves Him deeply enough and refuses to give up. The desire for His response must be with all one's heart." This is the Centre as the Inner Teacher.

In his introduction to the Vijnanabhairava Tantra, Singh (2003, p xviii) describes Abhinavagupta's exposition of *bhavana* from the Tantrasara. Thoughts are the nature of mind. So mentally grasp one pure (*shuddha*) thought (*vikalpa*), specifically that of the highest I-consciousness, the real Self as

Shiva. Imagine fervently with all faith that you are *Shiva.* This pure thought will eliminate all other thoughts and eventually even the pure thought also ceases. Then the empirical psychological small self dissolves and the identity shift puts you into your metempirical, metaphysical Self. First a Self-realized *sadguru* initiates the practitioner into the mysteries of the revealed texts (*agama*) to gain the irrefutable conviction that the essential Self is *Shiva.* Next comes *sat-tarka* – training the mind to being harmoniously one with the truth of the essential Self being *Shiva,* which will culminate in *bhavana.* "*Bhavana* is the power of spiritual attention, a total dedication of the mind to one central thought, a nostalgia of the soul, a spiritual thrust towards the source of one's being." This process of *bhavana* finally becomes a pure meditation and knowledge (*shuddha vidya*) that creates the identity shift in which the psychological small self or I is swallowed up into the essential metaphysical I. The process is discussed in verse 49 of the Vijnanabhairava Tantra.

An Inner Perceptual Paradox

There is an important paradox here. How is it that the aspirant first experiences the Centre of Consciousness as an object, if the ultimate realization is oneness with It? How is it possible for the self to see the Self as an object when all is a unity of consciousness?

An abstract way to think about it is to accept the experience as an aspect of normal subject-object consciousness in which the individual personality lives from day to day. It is an illusion of duality. Another way to consider it is that the Self sees Itself as a reflection in the inner surface of the *buddhi* like a mirror once the *buddhi* is clarified sufficiently through the purification of Yogic practice. How else can pure subjectivity experience itself except as a reflection? A reflection will give the illusion of duality, that the Centre of Consciousness is an object other than the observer. The texts put the same idea differently: *Shiva* (consciousness) recognizes Himself by his reflection in *Shakti* (energy; manifestation), and so *Shakti* is the path to *Shiva.*

The next step is to come to the realization that I (the observer) am That, as the Vedantic *maha-vakya* puts it: *Tat tvam asi.* This is done by the process of "as if," acting as if I and That are the same. This relates to the process of Ramana Maharshi's Who am I inquiry. In his introduction to Ramana Maharshi's pamphlet (1988), T.M.P. Mahadevan elegantly summarizes this Vedantic method as follows:

> The mind consists of thoughts. The "I" thought is the first to arise in the mind. When the inquiry "Who am I?" is persistently pursued, all other thoughts get destroyed, and finally the "I" thought itself vanishes leaving the supreme non-dual Self alone. The false identification of the Self with the phenomena of non-self such as the body and mind, thus ends, and there is illumination, *sakshatkara.* The process of enquiry, of course, is not an easy one. As one inquires "Who am I?", other thoughts will rise; but as these arise, one should not yield to them by following them; on the contrary, one should ask "To whom do they arise?" In order to do this, one has to be extremely vigilant. Through consistent enquiry one should make the mind stay in its source, without allowing it to

wander away and get lost in the mazes of thought created by itself. All other disciplines such as breath-control and meditation on the forms of God should be regarded as auxiliary practices. They are useful so far as they help the mind to become quiescent and one-pointed. For the mind that has gained skill in concentration Self-enquiry becomes comparatively easy. It is by ceaseless enquiry that the thoughts are destroyed and the Self realized – the plenary Reality in which there is not even the "I" thought, the experience which is referred to as "Silence."

Swami Niranjanananda (1995, p 135) has a Tantric version of this form of self-inquiry as follows:

- Sit in a comfortable posture with the eyes closed.
- Observe the body for areas of pain and pleasure, comfort and discomfort.
- After recognizing what is happening in the physical structure, say to yourself, "I am observing the body, but I am not the body. I am feeling the [identify the discomfort or comfort] in the body, but I am not identifying with either the state of comfort or discomfort." This should take no more than 5 minutes and dissociates you from the body.
- Now apply the same process to the mind (thoughts and feelings). Recognize states of comfort and discomfort in the mind. With each recognition dissociate yourself from the mind with, "I am not the mind, nor am I the experiences of pain and pleasure associated with the mind."
- "If I am not the body or the mind, then what am I?"
    At that moment focus the awareness either in *chidakasha* (the space at the eyebrow centre) or *hridayakasha* (the space at the heart centre), wherever you initially feel comfortable.
    Do not fight with yourself over which to use because this re-identifies you with the mind.
- When comfortable in your space, visualize and identify yourself with a flame or a point of white light. With the attention firmly fixed on the white light or flame, say to your self, "Light is my real nature. I am not the body; I am not the mind. I am not the experiences related with the body or the mind. Light is my nature." Identify with the light for no more than ten minutes.
- When you begin to focus on and identify with the light begin repeating your *mantra* or Om (can be chanted aloud) a few times or for a *mala* for however long you feel comfortable with the practice. With each chant of the *mantra* feel the mind merging with the *mantra* and the light.
- When the practice ends gradually begin to return to the mind and body again. This can be done just before going to sleep. In which case stretch out your legs and go to sleep.

Niranjanananda notes that this practice has several aspects: 1) gradual dissociation of the mind from the body; 2) awareness of the interaction between the mind and the body; 3) gradual dissociation of the consciousness from the mind; and 4) awareness of the nature of consciousness as a state of pure Being and harmony. If you begin with the *chidakasha*, he also advises that once stabilized in the head space and comfortable with concentration on the symbol there, you then move down and end up in *hridayakasha*, starting afresh to balance the heart space and focus yourself there. This is reminiscent of Aziz's relaxation into Presence and then energetic descent into Being.

Franklin Merrell-Wolff (1994, p 29) used concentration on the subject pole of subject-object consciousness.

> . . . I isolated the subjective moment from the relative manifold of objective consciousness, . . . and the result was Emptiness, darkness, and Silence, i.e., Consciousness with no object.

Now why is all this important? The *Yoga Vasishtha* repeatedly points out that Consciousness has an important and peculiar characteristic. If Consciousness holds a notion (a belief about what is real) for sufficiently long enough then that notion manifests as an experience. What the meditator believes about the experience will determine the outcome. The meditator has two choices to believe about the experience of the Centre of Consciousness. As the ego, the small self, I experience the Presence as an object as a background to the mind. The fundamental assumption here is that I and the Presence are separate and not one, and that is what will be experienced. This is a dualistic position and is characteristic of devotional approaches. By contrast Advaita is asking one to take a much bigger leap. If I believe I am seeing Myself as a reflection in *buddhi* then I am in reality That. *Tat tvam asi*, That Thou art. This moves me to transcend the mind into union with that Reality which is consciousness-without-an-object or nonduality and there is no need for an ego identification as the observer. The observed and the observer are one. This is why an accurate map of the journey is so necessary. The underlying beliefs and unquestioned assumptions of that map direct the outcome of the process. Working from this nondualistic set of assumptions will lead one with practice to realize union with the Self.

This perceptual paradox is referred to in the philosophy of Kashmir Shaivism. In *sutra* 14 of the Pratyabhijnahrdayam it is asked if *citi* is non-differentiating consciousness intrinsically, then why is it characterized by a sense of difference at the level of the individual (Singh, 1987, p 40)?

Kshemaraja addresses this paradox in his commentary on the ninth verse of section three of the Spanda Karikas, a text of Kashmir Shaivism (Singh, 1980, p 245). In his exposition on Kshemaraja's commentary, Singh writes:

> . . . when the mind is deeply engrossed in one thought, it is completely stilled, it is restricted from indulging in another thought. It is at such a moment that the met-empirical Self reveals itself. Mind is the slayer of the Real. When the slayer is slain, then the Real reveals itself.

This is a description of *dhyana*. Or more precisely, the method of effecting the identity shift – to use Classical Yoga terms, is by *samyama* (the integrated practice of *dharana, dhyana* and *samadhi*) on the Centre of Consciousness; at its height *samadhi* is absorption.

Singh goes on to comment on the paradox:

> . . . one has to be on one's guard in grasping the Real. If he wants to know it as an object, he will fail miserably, for it is the Eternal Subject which can never be reduced to an object. . . . since the meta-physical Self cannot be objectified, there has to be an effortless awareness of it as I-consciousness shorn of all its external trappings.

In support, Singh then quotes Ramakantha:

> This experience has to be regarded subjectively as "It is I, the Highest Self," the fount and source of every thing, distinct from anything else. Its nature cannot be grasped objectively as "this," like sound, etc.

The Centre of Consciousness and Death

It is worth a word or two on the implication of the opening of the Centre of Consciousness for death and dying. We have gone into this subject in more detail from the perspective of the Himalayan Tradition elsewhere (Jerry & Jerry, 2001; Veda Bharati, 1979b), especially around the idea that both sleep and meditation are considered to be models for the dying process. If you die with the awareness of the Presence, that is to say, if you die consciously, then you merely drop your body in exchange for a new one. But if you die as a small self, an ego, fully identified as an individualized personality and a body, then you truly experience a death. The reader should fully contemplate the implications of this idea. It makes a strong incentive for practice during life and a deep appreciation of the value of a human incarnation.

The Tibetan Buddhist tradition in particular has an extensive literature on various aspects of death, dying and the afterlife. Practices of consciousness transference are taught. With the awareness of the Presence as a direct experience this process is simplified. Elsewhere we have noted the oneness of the master's consciousness with the Centre of Consciousness (Jerry & Jerry, 2001). In meditation in the *guru chakra* a disciple may sense his or her master's presence as a kind of "flavor" or "coloring" within the Presence, so that the object of meditation becomes a kind of integration of *mantra*, master and Centre.

The whole point of our discussion of the key importance of *dharana* above is to gain the ability to hold the object of meditation effortlessly and without interruption – which is *dhyana*. Thus one is taught to enter sleep this way (as a meditation) and also to enter the dying process this way as a serene surrender into the integrated *mantra*/master/Presence awareness. The *guru's* grace is thereby invoked. To do so is to die consciously with the most auspicious final thought, for the Tradition says that one's final thoughts have the greatest influence on the character of the afterlife and rebirth.

To acquire the ability to concentrate and enter the spontaneous flow of meditation reliably can be the best practice in life to prepare for consciousness transference at death. The mastery also of *sumeru* breathing prepares one to lift the life energy up the spine and through the *brahmarandhra* at the crown of the head into that Presence. At the very least, the *mantra* will be your friend and guide. Practice it diligently into *ajapajapa* so that it pulses continuously and effortlessly all the time and thus is available at the critical moment of transition when the mind and personal will may be confused.

33

The Centre of Consciousness as Sound

It is said in the Tradition that some are led by light and some by sound. To this point we have emphasized the former, in keeping with a predominance of the visual sensory modality in most Westerners. Now we wish to comment on the latter for those in whom the auditory sensory modality is more dominant.

The Universe as Sound

We have described the individual, as well as the universe of which it is a holographic subset, as Consciousness (*Shiva*) enrobed in layers of vibrational energy (*Shakti*). Consciousness manifests in many degrees and can be experienced as sound, light, form and idea. Sound and light are physical vibrational energies while form and idea are constituents of thought in the vibrational mental field. *Shiva* and *Shakti* have both cosmic and individual aspects, and at the individual level appear as dual forces because of the obscuring power of *maya*, the force of the illusion which is inherent in the *Shakti* principle. Together *Shiva* and *Shakti* give rise to the unmanifest (*avyakta*) and manifest (*vyakta*). David Bohm's (1983) idea of the implicate and explicate realities is a more modern analogy.

The first manifestations of the cosmic process of creation are known in the Tantric tradition as *nada*, *bindu* and *kalaa*. *Nada* means vibration. In the unmanifest cosmos it exists as the cosmic vibration or *spandana* – the dynamic aspect of *Shiva* or primordial pulsation (Berendt, 1983). The doctrine of vibration or *Spanda* is a key aspect of the philosophy of Kashmir Shaivism (Dyczkowski, 1987). In manifest creation *nada* exists as sound of various frequencies. *Bindu* is a point or nucleus, a compact mass of *shakti* gathered into an undifferentiated point that serves as the source or substratum of the whole cosmos. It is a point of potential energy where descending Consciousness first emerges into diversity and multiplicity. The word is sometimes used as a symbol for creation and as a symbol of *Shiva*. *Kalaa* is a force or ray emanating from the nucleus or *bindu* because of vibrations created by *nada*. This cosmic manifestation of both *Shiva* and *Shakti*, of Consciousness and energy in the form of *nada*, *bindu* and *kalaa* mutually interact to give rise to all of the subtle and gross elements comprising the manifested universe as well as the human being. In Kashmir Shaivism (Lakshmanjoo, 2002) these *tattvas* or elements, principles, number thirty-six and cover the entire continuum of human existence and experience on causal, subtle and gross levels. The number of elements differs in various philosophical systems, for example, Samkhya (Larson, 1979), but the basic idea is similar.

According to Tantra, at the transcendental level Consciousness begins its expression from the primal point or *bindu* from which issues the primal sound or *nada*. The cosmic sound of *nada* is the first evolute in the scheme of creation. *Shiva*, the supreme Consciousness, creates by sending forth his creative power or *Shakti* who uses her inherent attributes of knowledge (*jnana*), action (*kriya*) and will (*iccha*) to create a *spandana* or vibration which gives rise to *nada*, the cosmic sound. Thus the primal sound *nada* is the first evolute to emerge from the *spandana* or vibration of the supreme consciousness and *bindu* is the nucleus from which this vibration emerges. This cosmic sound of vibration reverberates through the cosmos as the sound of OM, and within the individual as the unstruck sound or *anahata nada*.

The yogis described these unstruck sounds in many ways, as sounds emanating from the *chakras* such as the sounds of a flute, the call of a peacock or the roaring of thunder, and also as the various *mantras*. Among infinite possibilities the *nadas* that are most commonly heard during meditation are the sounds of bells, conch, lute, flute, cymbals and drum. But in addition to the subtle sounds from the *chakras*, *nada* gives rise to *mantra*, *akshara* and all forms of sound.

The concept of *akshara* is peculiar to Kashmir Shaivism and refers to the letters of the Sanskrit alphabet as being full of the indestructible divine creative energy of *shakti* which imbues the words and language as well as the letters written on the lotus petals of the *chakras* used for meditation. This creative energy is the power concealed in the *mantras* which is known as *matrika* (little mothers; the letters of the Sanskrit alphabet). When through initiation and proper practice the sound and the *mantra* become efficacious this hidden power is revealed to the aspirant. The *anahata nada* or unstruck sound lies in the *anahata chakra* or heart centre where it resonates unceasingly without any objective cause as would be the case for a struck or physical sound. All of the *akshara* or letters of the alphabet arise from this *anahata nada*, being formed by its various frequencies of vibrations. These vibrations form both sound (*dhvani*) and light (*jyotsma*).

Divine sound and light (*nada* and *bindu*) emerge from pure Consciousness as two inseparable streams which manifest outwardly as the world of diverse names and forms. The return inward journey can use either of these two equivalent vehicles: divine sound embodied in *mantra* or divine light embodied in forms like *yantras* (geometrical diagrams), *mandalas* (symbolic circular figures) and deities (personified subtle forces). Many spiritual traditions such as the Vedic, Talmudic and Biblical, tell of these two inseparable streams of light and sound, and eventually all paths converge to one with these two parallel tracks of *nada* and *bindu*. Paths using *mantra* are grounded in *nada*, while paths using sacred forms are grounded in *bindu*. The human body and personality is a crystallization and orchestration of both sound and light, "frozen" energy, a condensation of the spectrum of vibratory energy of the *shakti* principle, and thus the locus of both sound (*mantra*) and form (*yantra*, *mandala* and deity). The adepts of Sri Vidya know which of these energies lead to pure Consciousness.

The Descent of Divine Truth as Light and Sound

Light is the intrinsic nature of the absolute Truth (Tigunait, 1996, p 32). Revelation is the direct experience of that Divine Light, not the physical light seen with the eyes, but rather the light of knowledge revealed by intuition. This inner Light penetrates our consciousness with varying degrees of intensity depending on the density (*karmic* or mental impurities) or clarity of the mind field. It is brightest closest to the Source and dimmer when it reaches the mind. The descent of this Light occurs in three stages of revelation.

The first and highest level is *prajna* which is pure, complete and perfect spontaneous knowledge of Truth in its entirety. It is not subject-object knowledge but rather the experience of union and realization of truth in perfection and purity. There is complete oneness with the highest Truth, as exemplified by Christ's saying, "I and My Father are one."

Pratibha is the second stage of revelation at the level of exceptional intellectual revelation or genius. An aspect of truth is known in totality and perfection, but not the whole Truth. It involves instantaneous intuitive knowledge as a flash rather than as a continuous flow of inner light. One does not experience oneness with the highest Truth but has a sense of being a seer who can see the revealed knowledge.

Finally the third stage of revelation is *medha* or *dhi* which involves retentive power, the ability of the mind to store its experiences. The inner light illuminates experience over a wider realm than normal awareness encompasses to enable the intellect to make decisions based on previous experience and soul guidance. Communication with the Inner Teacher involves true intuition and occurs at the level of *pratibha* for the disciple, while the realized *guru* experiences *prajna*.

But there is also a descent of the Light of Truth as sound (Tigunait, 1996, p 40). Simultaneously with the manifestation of the Divine Light the Divine Sound manifests in three successive stages as *pashyanti*, *madhyama* and *vaikhari*. The highest stage is *pashyanti* where the Word embodies pure and perfect knowledge of Truth. It is not an articulate sound but the state of pure awareness experienced only in deep *samadhi*. This state has the potential of all the words with their meanings. It is said in the texts that without hearing, the hearer hears and that while hearing, the hearer never hears (Tigunait, 1996, p 41). In *pashyanti* the Divine Word is known as *shruti*, "that which is heard," and the one who hears is called a *rishi* or "seer." The seer is one with the Word in the same way that a sage with *prajna* is one with the highest Truth. "The knower of *Brahman* becomes *Brahman*, and the knower of *mantra* becomes *mantra*" (Tigunait, 1996, p 41). This is revelation in deep spiritual trance and is the way the words of the Vedas were heard by the seers who recorded them as revealed knowledge.

The second stage is *madhyama*. Here the Word contains clear knowledge about one aspect of the truth but not pure and perfect knowledge of all Truth. It is a vehicle for genius corresponding to *pratibha* and suddenly bursts forth in an intuitive flash containing a huge amount of nonverbal information in a concentrated flow of thought.

Articulation of thoughts into words occurs in the third stage of *vaikhari* where the Word is a focus for retentive power that allows the mind to store and express its experiences in language. *Pashyanti* is the source of all *mantras*, and if a *mantra* comes from that Source it eventually leads the consciousness of the meditator back toward that Source progressively from *vaikhari* through *madhyama* to *pashyanti*, for Divine Word comes forth from the Source and tends to return to the Source.

Nada Yoga

Nada Yoga is a system of concentration (*dharana*) that attunes the awareness to the inner subtle unstruck sounds (Sivananda, 1986a). Verses (*slokas*) 38 through 42 of the Vijnana Bhairava Tantra discuss these different meditations on *shabdabrahman* (verse 38), on *pranava* or *Aum* (verse 39), on the *matras* or letters of AUM (verse 40), on the *nada* itself (verse 41), and on the *bija* or seed *mantras* (verse 42) (Satyasangananda Saraswati, 2003). There is variation in the translation and precise interpretation of these verses (Singh, 2003).

Singh (2003, p 36) presents verse 38 as:

> *Anahate patrakarne'bhagnashabde sariddrute*
> *Shabdabrahmani nishnatah param brahmadhigacchati.*
>   "One who is steeped/immersed in *nada* which is *Brahman* in the form of sound
>   (*Shabdabrahman*), which is vibrating inside without any impact, which can be
>   heard only by the ear that becomes competent by yoga, which goes on sounding
>   uninterruptedly and which is rushing headlong like a river attains to *Brahman*."

In the tradition of Kashmir Shaivism this verse describes absorption in the unstruck sound (*anahata nada*) which vibrates spontaneously without any causative impact. Of the approximately ten kinds of *nada* (sound) that vibrate within, growing subtler and subtler, this verse refers to the subtlest of these *nadas* which vibrates in *pranashakti* (vital energy) within the central *sushumna* channel. At the universal level this *pranashakti* represents *parashakti*, the highest *shakti* (power) of the Divine or *citi* – the consciousness-power of the Absolute that brings about the world process. It is the *shakti* (power) of *Parama Shiva* – the Highest reality, the Absolute, the eternal energy of consciousness, the spiritual *spanda* (the dynamic aspect of *Shiva* (consciousness) or primordial creative pulsation).

The sound is heard as the *kundalini* begins to rise. It is made audible only to the aspirant who is made competent to hear it under *guru's* guidance and grace. The roll and thunder of this subtlest and primal *nada* is the auditory form of the opening of the Centre of Consciousness, the spontaneous vibration of OM. It is initially heard in the right ear and eventually spreads to parts and then to the whole body which can be felt to vibrate with the sound. It may be accompanied by visual effects of light filling a room at night, or of blue and gold light in the *ajna chakra*. Individual experiences vary. Tigunait (1996, p 145) refers to the white (*sushumna*), blue (*ida*) and red (*pingala*) dots. Muktananda (1992, p 54) describes the divine effulgence of the *sahasrara chakra* with its tiny central subtle blue light, the *nila bindu* or Blue pearl, which is the form and light of the Divine within, and contains the seed of the whole universe. Paramahansa Yogananda (2004, Vol 1, p 125) refers to a gold ring of light (the Holy Ghost) at the spiritual eye containing within it blue light (Christ Consciousness or God immanent) with a silver star in the centre (God transcendent) which must be pierced by the devotee's consciousness in turn.

To approach this subtlest level of *nada* the practitioner concentrates progressively on these inner sounds, moving from the gross to the subtler to the subtlest. The aspirant gradually becomes lost or absorbed in this internal sound, leaving the external world behind, and is finally absorbed in *chidakasha*, the vast expanse of consciousness (refer to our discussion of the Presence in Part One), which is also referred to as *shunya*, the Void. It is important to distinguish experiencing the space of consciousness from being absorbed in it; from experiencing the Self while remaining identified still as an individual small self to knowing one's true identity as the Self – the identity shift described earlier.

It is interesting that the commentary on all of these verses indicates that absorption in *nada* leads to awareness actually becoming that primal sound, to be absorbed in the source of all sound (*paravak*). Then the mind is gradually transcended and the Void is experienced. With the help of the power of the Void (*parashakti*) the Yogi becomes of the nature and form of the Void, identified as the Self freed from identification with the components of the personality such as *prana*, the body, etc. This is the identity shift described earlier. In Kashmir Shaivism, to attain the Void means to attain the nature of *Bhairava* (the Highest Reality) which is free of all difference, duality and *vikalpas* (thoughts). This *nirvikalpa* state of *shunya* is freedom from all external and internal objective support – consciousness-without-an-object.

The basic method itself is quite simple. It can be preceded with meditation on *so'ham* or one's *guru mantra* to allow the awareness to become interiorized and calm so that the inner sounds are easier to hear. Sitting erect, close the ears with the thumbs by pressing comfortably tight on each tragus (the cartilaginous fold of tissue in front of the opening of the ear) to close the openings to the external auditory canals. The little fingers are placed at the outer corners of the closed eyelids with the rest of the fingers resting on the forehead. The gaze is fixed at the point between the eyebrows (*ajna chakra*). Let all the awareness be on the inner sounds within the right ear, beginning with the loudest. Work with the unstruck inner sounds and not with physical sounds like the heart beat. Concentrate on only one sound at a time. As subtler sounds come forward listen to them one by one as each becomes prominent in turn, and follow them inward as they become progressively subtler. One can mentally chant "Om, Om" at the same time. This mental chanting and the gaze at the *ajna chakra* are relaxed and automatic, with all mental effort focused on the sound in the right ear.

With the opening of the Centre of Consciousness the primal sound of Om itself may be heard directly as a great rolling sound like thunder or surf. Concentrate on and be absorbed in that. You may notice light at the *ajna* centre (the point between the eyebrows), but the focus remains on the sound. Be one with and absorbed with reverence in whatever sound is heard. Remain relaxed with no feeling of strain. Intensity of mental effort and practice over long periods are needed to reach higher states of absorption in the Om vibration. As Om itself manifests, its prominence is such that the hand position is no longer needed. But in the early stages of the process the arms can fatigue. One can prop them on pillows on a table top or use a padded, adjustable, T-shaped elbow prop (*danda*) with its foot resting on the floor between the legs. Optimize the height so the hands and arms are supported but relaxed; one should not lean on them, but remain sitting erect.

Nada and *Mantra*

Nada is the source and true form of all *mantras*, not what is written or heard when a *mantra* is articulated (Tigunait, 1996, p 88; Alper, 1989). Here *nada* refers to the Word in the apostle John's "In the beginning was the Word, and the Word was with God, and the Word was God." (John 1:1). The entire universe in its potential or unmanifest form is contained in *nada*.

This pure, unstruck, eternal sound of *nada* is the essence of a *mantra*. A *mantra* is divinity enrobed in the energy of sound vibration. The power of a *mantra* can lead a meditator to the same state of consciousness that was held by the seer (*rishi*) who first heard and experienced it. During *mantra* initiation the Master articulates a *mantra* revealed through him or her in a deep meditative state. The power to give authentic *mantra* initiation is bestowed only by a *sadguru*. That *mantra* is essentially a manifestation of *nada*. Initiation plants the *mantra* as a seed of divine revelation at the core of the student's being. Correct and consistent *sadhana* of the practice of the *mantra* as given at the time of initiation nourishes that seed until it can grow, flower and give fruit at a rate dependent on the purity of the initiate's mind and body. With practice the sound vibration of the *mantra* becomes refined. One repeats it mentally and then one can hear it spontaneously (*ajapajapa*). As the practice deepens the vibration becomes even subtler until it is neither repeated nor heard but leads to its soundless sound. In this pristine state of the *mantra* one duplicates the original experience of the *mantra's* first seer. "Sooner or later the seed will blossom and produce inner illumination" (Tigunait, 1996, p 88).

The meditations using the unstruck sounds described in the Vijnana Bhairava Tantra (Satyasangananda Saraswati, 2003, pp 188–198; Singh, 2003, pp 36–41) deal with the following concentrations (*dharana*):

Verse (*sloka*)	Object of Concentration (*dharana*)	Outcome
38	*dharana* on *shabdabrahman* (unstruck sound)	*shunya* (void)
39	*dharana* on *pranava* (AUM) as *mantra*	*shunya* (void)
40	*dharana* on AUM *matras* (syllables)	*shunya* (void)
41	*dharana* on *nada* as musical sounds	*shunya* (void)
42	*dharana* on *bija mantra(s)*	*shunya* (void)

In the first *sloka* (38) the concentration is on the spontaneous, unstruck sound (*anahata nada*) itself arising from the *anahata chakra* (heart centre). It is the core of *nada* yoga and leads to the experience of the *shabdabrahman*, the supreme awareness and highest consciousness as sound. This is the *para* or highest (transcendental) cosmic level of sound (energy vibration), the AUM (OM), *Pranava* or *para nada* that vibrates at all times throughout the universe and is synonymous with the *Atman* or pure Self before it becomes qualified (associated) with manifest nature. Singh (2003,

246 Chariot of Sadhana

p 36) also calls this absorption into *chidakasha*, the space or vast expanse of consciousness, meaning that the yogi attains to *Brahman*.

In verse 39 *Aum* is repeated as a *mantra* for extended periods accompanied by focusing the awareness on the void (*shunya*) which is pure consciousness (*Shiva*) at the end of the protracted sound of the last letter M (Singh, 2003, p 37). The void here refers to freedom from all external or internal objective support – a mind that is made *nirvikalpa* or thought-free. The repetition must be technically perfect to influence the corresponding bodily energy centers (*chakras*) correctly.

In verse 40 the concentration is on the letters (*matras*) of AUM to awaken the three dimensions of consciousness that they represent: A for *jagrat* or wakefulness; U for *svapna* or dreaming; M for *sushupti* or deep sleep. This leads to the experience of the fourth state of *turiya* (the silence after the letter M), the transcendental state. Combined together these syllables represent the entire conscious field as addressed in the *Mandukya Upanishad*. Again the process leads to transcendence of the mind and the manifest dimensions with merging of the individual awareness into the source or void; one becomes the void, the space or vast expanse of consciousness.

In verse 41 the meditation is on the inner sounds generated from the *chakras* with the awakening of the *kundalini* as they resemble various musical instruments. Most commonly they are heard as bells, conch, lute, flute, cymbals and drum. Individuals experience them differently. They are often accompanied by images of light, color and form seen in the space of consciousness (*chidakasha*) at the point between the eyebrows. Again the end result is transcendence into the supreme consciousness as *shunya* (and here we identify the terms Void or *shunya*, Presence, or *turiya* as the Centre of Consciousness). Singh (2003, p 39) interprets this verse differently as a concentration on the echo or lasting resonance in the memory of a musical note played on a musical instrument, a sound that seems to arise out of eternity and finally to disappear into it. "Thereby the yogi is absorbed into the source of all sound (*paravak*) and acquires the nature of *Bhairava*."

Finally verse 42 describes concentration on one or more *bija* or seed *mantras* which often wholly or in part make up personal or *guru mantras* given in *mantra* initiation by an empowered teacher from the Tradition. *Bija* or seed *mantras* are letters of the Sanskrit alphabet with "M" (*makara*) at the end of each. Commonly used ones include *Aum, Aim, Hrim, Klim, Shrim, Vam, Lam, Ham* or *Ksham*. Some practitioners pronounce the terminal "m" sound of some of these *bijas* like the English "-ing" sound. Again they are used along with meditation on the void. With prolonged, continuous repetition of such a *mantra* the mind field attunes to and becomes stabilized in the frequencies of the sounds. Eventually the vibrations refine and become so subtle that the awareness attunes to the same sounds vibrating at the *paravak* level throughout the universe. At that point the aspirant can attune the cosmic sound of *nada* until the awareness becomes that sound. With further deepening the mind gradually transcends and the void is experienced.

All *mantras*, sounds and letters of the alphabet are contained within the *mantra*
Aum. This *mantra* represents all three states of awareness: *jagrat. svapna* and *sushupti*,
or conscious, subconscious and unconscious. These states can be experienced and

transcended by repetition of this *mantra* alone. If repeated for extended periods, it induces the experience of *turiya*, the transcendental state. The *mantra Aum* is none other than *Brahman*.

Swami Shivananda as quoted in Satyasangananda Saraswati, 2003, p 190.

In his revelatory commentary on the Lord's prayer, Yogananda (2004, Vol. II, p 1056) describes God contact "through communion with the Word or Holy Ghost – the Cosmic Sound of *Aum*, defined by Patanjali . . . as God's symbol or manifestation." He writes:

> Every devotee who enters interiorized silence, whether by the sheer intensity of devotion or by practice of a yoga technique, discovers, when the mind grows calm and the concentration is deep, the comforting vibratory presence of *Aum*, the Cosmic Sound. God's intelligence, immanent in the *Aum* Vibration, intimates divine guidance or inspiration through the devotee's intuitive feeling, hearing, or vision. *Aum* is the mother of all sounds in the universe, including all human languages; and also all types of rays in the cosmos. Any manifestation presupposes the inherent presence of the Cosmic Vibration. During the devotee's meditation, *Aum* can vibrate the response or wishes of the Divine in words of any intelligible language in audible form or in luminous letters revealed to the devotee's inner gaze. The etheric sounds or letters may be audible or visible to a single devotee or to a group of devotees, according to the wish of the Divine.

The *Hamsah Mantra* and the *Kundalini*. Verses 155 and 156 of the Vijnanabhairava Tantra give the process by which the *nada* manifests itself in the breath of every living creature (Singh, 2003, p xvii; pp 142–145). One exhales with the sound *sa* and inhales with the sound *ha* to recite the *mantra hamsah*. It occurs automatically with every cycle of expiration – inspiration and hence is called *ajapajapa* or automatic recitation. The *ha* represents *shakti* (the divine energy as imperceptible and spontaneous sound in a living being) and *sah* represents *Shiva*. The *am* in *hamsah* represents the *jiva* (*nara*) or empirical individual. Hence it is called the *trika* (triad or threefold) *mantra* including within itself the three realities of *Shiva*, *shakti* and *nara* or *jiva*. Concentration is on the *am* or junction point of *ha* and *sah*. If one cycle of inspiration-expiration takes 4 seconds then *hamsah* repeats itself 15 times in a minute. There are (15×60) or 900 repetitions in an hour and (900×24) or 21,600 repetitions in a full twenty-four hour day. This *hamsah mantra* (I am He, meaning I am Shiva or the Divine) is described as the *adi prana* or initial or primal *prana* which is the first evolute or transformation of consciousness.

When this automatic *pranic mantra* is consciously and repeatedly concentrated on it automatically becomes *so'ham* (That am I). By constant concentration on this *mantra* the *kundalini* awakens and rises upwards. The *mantra* can be used to awaken *kundalini* in two ways (Singh, 2003, p xvii). One is through prolonged mental awareness of the automatic process (*anusandhana*) and the other is by conscious *japa* or repetition of the *mantra* as *so'ham* or just *Aum*. *Japa* begins in the *vaikhari* form as willful vocal muttering, and then becomes mental. After constant practice for some years it becomes *ajapajapa* and goes on automatically inwardly with no effort. When *ajapajapa* proceeds for a long time the *prana* and *apana* currents that normally flow in *ida* and *pingala nadis* equilibrate. *Kundalini* now awakens and the equilibrated current flows upward in the *sushumna* channel in the centre of the spine. As it rises the practitioner experiences the automatic unstruck sounds (*anahata nada*) as it passes through the *chakras*. When it finally reaches the *Brahmarandhra* or *Sahasrara chakra* at the top of the head the *nada* ceases and it is converted into light (*jyoti*). Paramahamsa Niranjanananda describes the practice of *ajapa dharana* in great detail in his book *Dharana Darshan* (1993b, pp 68–154).

Part Six

Grace and the Inner Teacher

34

Awakening the Inner Teacher: A Recapitulation

Our first meeting with our spiritual preceptor, the late H.H. Sri Swami Rama of the Himalayas, left us with powerful memories. He was an imposing figure, over six feet in height in dark red robes, who towered over us. Taking our hands, he held our eyes with his and said three times, "I will answer all your questions." We did not realize until very much later that this was our first introduction to the Inner Teacher and to the ultimate promise of *samadhi*. For Swamiji defined *samadhi* as the state in which all questions are answered and no questions remain. "The word *samadhi* means *samahitam* – no question remains unanswered, no mystery remains unsolved." (Rama, 1999a).

Discipleship, authority and self-transcendence form a triad that has its basis in the awakening of the Inner Teacher. But three more components could be added: *guru*, initiation and the awakening of the intuitive faculty. Like constellations in the night sky revolving around the polestar, these six factors point the new disciple in an authentic spiritual tradition towards the Inner Teacher and map the process and curriculum of that interaction. The awakening of the Inner Teacher integrates these six factors and gives them meaning on the spiritual path.

Let us review briefly this concept of the Inner Teacher which unifies these six factors and gives them meaning for the new disciple (Jerry & Jerry, 2001). The role of the sage in the Himalayan Tradition of Yoga is to awaken within the qualified student the divine flame, that spark of divinity that all human beings carry within them, and which Sri Swami Rama called the Teacher within, or the Centre of Consciousness. Swamiji described the Centre of Consciousness as the divine core within the personality from which consciousness flows in various degrees and grades. He was referring to *turiya*, the Fourth, and by various degrees and grades he meant the three states of Consciousness of waking (*jagrat*), dreaming (*svapna*) and deep sleep (*sushupti*) as described in the *Mandukya Upanishad* (Rama, 1982b; Nikhilananda, 1987a; Fort, 1990). He called himself a messenger, delivering the wisdom of the Himalayan sages of his tradition. His job was to introduce the student to the Teacher within. "*Hiranyagarbha* alone is the teacher of Yoga, and no other." (*Brhad-yogi-yajnavalkya-smrti* XII.5).

Swami Veda Bharati identifies the Inner Teacher or Inner *Guru* with *Hiranyagarbha* or *Ishvara*, and points to parallels in the Buddhist concept of *Sambhogakaya* (Veda Bharati, 1979a) and the Christian Holy Ghost or Teaching Spirit in the universe. But the new disciple also wants to know about the inner mystical experience of this Centre of Consciousness.

The awakening of the Centre is a qualitatively new and unique experience in the disciple's inner world. While the many descriptions of it are quite literal, one cannot imagine it from those descriptions. It is like the awakening of the faculty of sight in the blind: it simply cannot be imagined beforehand. For that reason Swami Veda Bharati calls it a secret that once revealed remains a secret. Indeed this unexpected recognition of something qualitatively new in the mind, however subtle, can be initially quite disconcerting.

In the *Upanishads* the sages use words like "That" or "It" as does Merrell-Wolff (1994, p 82), along with the term Consciousness-Without-an-Object (1994, p 85). One finds the terms "Void" (*Yoga Vasishtha* VI.2:29) or "Space" (*Tripura Rahasya* XVIII:72–79) often used. Space is Self and Self is Space. In inner space the wise find the Intelligence of pure Consciousness, and ultimate Truth in the effulgent Void. Another term that is commonly used, and one that we are coming to prefer, is "Presence." Elsewhere we have defined It experientially as: "the Centre of Consciousness is a still, but effulgent, Conscious Presence, Silence or 'Thatness.' It is that Void or Emptiness that paradoxically is also a Plenum or Fullness. It pervades all of inner space and holds all manifestation, all inner mental content within Itself like space pervades and holds the contents of a room, and yet is unaffected by them." (Jerry & Jerry, 2001, p 82). Perhaps the best experiential description of the phenomenon and how to interact with It that we have found is in the writings of the modern sage Aziz Kristof (Kristof, 2000), presented in Part One. The Presence is the first inner glimpse of the background Awareness of what he calls Presence, Being and Heart which we interpret as analogous to the *cit, sat* and *ananda* aspects respectively of *Brahman*. His writings provide a detailed evolutionary typology of the unfolding of this inner experience through its many levels into completeness and unity to reach full human evolution (Kristof & Emami, 1999; Kristof, 1999). Another description of the Centre and how to work with it is the passage on the Warrior Within in the Theosophical text, *Light on the Path*. (Collins, 1976, p 9) given in chapter 5, Part One. This is not a momentary experience, but rather a consistent and evolving change in the disciple's inner space, although it may vary in the degree of its expression from time to time.

From this Centre of Consciousness comes the gentle intuitive whisperings of the Inner Teacher, a wordless flow of the purest knowing that Swamiji identified as having the characteristics of self-consistency and certainty (Rama, 1982b, p 4). One knows, one knows that one knows, and one is certain of that knowledge. This flow of communication is extremely subtle and doubt can be a serious obstacle. A noisy mental field can also obscure that communication. One must be capable of the still, one-pointed concentration that evolves gradually through the regular and systematic practice of *dharana* and *dhyana* to work productively with It. The process is initially intermittent but as the experience of the Centre becomes natural and spontaneous, the flow becomes continuous whenever the mind turns inward and is relatively still. The communication flows both ways between the disciple and the Inner Teacher like a quiet, metaphorical wordless whispering, a flow of pure meaning and understanding. But more than the whisperings of knowledge flow into the mind from that Centre. There are also the whisperings of love, and much more.

This inner force is also called *atma shakti* (Tigunait, 1996, p 65), the power of the soul. Indeed the only sin in the Himalayan Tradition is to kill one's conscience. Swamiji often referred to the Centre of Consciousness as the Conscience. Not to listen to and heed its whisperings is to kill the conscience. But when we listen and comply we receive *atma kripa* (the grace of oneself), and if that flows freely without obstruction, one can obtain the highest illumination without help from any other source (Tigunait, 1996, p 65). And from that blessing with the grace of our inner Self (*atman kripa*) eventually flows the other three forms of grace: the grace of the scriptures (*shastra kripa*), the grace of God (*Ishvara kripa*), and the grace of the *guru* (*guru kripa*) with the possibility of spiritual initiation. One form of grace invites the other forms of grace into our life. And all of this is because the Teacher Within (*atma shakti*) has led us to the teacher without, and paradoxically the teacher without has lovingly introduced us to the Teacher Within!

Now what of the first of the six factors, **discipleship**? This leads immediately to the *guru*-disciple relationship and even the question of how does one know if one is a disciple? Answers to these questions come from the significance at this stage on the spiritual path of the awakening of this Centre of Consciousness as an inner experience. One soon learns that the outer teacher, the *guru*, is but an expression of the Inner Teacher. In consciousness they are one and the same. The new disciple is shown this unequivocally as an inner experience. One learns that communication to the Inner Teacher is communication to the outer master. Teaching from the Inner Teacher is teaching from the outer master, and vice versa. The Inner Ashram has opened. The student has been fully tested and is now accepted as a disciple. We remember standing with Swamiji in the gardens of his ashram by the Ganges in Rishikesh with everything washed in the light of a full moon. In the midst of a conversation about other things he suddenly paused, turned to us, and said, "Our relationship is eternal."

The student has asked through yearning and long preparation. The Inner Teacher has responded with the grace of a master. In the Yoga Tradition we say that when the student is ready the master will appear. "Ask, and it shall be given you; seek, and ye shall find; knock, and it shall be opened unto you." (Matthew 7:7). We did not deliberately search for a master, but ever since we met in our late teens, we have shared a yearning for Truth and the search for spirituality as the motivating factor at the core of our lives. And incidentally what a blessing it is when one's life companion shares that search fully. Our long journey to Sri Swamiji was an unfolding sequence of synchronicities, doors opening at the right time and place. Looking back on it now it felt guided; perhaps the Inner Teacher was already at work throughout. We passed through many traditions on the way but prevailing circumstances always blocked initiation. When one is ready, apparently not only is one led to the outer teacher, but one is led to the right one! But at each step free will was preserved. We had to be sufficiently qualified to recognize the synchronicity and then to take the initiative to walk through the open door.

The entry to the Path has at last been found. Now the Centre of Consciousness calls the student to discipleship. But to answer this call, to cross over the threshold and begin to tread the Path in earnest, the student must die to the world, and a slow death it can be! The new disciple must be strong enough to leave behind worldly attractions and attachments. If he or she is not strong enough, not yet ready, the portal will close. But it does so only for a while until the student gains detachment through further worldly experience and tires of worldly attractions through the pain of that experience. For once the door has opened, the relationship is eternal. It is always possible to learn, even though the student waivers, hesitates and turns aside. "The voice of the silence remains within him, and though he leave the path utterly, yet one day it will resound and rend him asunder and separate his passions from his divine possibilities. Then with pain and desperate cries from the deserted lower self he will return." (Collins, 1976, p 58). To answer this call, total surrender on the part of the disciple and total commitment are required. For the Inner Teacher ultimately is one's own Self.

Discipleship also raises the issues of discipline and qualification. In the West where freedom of speech and action are so highly valued, the idea of discipline can have unhappy associations. But discipline here is not something imposed from without that limits freedom of expression. Rather it is the discipline of the Olympic athlete, the surgeon or the concert pianist which is long, rigorous but willingly self-imposed, and which leads to the creative freedom that comes from complete mastery of one's medium of expression. After high school this can be sixteen years in graduate and postgraduate training for a physician-scientist who would accept that very demanding experience without protest. Why then would one think that the spiritual path would require any less a commitment?

Qualification (*adhikara*) (Veda Bharati, 1986, p 66) is also a critical aspect of discipleship for the Centre of Consciousness awakens only in the qualified student. Only the qualified student can receive the higher initiation (*shaktipata*) from the *Guru* that awakens the Centre of Consciousness. We think of this as sowing seed on fertile ground and the practices that bestow qualification as both preparing that fertile ground and nurturing the seed that has been sown (for example, *mantra initiation*), like a kind of gardening of the soul.

The philosophical texts of Vedanta define the qualified student as one who has practiced the six treasures (*shat-sampat*) of *shama, dama, uparati, titiksha, samadhana* and *shraddha*. (Veda Bharati, 1986, p 67). In the Tantric tradition an analogous set of qualifications exist (Johari, 1986, p 9). The first six are said to give control over one's animal or biological nature and include *daksha, jitendriya, sarva hinsa vinirmukta, sarva prani hitrata, shuchi,* and *astik,* and the remaining qualifications are the same six treasures of Vedanta.

In the Tradition there are preparations that are prerequisites to imparting a teaching (Veda Bharati, 1986, p 68). How seriously does the student apply himself and what questions does he or she raise? What is the quality and extent of practice, ascetic observances and purifications? What is the preparation of the body, including lifestyle issues such as exercise and diet? The point is that in addition to moral behavior there are deeper issues of qualification here about the readiness of biology to contain the higher energies of advanced spiritual initiation and realization.

Now what of **authority**, yet another unwelcome term in Western society? In English the word has a number of connotations. It often conveys the power or right to give commands, and force obedience, take action, or make final decisions. It has been pointed out in the Yoga Tradition (Feuerstein, 2001, p 14) that the Sanskrit word for "student" is *shishya* which comes from a verb root *shas*, meaning both "to instruct" and "to chastise." Respect for the authority of the master is expected from students. The master will not hesitate to reprimand to correct a student's behavior. With Swami Rama this process was always verbal and never involved physical abuse. With disciples his favorite method was to stop talking to them and ignore them completely. This distressing and puzzling situation soon brought the aspirant around when he or she began to realize that his or her behavior was blocking communication with the Inner Teacher which Swamiji's ignoring them symbolized. Actual physical abuse would never be tolerated in this relationship.

The word also has the meaning of an expert, and both the teacher and the master are certainly experts to the disciple in conveying the teachings. The master assigns a senior teacher to the new disciple to give the practical and theoretical details of the teachings in the Tradition. The master teaches the basics to groups, but the teaching interaction with the individual disciple is at the level of silent transmission – something that takes some considerable adjustment to get used to.

Yet another meaning of the word has to do with power of influence resulting from knowledge, prestige, and so on. A *sadguru* enjoys continuous *Brahman*-Consciousness and all that that implies. Such an individual is larger-than-life and has no difficulty with commanding beneficial influence. Such masters have *siddhis*, but a *sadguru* does not display these openly or use them for control. Swami Rama had them all in abundance, but they were rarely displayed except in private to selected senior disciples for the purpose of teaching and testing. However, he often healed many people silently and they were never aware of his intervention until afterward. There are many stories of his interventions and we have experienced our own. He would respond generously to requests for healing, but not to all. He frequently did so by taking serious diseases like cancer onto himself and then discharging them somehow into nature. Such activities have serious *karmic* implications and he always respected this natural order of things.

Another aspect of authority is scriptural authority, or the authenticity of teachings. Swamiji was given the mission by his own *guru* to teach only what is in the revealed scriptures and what he had personally experienced, provided it agreed with the scriptures. If there were experiences that did not agree with the scriptures, he was to resolve the conflict first before teaching. He taught Yoga as a spiritual science with an authenticity that came both from the revealed scriptures like the *Upanishads* and his own inner state of Self-realization. He did not teach his own version of Yoga. Authenticity here always meant *shruti*, divine revelation, teachings that flowed undistorted from the Inner Teacher.

We searched a long time to find an authentic tradition. The aspiring student should beware and should be prepared to assess carefully any teaching or teacher/*guru* for authenticity, just as the *guru* will test the disciple. Some texts even suggest that the student observe the teacher for twelve years before committing! Access to the Inner Teacher will allow the student to be guided without fail to an authentic Tradition and to authentic texts despite the chaos, the cacophony and the commercialism of what passes as Yoga in the modern West.

We have discussed above the role of the *guru* and the *guru*-disciple relationship. But a word must be said about the opening of **intuition**, for intuition is the modality by which the whisperings from the Inner Teacher are transmitted to the disciple. We all have intuitions at times but few of us seem to be able to recognize them. Either they are devalued by the Western worship of rationality, or they are confused with instinct or with material welling up from the unconscious, or they are lost in the confusion of the flow of thoughts, images, feelings, emotions, memories, etc. that overwhelm the untrained mind. Thus the training in concentration and meditation as well as other aspects of Patanjali's Raja Yoga that lead to control of the modifications and stilling of the mind become essential for the cultivation of intuition flowing from the higher mind or *buddhi*, the mind used as a sixth sense for direct apperception of higher Reality. The light of intuition is to the Centre of Consciousness as light is to the sun, illuminating directly all it touches.

It is said in the Tradition that some are led by Light, some by Sound, and some by both. Light is the intrinsic nature of the absolute Truth (Tigunait, 1996, p 32). It animates us, but mind stands between it and our individual consciousness. Revelation is the direct experience of Divine Light. By Light we mean not physical light seen with the eyes, but rather the light of knowledge that reveals the mystery of the unknown and unseen. It is always complete and there is no higher or lower revelation. The Light of inner being penetrates our consciousness with varying degrees of intensity depending on the density (*karmic* or mental impurities) or clarity of the mind. It is brightest closest to the Source and dimmer when it reaches the mind field. Thus in chapter 33, Part Five we described the descent of Light as occurring in three stages of revelation: *prajna*, *pratibha* and *medha* or *dhi*. Communication with the Inner Teacher involves true intuition and occurs at the level of *pratibha* for the disciple, while the realized *guru* experiences *prajna*.

But there is also a descent of the Light as sound (Tigunait, 1996, p 40). Simultaneously with the manifestation of the Divine Light in three successive stages, in chapter 33 we described how the Divine Sound manifests successively as *pashyanti*, *madhyama* and *vaikhari*. The highest stage is *pashyanti* where the Word embodies pure and perfect knowledge of Truth in a state of pure awareness experienced only in deep *samadhi* This is revelation in deep spiritual trance and is the way the words of the Vedas were heard by the seers who recorded them as revealed knowledge.

The second stage is *madhyama*. It is a vehicle for genius corresponding to *pratibha* and suddenly bursts forth in an intuitive flash containing a huge amount of nonverbal information in a concentrated flow of thought. Articulation of thoughts into words occurs in the third stage of *vaikhari* where the Word is a focus for retentive power that allows the mind to store and express its experiences in language. *Pashyanti* is the source of all *mantras*, and if a *mantra* comes from that Source it eventually leads the consciousness of the meditator back toward that Source progressively from *vaikhari* through *madhyama* to *pashyanti*, for Divine Word comes forth from the Source and tends to return to the Source.

The role of the *guru* and the *guru*-disciple relationship has been discussed above, but a key factor in this relationship is the role of **initiation** (*diksha*). The Himalayan Tradition is also an initiatory Tradition. The process is called transmission (Veda Bharati, 1998). The Tradition is based in Patanjali's Raja Yoga, but meditation is taught as Mantra Yoga, initially using the universal *mantra*, so'ham with the breath. "Ceaseless awareness of so'ham is the luminous flame in the lamp of meditation. In the blissful light of Self-realization radiating from this flame, delusion rooted in dualism – the cause of bondage – is forever annihilated." (*Ramcharit Manas, Uttar Khanda* 118).

The first initiation is *mantra* initiation using awakened (*jagrata*) *mantras* received from the lineage, and only they have the power to awaken the student (Tigunait, 1996, p 93). This is a form of *krama diksha* which is a process of gradual unfoldment of the inner *shakti*. The power to initiate is bestowed by the master and cannot be passed on to someone else by the initiator. The flow of compassion (*karuna* or *anugraha shakti*) is the medium through which the *guru mantra* descends and in the process the intuitive wisdom *prajna* comes forth in the form of *mantra shakti* so that the specific *mantra* appropriate for the student being initiated appears from the pool of the lineage. During initiation a genuine teacher is nonexistent as a person. S/he has lost his or her individuality in the master and can only impart what has been willed by the master.

Higher initiations are described by the term *shaktipata* which signifies "bestowing the energy," "lighting the lamp" or the "descent of power" (Rama, 1996, p 88). A power comes from above, of its own, to a vessel that is cleaned, purified and is prepared to receive it. It is the grace of God and uses the master as its instrument of transmission. This grace is possible only with the disciple who has undergone a long period of discipline, austerity and spiritual practices. Then the subtlest obstacles are removed by the master. Swami Rama would say that when all possible sincere efforts have been made then grace is the fruit the disciple receives from faithful and sincere effort. "When you have done your duties skillfully and wholeheartedly, you reap the fruits gracefully." *Shaktipata* is the grace of God transmitted through the master. There are many different kinds of *shaktipata* and many different ways it is transmitted. In the Tradition they fall into two major categories: *maha diksha* (the rarest and highest level of initiation where the spiritual energy is delivered with full force through an adept to a perfectly prepared disciple), and *krama diksha* (initiation step by step).

In addition to accessing higher states of consciousness, spiritual knowledge and wisdom are also passed on by transmission. It is said in the Tradition that an enlightened master can pass on the full wisdom and power of the Tradition to his or her successor in the silence of deepest meditation during the course of one night. Thus initiation/transmission together with the awakening of intuition forms the bridge between the disciple and the higher states of self-transcendence.

The end of Yoga, the ultimate goal of life, is the union of the individual self with the transcendental Self. But before **self-transcendence** comes self-transformation. Paramahamsa Satyananda once said that Yoga is not about enlightenment (Niranjanananda, 1993a). What he meant was that a transcendental reality can not be appreciated by an un-transcendental mind and personality. The aim of spiritual practices is to convert the self into a transcendental being. Their aim is not to provide realization. Once the mind, the brain, the body and the senses all become transcendental, then the transcendental awareness will merge with the disciple. The practices provide the means to become transcendental.

If one accepts the modern energetic conception of the universe as described in quantum mechanics, then the process of spiritual *sadhana* can be thought of as raising the set point or fundamental vibration of the whole personality, until it can attune to and contain higher spiritual energies. Here the *guru* and initiation play a critical role by entraining the disciple's vibration and raising it to the *guru*'s faster vibratory rate.

May the universe in some strange sense be "brought into being" by the participation of those who participate? "Participation" is the incontrovertible new concept given by quantum mechanics. It strikes down the "observer" of classical theory, the man who stands safely behind the thick glass wall and watches what goes on without taking part.

John Wheeler as quoted by Hey and Walters (2003, p 299).

Part of this transformation involves emotional purification which is a major part of the practices of the Himalayan Tradition (Veda Bharati, 1998, p 3). It also involves fundamental change in the disciple's model of the world or *weltanschauung*, as indicated by changes in values, attitudes and criteria, to a configuration more in harmony with higher states of consciousness. The moral practices of the *yamas* and *niyamas* as well as a six treasures of Vedanta help to accomplish this transformational change, as does the study of revealed texts like the *Upanishads* with an enlightened master and the practices of Vedantic contemplation of the *mahavakyas* under a master's instruction. But ultimately self-transformation must lead to self-transcendence and to Self-realization. We think of this as an identity shift.

For the new disciple for whom the Centre of Consciousness has awakened the nature of *sadhana* begins to change significantly to a more subtle level. Spiritual practices are still based in Patanjali's Raja Yoga, but now the disciple "graduates" his or her focus from *pada* two of the *Yoga-Sutra* to *pada* one where the twin processes of *abhyasa* and *vairagya* begin to predominate (YS I.12). Sri Swami Rama called these two the wheels of the Chariot of *Sadhana*. A chariot cannot move forward unless the two wheels turn together. Through the practices of *vairagya* the aspirant lets go of, releases and moves away from what holds him or her back, and through *abhyasa* he or she moves toward the goal in a much more conscious and deliberate way. This becomes possible with the awakening of the Centre of Consciousness towards which one can move as an actual experience.

All of the Yogas of life begin to converge in the Centre, for the Centre has an outward arc and an inward arc. Jnana Yoga develops with the outward wisdom flow of intuition and Karma Yoga becomes action flowing from the Centre of Consciousness through a surrendered personality (a kind of self or ego-transcendence) as a conscious experience. One knows and performs right action in any given situation as duty because, simply, it is to be done. One would try to thank Sri Swami Rama for all of his love and generosity. He would simply reply, "I'm only doing my duty." One then realized that this interaction was not personal. This outward arc or manifestation of the Centre into doing is a co-creative process between the individual self and the Centre and results in attunement and alignment of all parts of the personality with the Centre, which is a psychological way of talking about the elevation of vibratory set point.

But the inward arc, or absorption into Being, becomes a flow of surrender and absorption into the Presence. It becomes a process of *ishvara pranidhana* or of practicing the presence of God (or the Centre) in every moment which is the essence of Bhakti. *Pranidhana* has the significance of placing the mind within, dwelling near and close to God. It is *bhavana*, impressing the object of concentration repeatedly on the mind in meditation and in daily life (Veda Bharati, 1986, pp 220,

228, 316). Practicing the presence of God is continual remembrance of the Centre/Presence as a constant background of silent, witnessing Awareness in every moment and situation of daily life until that Presence is perfectly stabilized so that the absorption into Being can occur. Clearly this involves a shift in self identity from that of a limited ego to the transcendental Self. It becomes the ultimate answer to the question, "Who am I?" Since the Presence and the master are one and the same in consciousness, surrender to the physical *guru* is connection to the Supreme *guru* or Inner Teacher. They are one and the same. Patanjali is clear that the consequence of this process of *ishvara pranidhana* is *samadhi* (YS II.45).

The identity shift of self-transcendence into Self-realization becomes an evolving dialogue with the Presence, a movement from duality to non-duality and from doing to being. This interaction between the individual self of the new disciple and the newly awakened Centre of Consciousness begins as a conversation, a relationship that progresses through attitudes of praise and gratitude into trust. With time the conversation moves into friendship and the relationship into love and reverence. The relationship then moves to intimacy and communion. Finally there is absorption and full union, "I am That," and the identity shift of self into Self is complete, of duality and subject-object consciousness into the non-duality of consciousness-without-an-object (Jerry & Jerry, 2001, pp 163–166).

The components of discipleship, authority, intuition, *guru*, initiation and self-transcendence are all unified in the experience of the Inner Teacher or awakened Presence. True discipleship is centered in the relationship with the awakened Inner Teacher. True authority is surrender through the *guru* to the Inner Teacher which is the source of intuitive revelatory authenticity in a flow of love, trust and grace. This leads ultimately to self-transcendence and to the identity shift of self to Self. Until that ultimate climax the essential work with the Centre of Consciousness is to follow Spirit without hesitation in all things. As to that higher climax:

> It is written that for him who is on the threshold of divinity no law can be framed, no guide can exist. Yet to enlighten the disciple, the final struggle may be thus expressed: hold fast to that which has neither substance nor existence. Listen only to the voice which is soundless. Look only on that which is invisible alike to the inner and the outer sense.
>
> Collins, 1976, p 18.

35

The Nondualist Vision – NIRVANA *Equals* SAMSARA

Row, row, row your boat
Gently down the stream.
Merrily, merrily, merrily, merrily
Life is but a dream.

Although we have referred extensively in Parts Two, Three and Four to Patanjali's *Yoga-Sutra* which is considered to be a dualistic text, the philosophy on which this book rests is solidly nondualistic (*advaita*). The idea is captured by the phrase, *nirvana* equals *samsara*; immanence equals transcendence. This is the great dictum of Tantrism which straddles Hinduism and Buddhism. The transcendental Reality is coessential with the conditioned manifested world. The Mahayana Buddhist master Nagarjuna would vigorously say that *nirvana* is *samsara* and *samsara* is *nirvana* (Feuerstein, 2003, p 111). If Reality is anywhere, then it must be everywhere and not exclusively inside the human psyche. Spiritual concerns and material existence become integrated in a way that is philosophically relevant today. This paradigm contrasts with Indian psychospiritual technology which has been described as verticalism (Feuerstein, 2001, p xxix). Realization comes about by directing the attention inward and then upward through a series of higher and higher states of consciousness in an inner hierarchy until all is transcended. The focus of Indian Yoga has been described as "in, up and out."

Samsara equals *nirvana* is crazy wisdom in Mahayana Buddhist terms. It is a paradox that the enlightened adept dwells in spaceless and timeless Being-Consciousness-Bliss and yet appears to inhabit a particular body-mind in space-time. In nondualist Advaita Vedanta enlightenment is the realization that the innermost self (*adhyatman*) is the same as the transcendental Self (*parama-atman*), and that the ultimate Ground of Being (*Brahman*) is identical with the cosmos in all its levels of manifestation including the personal self. In his description of the descent of the Supermind, Sri Aurobindo experienced a silent "world of forms, materialized shadows without true substance" (Aurobindo, 1953, pp. 154–155). He described a cinematic or shadow world of illusion that was a small surface phenomenon resting on an immense Divine Reality that lay behind and above it, and at the very heart of everything.

Samsara equals *nirvana* is also a formula of Mahayana Buddhism. The world of change is the changeless Reality. The transcendental Reality is identical with the world of impermanence and vice versa. The changeable world of forms is inherently empty (*shunya*) and *nirvana* must not be sought outside of *samsara*. This doctrine was first elaborated in the *Prajna-Paramita-Sutras* around 200 B.C.E. and was later established in the *Vijnanavada* and *Yogacara* schools in the fourth century C.E. (Feuerstein, 2001, p 157). The best known is the Heart *Sutra* (*Prajna-Paramita-Hridaya-Sutra*) composed about 300 C.E. which deals with the key Mahayana doctrine of emptiness or voidness. Although all things and beings are empty of essence the *bodhisattva* seeks to liberate these phantom beings. All suffering and finite experience is empty but beings experience pain and suffering because their minds are clouded by ignorance of the ultimate Reality beyond all appearance. With enlightenment suffering is transcended along with the deluded mind and all phenomena. The Tantra of Vajrayana Buddhism is a practical path for transforming human consciousness until the Ultimate Truth becomes obvious. Indeed all Tantra is intensely practical. It is a *sadhana*, a practice of realization to which Yoga is central. It has been called a dialectical response to the abstract approach of Advaita Vedanta, the dominant philosophy of the Hindu elite (Feuerstein, 2001, p 343). All Tantric schools affirm that this transcendental Truth is to be found in the human body and not somewhere else.

Nirvana (*nibbana*) is variously rendered as extinction, the unconditioned, perfection or the Great Peace (Grimes, 1989, p 224). It is the goal of life for Buddhists, the cessation of suffering (Gethin, 1998, pp 74–79; Mizuno, 1996, pp 132–134). There are various versions in the different Buddhist schools, but in Mahayana it is becoming conscious of one's own suchness with its four characteristics of bliss, permanence, freedom and purity. It is a state of peace that the Buddha described as unknown, unique, uncreated and uncultured. For the most part he declined to speculate on it. It has been called unborn, absolute freedom, unconditional, *tathata* or suchness, unchangeable, indescribable, *Dharma-kaya*, and non-attachment to either being or non-being (Cheethan, 1994, p 270). It is the blowing out of the fires of greed, hatred and delusion. According to Mahayana *nirvana* is both immanent and transcendental, and not just something external to the phenomenal universe. Suffering is an illusion that is not avoided by leaving the world, but is corrected by proper insight – a nondualistic conception of reality like that of the *Upanishads*. The One appears as many. Phenomena are void (*shunya*) because they lack essence: there is only universal voidness or emptiness (*shunyata*), which itself is void. This concept of emptiness is also found in the tenth-century *Yoga-Vasishtha*. This emptiness is not nothingness, but no-thing-ness, that is to say, illusion. Anything one could possibly point to, speak or think about is a conceptual construct. Thus nothing that is composite has any essence (*svabhava*) and everything is "without self" (*nairatmya*). In the practical world phenomena provide the content of our experiences. But actually both *nirvana* and *samsara* are constructions of an unillumined mind beyond which the aspirant must rise (Feuerstein, 2001, p 164). In Nagarjuna's Madhyamaka school the teaching means that nothing is independently real (Feuerstein, 2003, p 368).

Feuerstein (2003, p 110) describes *samsara* as "running around in circles." It is conditional existence, the state of being unenlightened. He points out that the word means "confluence" in the sense of a flowing together of the *karmic* conditions that shape our lives. *Samsara* is conditioned existence in which unenlightened beings repeat themselves by endlessly duplicating their *karmic* patterning. It describes the sum total of the habitual behaviors of all beings and things. It is predictable behavioral rigidity and it is in this sense that the unenlightened are masters of limitation. We fear change and we fear the freedom that threatens the ego, which is a homeostatic mechanism, as death itself. Our ignorance (*avidya*) of our true nature through misidentification with the individuality of a particular body-mind prevents the recognition of our reality as transcendental Spirit which is in every being and thing and which is our inalienable nature.

The Kaula school, a branch of Tantrism, follows the principle of reversal (*paravritti*) in which apparently unspiritual activities are considered to be spiritual. Thus enlightenment is not a matter of abandoning the world or of killing one's natural impulses, but a process of visualizing the lower manifested reality as contained in and fusing with the higher Reality. The higher Reality transforms the lower reality. The idea is integration: the self with the Self (what we have termed the identity shift (Jerry & Jerry, 2001, pp 147–156)), and bodily existence with spiritual Reality. Ananda Coomaraswamy (1948, p 40) writes of the "identity of spirit and matter, subject and object" and that "this very world of birth and death is also the great Abyss." The Tantric schools also share the doctrine that from a practical viewpoint this one Reality manifests as a polarity: a static male principle (*Shiva* or *prajna*) of pure Consciousness and a dynamic female principle (*Shakti* or *karuna*) of creative Energy. They are like two sides of the same coin. The universe can be conceptualized as Consciousness enrobed in energy which manifests as a vibrational spectrum layer after layer down to matter.

There are some parallels in modern science. The equivalence of matter and energy is well known in special relativity as described by Einstein's famous equation, $E = mc^2$ (French, 1968), and in quantum mechanics the inseparability of the observer and the observed is now understood in terms of the measurement problem, Heisenberg's uncertainty principle and the phenomenon of non-locality arising from Bell's theorem (Nadeau & Kafatos, 1999; Schwabl, 1995; Griffiths, 1995). Kafetos and Nadeau (1999) see in nonlocality evidence that the universe is conscious. Physics and biology are still firmly rooted in materialism. There are some attempts to assert the primacy of consciousness in the universe by idealist physicists (Goswami, 1993); the relationship between energy and matter becomes the equation: consciousness → energy → matter. But in neuroscience consciousness is still considered to be an emergent property of neural networks in the brain (Blackmore, 2004). Physics conceptualizes two basic kinds of energy: potential and dynamic. The latter includes all of its manifested forms such as kinetic, chemical, heat, electromagnetic, nuclear, etc. The descriptions of *Shakti* seem analogous, with most in potential form (at the individual level the unawakened coiled *kundalini*). The idea resembles David Bohm's implicate (potential) and explicate (manifested) realties in quantum physics (Bohm, 1983). However, modern theory indicates that hidden variables theories such as this one are no longer tenable.

36

The Practice of Nondualistic Tantra in Daily Life

The nondualistic paradigm sketched in chapter 35 has a profound impact on the practice of Tantra in daily life, particularly on the attitudes one brings to one's practice, and how they influence how one practices. The effect is total and pervasive – a new world view.

Tantric Practice in Daily Life

The Himalayan Tradition is an integrated system that progresses seamlessly from Raja Yoga as embodied in Patanjali's Classical Yoga through Vedanta (Shankara is a master in the direct lineage of the Himalayan Tradition), and then to the *samaya* Tantra of Sri Vidya. All these levels depend on the student's spiritual qualification (*adhikara*). The process is an ever inclusive and expanding hierarchy of knowledge and awareness. Transmission (initiation) by the enlightened *guru* is key to the process. Sri Swami Rama (1989; 2002e) outlines the basic curriculum which is founded on the eight rungs of Classical Yoga. In addition it includes developing a personal philosophy of life, working with the four primitive fountains (food, sex, sleep and self-preservation), emotional purification, the use of *mantra*, meditation, prayer and contemplation, the selfless action of Karma Yoga, working with everyday relationships, and some special techniques such as *yoga nidra*, *agni sara*, exercises without movement, *bhuta shuddhi*, and the application of *sushumna*. From the Tantric perspective the first initiation is *mantra*, the second is *yantra* and the third is *chakra puja* (Tigunait, 1999). Swami Veda Bharati (1998) has summarized the components of the Himalayan Tradition of Yoga meditation.

As opposed to the verticalism described above in chapter 35 (Feuerstein, 2001, p xxix), this is a path of integralism that is designed to express divine potential here and now. We are all masters of limitation. We say "mastery" of limitation because of the masterful way in which we manage day to day to make a mess of our own lives and of the lives of others! Tantric practice in daily life is about recreating ourselves as Masters of Divine Expression. Sri Swami Rama would tell us to never mind about God and enlightenment after death. You need Him right here and now.

With the opening of the Centre of Consciousness into direct awareness all daily practice changes radically (Jerry & Jerry, 2001, pp 161–180). Practices like *hatha* and *pranayama* are now done as meditation in action, that is, immersed in and flowing from that Centre. Meditation changes radically as the Presence becomes the object of *bhavana*: practicing the presence of God or *ishvara pranidhana* as described in the *Yoga-Sutra*. The objective becomes to crystallize that Presence into a stable background of awareness in all things (Kristof, 2000, pp 162–182). All life is lived mindfully and not mechanically. What Swami Rama called the Chariot of *Sadhana* – *abhyasa* and *vairagya* as described in the first *pada* of the *Yoga-Sutra* – becomes the core of practice. The task is to raise one's life to the level of one's meditation.

Figure and Ground

Like the proverbial elephant in the tent this new model of the world takes over one's life. It is like a figure-ground reversal. For most students Yoga is something one does occasionally during the day or during the week. The demands of life are front and centre. But gradually Yoga moves from the periphery to the centre in a complete reversal of priorities that deepens one's life purpose. In a new way you know who you are, why you are here, and the task to be done.

As Lord Krishna (representing the Inner Teacher) explains to Arjuna (the qualified disciple) in the second chapter of the *Bhagavad Gita*, a realized being is one who is established in *sthita prajna* – stable wisdom or stabilized consciousness, equipoise, *aequanimitas*. Only when one is anchored in this way in the Centre of Consciousness is one stable and unreactive, unable to be tipped out by anything. Only when one's sense of identity is stably centered in this way beyond the everyday ego awareness can one begin the journey with *guru*'s guidance to the other shore and not get lost or fall into insanity as the familiar world collapses into higher states of Consciousness.

Mastery of *dharana* is essential to this achievement (Satyasangananda Saraswati, 2003, p 64). There are many realized beings who have no control over their external functions, and who require someone to help feed and clothe them and to direct their physical functioning because they remain immersed in a trance-like state unaware of the body and its needs. One established in stable wisdom is unconflicted, in total control over life and personality with no aberration of thought, speech, action or behavior. A master can hold the bliss and ecstasy of the highest realization without being overwhelmed and still remember his telephone number and zip code and how to function in a bank or grocery store. "Perform actions dwelling in Yoga, abandoning attachment, O Conqueror of Wealth, being alike to success and failure. Equanimity is called yoga." (*Bhagavad Gita* II.48: Rama, 1985, p 84).

The Unity of All Life

The unity of *nirvana* and *samsara* leads to a profound change in how life is experienced and lived. From this nondualist position there can be no "other." In Tantra there is reverence for the body as a temple of God. Unfortunately many of us dislike or even hate our physical body and see it as imperfect. This keeps the cosmetic plastic surgeons very busy! But now the body is to be treated with respect and looked after as a vehicle for enlightenment. This means a holistic approach to exercise, cleansing practices, diet, supplements, stress management, emotional purification, learning to be still, self-training, management of the instinctual urges, avoiding substance abuse, etc. (Rama, 1980). The Inner critic must be silenced. One abandons self abuse, physical, verbal or mental. One can no longer afford the luxury of negative thinking. The concept extends to relationships, for now the "other" is also God, and what I do to another also hurts me. The practice of the *yamas* and *niyamas* in daily life, especially *ahimsa*, is raised to a new level of intensity.

These changes do not happen overnight in a burst of inner light. Rather they ferment and emerge gradually over many years. But the process is inexorable. Once the Divine Flame has been lit there is no going back. Like a tender young plant struggling towards the light each and every advance has to be integrated from practice into being at every level of the personality before the flower can bloom. It is a long and arduous journey, but its ultimate end is the birth of a fully realized being, the spiritualization of matter.

Karma and Creativity

We were always astounded by Swami Rama's capacity to manifest in the physical world – organizations, resources of all kinds, physical structures, cultural and artistic endeavors. "Yoga is skillfulness in action." (*Bhagavad Gita* II.50). Swamiji was a devotee of the Divine Mother Who blessed his every move with grace and abundance (he was a master of Sri Vidya which is a branch of Shakta Tantrism (Tigunait, 1998b, p 41)). The new paradigm means that one's interactions are with a universe of living energy and become co-creative rather than the usual relationship of control and exploitation of a dead material world.

One learns that human beings are continuously creative with no off switch, continuously engaging the laws of *karma* in an ongoing dance of interactions. The experience of Karma Yoga becomes one of action flowing from the Centre of Consciousness. One is doing right action in the moment in the right place, at the right time, with the right people.

One begins to understand that the laws of *karma* are not retributive or punitive, but actually the laws of creativity, of manifestation in the world. Manifestation cannot happen without the play of cause and effect, and the laws of *karma* are the laws of cause and effect extended into the moral and psychic realm. Choice is in the moment, but once a choice is made its consequences must be experienced according to those laws.

Our language through nominalization has reified the universe into a thing, but actually it is a process. As a thing we project imperfection onto it, but in fact it is a perfect process which operates truly according to its laws of time, space and causation. A child makes a mess with a lump of clay, but a skilled artist creates a masterpiece of sculpture. The clay performs perfectly in both cases according to the causal laws of that medium. But the artist knows how to guide those laws into artistic manifestation. So much of the training of an artist or musician is learning to master one's expressive medium. Paradoxically the discipline of that mastery unleashes the freedom of artistic expression of the master. Living life in relationship to *Shakti* in this way turns life into an art.

Speaking metaphorically (Jerry & Jerry, 2001, pp 139–160), one learns to experience how the universe seems to mirror one's pictures of reality, one's model of the world, faithfully following the point of attention and intention behind actions. Paradigms have creative power and to radically change your life the most powerful thing you can do is to change your models of reality with their beliefs, values, attitudes, criteria and cause-effects, desires and expectations. One learns how to interact co-creatively with this process to manifest desires and visions. One also realizes that the grand creation of a master of divine expression, which is enlightenment, is an extension of this same process.

This is a kind of transpersonal visioning (for you can only create what you can imagine) in which you generate a life vision of extraordinary beingness under the guidance of the Inner Teacher. By performing actions established in Yoga (following your Centre without hesitation) you re-create yourself over and over, step by step into the highest vision that you can have of yourself until that pinnacle of perfection is reached. In the process you transform your identity, recreate your life context and alter your way of evaluating what is real. The universe responds by restructuring itself to fit your expanding new models of reality.

This is not a *siddhi* (power); we all do it all of the time. But now the process becomes more conscious and hence more intentional. But to function this way in the world requires a sense of the universe as *Shakti*, as live, intelligent and dynamic creative energy. The *Shiva/Shakti* polarity of Tantra lies at the base of this process, the one acting as Guide and the other as co-creative movement.

One of the striking aspects of this process is synchronicity. One learns to recognize synchronicities and to distinguish them from serendipity and chance occurrences. One also learns to walk fearlessly through these doors when they open.

> If you have within you ... (an Inner Being) ... sufficiently awake to watch over you, to prepare your path, it can draw towards you things which help you, draw people, books, circumstances, all sorts of little coincidences which come to you as though brought by some benevolent will and give you an indication, a help, a support to take decisions and turn you in the right direction. But once you have taken this decision, once you have decided to find the truth of your being, once you start sincerely on the road, then everything seems to conspire to help you in your advance.
>
> The Mother, 1972, p 233

Existential Crisis

This nondual Tantric paradigm can precipitate a deep existential crisis when the disciple recognizes that the universe is not an independent reality. This can also occur during retirement (*vanaprastha*) when an individual begins to commit seriously to spiritual search and can step back from the world. One begins to see it all as a game, a *karmic* pool, and one stops wanting to participate. One realizes that to step back into worldly activities will only reactivate the same worldly conflicts and frustrations. Desires and visions are attractive at first but they soon draw one back into the worldly fray. In the unprepared individual this can produce a severe depression and apathy as an existential crisis.

Perhaps the longest and deepest example of such a crisis in the texts is Rama's lament to Vasishtha in the Yoga Vasishtha (Venkatesananda, 1993, pp 8–19). But for the disciple this experience is a blessing in disguise for it indicates his or her readiness for spiritual instruction, having attained a degree of non-attachment. The disciple has lost interest in worldly activities, achieved some detachment and now can turn inwards for the spiritual journey. This is true detachment, a position of spiritual strength. It is not the weakness of old-age, sickness, depression or apathy.

Virtual Reality

Perhaps as an extension of the above one can talk about the existential crisis of a virtual reality. In the modern world we are all very familiar with the idea of a virtual reality. Computer games are perhaps the best example. Simulators are used to train pilots and surgeons. But for a fully absorbed participant even movies, television or a good book (e.g., Sagan 2003), can provide a virtual reality. New Age philosophy says that we create our own reality. We think it is more accurate to say that we construct our own experience of reality. The idealistic position that there is no reality "out there" and all that we experience is just projection from the mind is less tenable than a position that there is a reality of some kind "out there" which can be studied by science and that we construct our personal experience of it using our nervous system and mind. Science describes that reality in terms of mostly space containing energy fields of various kinds (including particles).

Cognitive neuroscience describes in great detail how the five senses transmit information from that external reality to the central nervous system and brain, which, in turn, constructs our sensory experience (perception) (Gazzaniga et al, 1998; Purves et al, 2001). In the process of cognition the mind then uses about 20% of that information to construct through generalization, deletion and distortion a model of that world consisting of beliefs, values, attitudes, etc., which it codes in language and stores in memory (Grinder & Bandler, 1976). Whatever may actually be "out there," our experience of it is a virtual reality produced by our mind and nervous system. While models of the world share with others commonalities of culture and experience they are ultimately relative, changeable and highly individualistic. Using the methods of qualitative analysis the postmodern movement has asserted the relativity of truth as produced by our models of the world.

These considerations address the nature of the universe as *maya*, as a manifestation of *Shakti*. Whatever our experience of it, is the universe essentially real or unreal? Do we live in a virtual reality? Perhaps the best example of this kind of illusion is a dream. Is the universe God's dream and do we participate in it also as part of that dream? Apart from the phenomenon of lucid dreaming, most of us realize that a dream is unreal after we awaken from it. A related issue is how do we know that something is real? The perennial wisdom defines real as eternally unchanging, a criterion that can be met only by Consciousness, and one that makes the entire manifested and changing universe unreal. Recent research in psychology suggests that at the everyday level we decide what is real by how the mind uses and assigns sensory submodalities to internal imagery (Andreas & Andreas, 1987). By analogy then do we realize that the world is unreal, a dream, when we wake up from it with enlightenment? "Viewing the centers (the *chakras*) in deep meditation, and ascending his consciousness through them in the various stages of *samadhi* or deep meditation, the Yogi has solved the mystery of the body. He knows it as a manipulatable form of light vibrations." (Yogananda, 1995).

Dream Yoga addresses this paradox as a direct *sadhana*. It is not part of the Himalayan Tradition, but it is one of the six Yogas of Naropa in Tibetan Buddhism (Feuerstein, 2001, p 180) which is Vajrayana (Tantric) Buddhism. The Yoga of the dream state (*milam*) is used to uncover the illusory nature of the waking and dream states (Norbu, 1992; Wangyal Rinpoche, 1998). It leads to lucid dreaming in which practitioners can enter the dream state at will and with full self awareness and learn to control dream events. Part of the practice consists of constantly inquiring whether conscious experience is dreaming or waking. The Yoga of the Illusory Body is another of these six Yogas that also addresses the ultimate illusoriness or voidness of the body, eventually allowing identification with absolute Reality.

Practicing Nonduality

Tantrism has basically a nondualist orientation (Feuerstein, 1998, pp 66–68). Its keynote is integration – of self with Self, and of bodily existence with spiritual Reality. In Hindu Tantra *Shiva* is the primordial, unqualified Reality as pure Consciousness or Light. *Shakti* is the same Reality in dynamic movement and expression into manifestation. *Shakti* is the Life Force, the Universal Energy of Consciousness and the driving force behind all change and evolution. Ultimate Reality is One, expressing as a bipolar process like two sides of the same coin. Creation occurs when the feminine or *Shakti* pole predominates. But dominance of the masculine or *Shiva* pole results in transcendence. The previous section on virtual reality addresses something of the practical aspects of working with the *Shakti* side of the polarity. What about working with the *Shiva* pole?

As a practical example of Tantra's nondualistic metaphysics Feuerstein (1998, p 126) notes that the *Sharada-Tilaka-Tantra* defines *samadhi* as the constant contemplation of the sameness between the small self and Self. As a further example, in the *Tantrasara* Abhinavagupta describes the practice of *bhavana* or creative contemplation of one's essential self as being the same as *Shiva* (Singh, 2003, p xix). According to Singh the method is also given in *sutra* 49 of the Vijnana-Bhairava-Tantra (Singh, 2003, p 45; Satyasangananda Saraswati, 2003, p 209) in the form of *dharana* on the *mantra* in the heart space. *Sutra* 54 is a subtler practice of *tattva dharana*, a *bhavana* of *laya* or dissolution of the various *tattvas* (subtle principles) in regressive order from gross to subtle to transcendence (Singh, 2003, p xix).

This resembles Brunton's Short Path (Brunton, 1988) of constantly reminding ourselves of our true nature. "By incessantly remembering what we really are . . . we set ourselves free. Why wait for what already is?" This approach attests to the philosophy and co-creative power of imagination and the practice of "as if." But without first establishing a solid foundation of the basics one can deceive oneself or be deceived by others. Carl Jung warned about this fatal error of identifying with the unconscious archetype of the god-man with a resultant inflation of the personality, instead of with the transcendental Reality (Jerry & Jerry, 2001, p 149). This danger is averted by the awakening of the Centre of Consciousness or Presence with its accompanying guidance from the Inner Teacher. Now the process becomes one of surrender to that Presence through constant remembrance to bring about the identity shift naturally and in right timing. The Presence is real and not something imaginary conjured up by the mind in an "as if" process. This daily practice of the Presence becomes meditation in action with the goal of crystallizing that Presence as a constant background Awareness (Kristof, 2000, pp 162–182).

This section began with the quotation of a popular musical round familiar to every small Western child. What does it have to do with an obscure and erudite philosophy like *nirvana* equals *samsara*? The song exhorts the singer to row his or her boat down life's stream. The boat might represent the personality (of which the body is only a small part in the Vedantic model of the *koshas*), the vehicle necessary to negotiate the flow of life's stream. But the instruction is "gently" and "down." The rower is to "go with the flow" without resistance – to let life unfold in all of its mystery and wonder in full surrender and acceptance. To do this the rower must live in the internal Now, the ultimate Reality beyond time, space and causation, and yet be intimately one with that changing flow of manifestation.

But the instruction goes further. The journey is to be done "merrily." Swami Rama would repeatedly exhort students to be happy and to enjoy their lives. He would say that hurry, worry and curry were the obstacles to enjoyment. (It reminds one of a popular song of the 1970s called "Don't worry, be happy.") But this is an unconditional happiness, a happiness-without-object rooted in *nirvana*, from identification beyond time, space and causation, from the Fullness (*purna*) and Bliss of the Being-Consciousness of the ultimate Reality. And with this identification also comes the realization that "Life is but a dream" – the *maya* of *samsara*, the ever changing cosmos. The shadowy unreality of a dream cannot disturb that eternal happiness. But that happiness (as positive thinking) has additional significance if the New Age idealists who claim that you create your reality are correct. Their Law of Attraction means the universe, like a live energy, will rearrange itself to accommodate and match one's pictures of reality. Under these circumstances one cannot allow oneself the luxury of negative thinking. Hidden depths within a simple ditty! Could it be that this simple lyric symbolizes the essence of the phrase "*nirvana* equals *samsara*"? We think so!

37

The Role of Grace

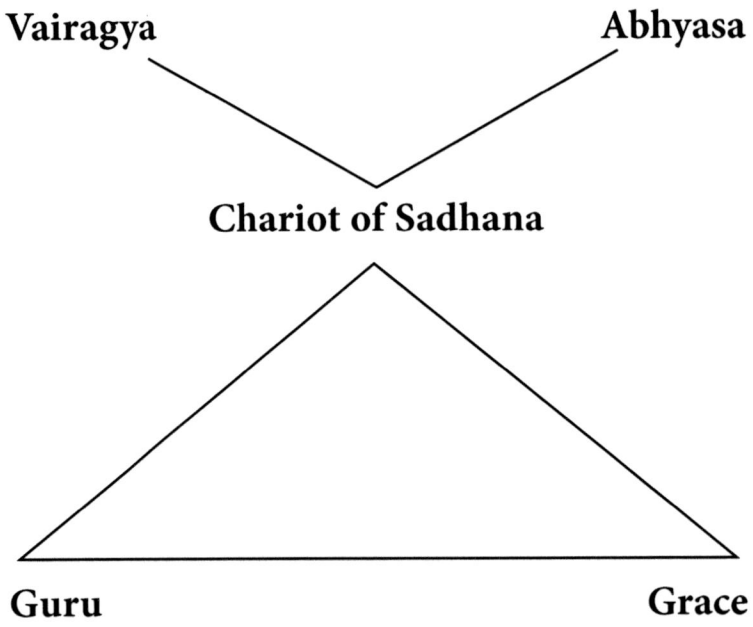

Figure 37.1 *Guru*, Grace and the *Chariot of Sadhana*

In the chapter on Divine Grace in his book *Sacred Journey* (1996) Sri Swami Rama discusses the essential role of grace on the spiritual path. He describes it as the impulse of the divine energy to dispel darkness. It comes in many forms. One is the grace of the scriptures which contains the revealed wisdom passed down from the sages. The grace of the teacher brings that wisdom to life in the student. The grace of God, pure Consciousness, is always present in the life of all of us. But central to all of these is the grace of the student who undertakes spiritual *sadhana* and preparation with the commitment to walk the spiritual path in life with purpose.

Initiation as Grace

In the Himalayan Tradition grace is bestowed through the Master by transmission or initiation. The process is called *shaktipata*, from the words *shakti* (energy) and *pata* (bestowing). Swami Rama translates it as "bestowing the energy" or "lighting the lamp." In the Himalayan Tradition of Yoga, the role of the sage is to awaken within the student the divine flame, that spark of divinity that all human beings carry within. Swami Rama called this the "Teacher within," or the Centre of

Consciousness. Lighting that divine flame is carried out through the grace of God as *shaktipata*. He points out that the term is sometimes translated as "descent of power." Swamiji says that "a power comes from above, of its own, to a vessel that is cleaned, purified, and is prepared to receive it." The student has followed and carried out the *guru's* instructions and has become accomplished in surrender and selflessness. The unconscious residues or *samskaras* have been burned. At this point that grace comes.

In that chapter on Divine Grace in his book *Sacred Journey* (1996) Swami Rama describes his own experience of *shaktipata*, and then asks his master a question. "I wondered if this experience came about because of my effort or my Master's. His answer was simply, 'Grace. A human being,' he explained, 'should make all possible sincere efforts. When he has become exhausted and cries out in despair, in the highest state of devotional emotion, he will attain ecstasy. That is the grace of God. Grace is the fruit that you receive from your faithful and sincere efforts.' "

That means that grace is only possible when a disciple goes through a long period of austerity and spiritual disciplines. He or she must do the assigned practices and follow the teacher's instructions faithfully with truthfulness and sincerity. Then the Master can remove the subtlest obstacle. The experience of enlightenment requires the sincere effort of both Master and disciple. "When you have done your duties skillfully and wholeheartedly, you reap the fruits gracefully. Grace dawns when action ends. *Shaktipata* is the grace of God transmitted through the Master."

The Relationship between the Chariot of *Sadhana* and the Inner Teacher

In the figure above notice the triangle formed by the words Chariot, *guru* and Grace. The practices of *vairagya* and *abhyasa* are the responsibility of the disciple, and thereby he or she begins to understand life and learns how to approach death meaningfully. If the Chariot is practiced sincerely then it invokes additional help. This comes as the *guru* and grace. Swami Rama points out that each is linked to the other, "each so beautiful and comforting, each so powerful. Unfortunately, each is so frequently misunderstood."

The Master sometimes teaches without words or actions. By learning to surrender and moving the ego aside the disciple grows more selfless and gains the ability to learn intuitively from the *guru*. This is the role of the *guru* as an external manifestation of the Inner Teacher or Centre of Consciousness with which he or she is one. The disciple learns in the "cave of silence" as though tuning into the *guru's* frequency and into that stream of knowledge. The *guru* always works from that Centre and the disciple's job is also to learn to work from that same Centre. Swamiji said that this is learned by "doing all duties with love, by being nonattached, and by surrendering." The disciple strives continually for purification and to be prepared for more and greater knowledge. Then Swamiji writes, "Then God will say, 'I want to enter this living temple that you are.' Remove the impurities and you will find that the one who wants to know reality is the source of reality." As disciples our relationship to the Master is eternal. Swamiji puts it this way: "*guru* is the disciple's guide through life, through the mysterious terrain of the spiritual heart, and into and beyond the realm of death." (Rama, 1999b).

Understand this if nothing else: spiritual freedom and oneness with the Tao are not randomly bestowed gifts, but the rewards of conscious self-transformation and self-evolution.

Lao Tzu (Walker, 1992, p 90)

Glossary

abhi-dhyana directing the will, thought or concentration towards (God)

abhinivesha fear of death; "May I not cease to be." One of the *kleshas* (afflictions)

abhyasa regular practice; repetition of the same thing again and again to form a strong habit; the endeavor to make the mind stable and still

acharya Self-realized teacher; a scholar and commentator

adhibhautika caused by other beings such as beasts of prey or one's enemies; one of the three kinds of pain

adhidaivika caused by deities or by natural forces like planetary influences or heat and cold, or by conscious powers of the subtler worlds; one of the three kinds of pain

adhikara a student's qualification

adhikarin qualified; one who is qualified for a study

adhyatman spiritual; pertaining to *Atman*, the innermost self

adhyatma-vidya pursuit of a spiritual science

adhyatmika within one's self; internal to oneself; one of the three kinds of pain from physical sources (illness) or from mental sources (desire, passion, jealousy, greed, fear or depression)

adhyaya formal study of the Vedas

advaita non-dual, not two

agama revealed scriptures or revealed authority

agape highest form of disinterested love in Christianity

agni sara also known as the abdominal lift, is a Yogic *kriya* which lifts the abdominal muscles and pulls up the pelvis gradually to strengthen the navel centre

ahamkara I-maker, ego, ego process

ahara food

ahimsa non-harming, non-violence

aishvarya sovereignty and spiritual freedom; lordship; worldly success; power, luxury and affluence

ajapajapa spontaneous repetition of the *mantra*

akshara letters of the Sanskrit alphabet full of the indestructible divine creative energy of *shakti* which imbues the words and language as well as the letters written on the lotus petals of the *chakras* used for meditation

alabdha-bhumikatva failure to gain the ground of a state of consciousness

aladani transition state between dreaming and deep sleep

alambana object, focus or support for the mind in meditation or concentration

alasya sloth, laziness, languor from *tamas*

amatra without a letter or corresponding sound

anahad nada, anahata nada unstruck subtle sounds in the heart centre

ananda shakti the energy of bliss

ananda, anandam bliss

anandamayakosha blissful sheath or body

ananta infinite, limitless

anapana-sati (Pali) Buddhist meditation using breath awareness at the nostrils; measured breathing

an-avasthitatva instability; having gained a higher ground, one falls from it

angam-ejayatva moving and twitching of limbs in meditation; unsteadiness or shaking of the body

angas the eight limbs of Raja Yoga

annamayakosha food sheath, physical body

antahkarana inner mental instrument (*manas, chitta, buddhi* and *ahamkara*); psyche

antar internal

antar mouna the practice of inner silence

antarayas impediments, obstructions or obstacles

antaryamin the indweller (inner teacher or *guru*); pervading within all things and beings

anugraha grace, benevolence, kindness

anugraha shakti the flow of grace

anumana inference (a valid proof); logical, rational inferential process leading to a conclusion

apara-vairagya relative renunciation; preliminary detachment; the lower dispassion relating to worldly objects, and falling within *samprajnata samadhi*

aparigraha nonindulgence, non-possessiveness

arca sacred icons

arjava moral integrity

asamprajnata the *samadhi* which is acognitive, with total control and cessation of *vrittis*, and seedless (*nirbija*), in which the self dwells in the Self

asana Yogic posture

ashram hermitage

ashrama stage of life; traditional Hinduism distinguishes four: student (*brahmacharya*), house-holder (*grihastha*), forest dweller (*vanaprastha*) and renunciate (*sannyasa*)

ashtanga eightfold; Patanjali's Classical or Raja Yoga as described in his *Yoga-Sutra*

asmita ego, I-sense as doer, I-am-ness; reflected spirit (*purusha*) in matter (*prakriti*)

asteya non-stealing

astikya belief in truth as *vidya* (knowledge) *veda* (body of knowledge) and God

atma kripa the grace of the inner Self

atma shakti the power of the soul; spiritual energy or force

atman the inner Divine Self; the self; the spiritual self; oneself

AUM, OM see *pranava*

avastha state

avatara incarnation of a deity

avidya primal ignorance

avikalpa thoughtless

a-virati non-abstention

aviveka indiscrimination

avyakta unmanifest

bahir external

bala strength

bhairava see *Shiva*

bhairavi see *Shakti*

bhakti love, devotion

bhavana contemplating a meaning by cultivating it and impressing it upon oneself until it becomes one's own nature

bhava mental-emotional attitude

bhavya object of concentration

bhaya self-preservation

bhranti-darshana confused philosophies

bhumi ground, level or plateau on the way to *samadhi*

bhur, bhuvah, svah in earth, sky and heaven

bhuta shuddhi purification of the elements

bija mantras see *mantras*

bindu a drop, point or nucleus; infinite point, dot; a compact mass of *shakti* gathered into an undifferentiated point that serves as the source or substratum of the whole cosmos; a point of potential energy where descending Consciousness first emerges into diversity and multiplicity

bodhi awareness of experience

bodhisattva "enlightenment being;" the spiritual practitioner in Mahayana Buddhism who vows to practice for the liberation of all sentient beings

Brahma the Creator

brahma-atma-pranidhana: maintaining the self in *Brahman*

brahmacarya, brahmacharya continence, celibacy; moderation of the senses

Brahman the ultimate Reality; God the Father; Logos, the transcendental Reality

brahma-nadi see *sushumna-nadi*

brahmanda Cosmic Egg of *Brahma* (solar systems, galaxies)

brahmarandhra the soft spot at the crown of the head

brahma-viharas Frolicking in God; the four right attitudes (friendliness toward the happy, compassion for the unhappy, delight in the virtuous, and indifference toward the wicked)

buddhi higher intellect, intuition, intelligence, understanding

catur four

chakra, cakra wheel, plexus, centre

chakra puja worship using the *chakras*

chankramanam walking meditation

chatushpad four foot or part

chetana consciousness; faculty of awareness

chidakasha, cidakasha inner or mental space; the inner screen of awareness behind the eyes and forehead; the space of consciousness

chitta, citta mind field, mind, memory

chitta shakti mental energy

chitta prasadhana clarity and pleasantness to the mind field ; a tranquil, even-mindedness

cit consciousness; awareness

cit shakti the energy of consciousness

citi non-differentiating consciousness; the consciousness-power of the Absolute that brings about the world process

daksha intelligence

dama temperance, restraint of the senses

danda T-shaped elbow prop for meditation in Nada Yoga

darshan audience with a holy individual

darshana seeing

daur-manasya ill-mindedness

daya compassion

devas deities, personified subtle forces

dhairya steadfastness and patience

dharana concentration

dharma law, duty, righteousness, ethical or moral issues, life philosophy or mission

dharma-megha, the *samadhi* of the rain cloud of virtue and of the knowledge of the nature of all things

dhatus bodily constituents

dhi see *medha*

dhriti steadfastness in being true to one's principles

dhvani sound

dhyana meditation

diksha initiation

drashta Seer

duhkha pain

dvaita dualistic

dvandva the pairs of opposites

dvesha aversion

ekagra concentrated, one-pointed

ekagrata one-pointedness

ekendriya third stage in *vairagya*

gunas qualities; attributes, characteristics or constituents of unmanifest *prakriti* (primal nature) which are in equilibrium; their disequilibrium produces the process of creation in which all material entities or evolutes including the mind are composed of the three *gunas* in various degrees and combinations in an evolving hierarchy

guru kripa the grace of the *guru*

guru mantra personal *mantra* received by initiation

guru teacher, master, one who removes (*ru*) darkness (*gu*)

hamsa vidya, the science of *Hamsa*

hara (centre) vital energy centre four cm. below the navel

hatha physical yoga embodying interior, subtle forces

Hiranyagarbha the Golden Womb; God as the immanent spirit of the universe

hitam, mitam, priyam: cultivating a speech that is beneficial, measured, and pleasant

hridayakasha the space at the heart centre

iccha shakti the energy of will

iccha will

ida subtle *nadi* running parallel to the spinal column on the left side; it controls the breath in the left nostril, and when dominant, one's behavior is intuitive and passive

indriyas the ten senses

ishta-devata a spiritual practitioner's chosen or favored deity

Ishvara kripa the grace of God

ishvara pranidhana practicing the presence of God; surrender or devotion to the Lord

Ishvara the Lord or personal God; Divine with form (*saguna-brahman*); *parama-atman*

jagrat, jagriti waking state

jagrata mantra awakened *mantra*

japa repetition of a *mantra*

jitendriya sensory control

jiva individual soul

jivanmukta liberated while living; *jivanmukti* liberation while living

jiva-tattva life principle

jnana knowledge, wisdom or comprehension

jnana shakti the energy of knowledge

jnanendriyas the five cognitive senses

jnani one who knows

jyotsma light

kaivalya liberation, isolation

kalaa a force or ray emanating from the nucleus or *bindu* because of vibrations created by *nada*

kalyana beautiful

karana causal dimension or body (*karana sharira*); cosmic mind; instrument; sense

karanas active and cognitive senses plus the mind

karika verse

karma action that leads to results through the law of cause and effect

karmashaya the storehouse or field of *karma* as *samskaras* and *vasanas*

karmendriyas the five active senses

karuna compassion; dynamic female principle – see *Shakti*

kashayas disrupting emotions

kaya sthairyam body steadiness

kevala-kumbhaka breath suspension; "solo-retention"

khyati discriminating awareness, discernment

klesha affliction

kosha sheath, body

krama diksha gradual unfoldment of the inner *shakti* by initiation; initiation step by step

kritya divine action

kriya action, activity

kriya shakti the energy of action

Kriya Yoga Yoga of transformative action; a path of action

kriyamana karma potential karma

kriyas Yoga practices and other acts

kshama patience

kshipta, kshiptum disturbed, turbulent

kundalini "the serpent power;" spiritual or evolutionary energy

kutastha or Christ center; the *ajna chakra*

lakshana-sutra definition *sutra*

laya dissolution

lila God's play in creation; the divine game of God who creates the worlds in play

lokas planes called *bhu, bhvah, svah, mahah, janah, tapa* and *satya*

madhya centre; consciousness of central reality

madhyama mental level; second stage of descent of Divine Truth as sound

madhyama-nadi see *sushumna-nadi*

madhya-vikasa the development or unfoldment of the centre

maha diksha the rarest and highest level of initiation where the spiritual energy is delivered with full force through an adept to a perfectly prepared disciple

maha-seva service to the *guru* or Master

mahavakya the great sayings of the *Upanishads* used for contemplation in Vedanta

maha-vrata great vow

Maheshvara the Supreme Lord

maithunancha sex

mala blemish; string of 108 beads used as a counter and timer for one's practice of *mantra*

manas sensory-motor mind; lower mind that registers and stores sensory impressions

manasa-putra mental offspring

mandalas symbolic circular figures

manipura "filled with jewels;" the third chakra, the centre of fire, the navel centre

manomayakosha mental sheath or body

mantra, mantram a holy phrase or spiritual formula; combination of syllables or words corresponding to a particular energy vibration and used as an object for meditation

mantra shakti power of a *mantra*

maranatha Come Lord, Come Lord Jesus or *the Lord comes*; *mantra* used in Christian meditation *marma* vital points on the body which are the junction of the body and mind; anatomical sites where muscle, veins, ligaments, bones and joints meet together

matra letter or sound; syllable

matrika little mothers; the letters of the Sanskrit alphabet

maya worldly illusion

medha third stage of revelation of Divine Light as retentive power, the ability of the mind to store its experiences

milam Yoga of the dream state

mitahara a meager diet

mora silent half that follows AUM

mudha, *mudham* somnolent, stupified

muladhara first or root support *chakra* at the base of the spine

mumukshutva drive or desire to enlightenment or liberation

nada vibration; see *spanda*

nadi subtle energy channel

nadi shodhana alternate nostril breathing

nairatmya without self

nasagra point where the bridge of the nose joins the upper lip

neti neti not this, not that

nibbana (Pali) *nirvana*

nidra sleep

nila bindu blue pearl

nirbija without seed

nirguna without attributes; free from all limiting conditions

nirmana-chitta lineage of produced minds forming a Tradition

Nirmanakaya an incarnate form; historical, physical body of a Buddha

nirodha, *nirodhah* control, cessation

niruddha, *niruddhah* totally controlled, arrested state: related to the word *nirodhah*

nirvana "extinction;" transcendence of the ego-self in Buddhism into a Reality beyond space and time; liberation

nir-vitarka without a gross thought; *samadhi* without *vitarkas* or thoughts

nishkama desireless; without desire for fruits

niyamas observances of Yoga

nyasa to place; to take the mind to a point

OM see *pranava*

pada chapter, quarter

para supreme absorption in the transcendent, the supreme Silence; transcendent, transcendental, supreme, beyond

para-atman transcendental self

parabrahman God transcendent

parama Shiva the Highest reality, the Absolute

parama-atman Supreme Self; *Brahman*; *Ishvara*

parashakti the Void; the highest *shakti* (power) of the Divine; see *citi*

para-vairagya absolute renunciation, superior or supreme detachment

paravak source of all sound

paravritti reversal

pashyanti revelation; first stage of descent of Divine Truth as sound

phala fruit

pingala subtle *nadi* running parallel to the spinal column on the right side. It controls the flow of the breath in the right nostril, and when dominant, one's behavior is rational, active and energetic

Prajapati the Progenitor

prajna see *sushupti*; realized wisdom; intuition; the intuitive realization of the true nature of the objects in meditation; process of awakening of wisdom and the wisdom itself

prakarana chapter

prakriti primal nature; matter-energy

pramada negligence

prana vital force

pranamayakosha subtle energy sheath or body

pranapana-smrti breath awareness at the nostrils

pranashakti vital energy or life force

pranava AUM or OM

prana-vyutthana arousal of life force (*prana*) in Yoga

pranayama breath control; voluntary control or expansion of the *pranic* force

pranidhana placing the mind in; to place the mind within

pra-ni-dhatrs those who practice His presence

prarabdha karma active *karma*

prasada clear with a mental state of happiness, joyfulness and intense pleasantness

prasara see *vikasa*

pra-shvasa involuntary exhalation

pratibha flash of light (insight, intuition); second stage of revelation of Divine Truth

pratyahara sensory withdrawal

praxis method

prayoga-shastra, a text or science that teaches a practical method

puja worship

puraka controlled inhalation

purashcharana special intensive practice of a *mantra* for self-purification and liberation, to attain a desired result, or to obtain the *siddhis* of that *mantra* – usually the number of syllables multiplied by a hundred thousand plus twenty percent

purusha see *Shiva*; Spirit; individual soul, roughly interchangeable with the *Atman*

raga attraction, attachment

rajas activity; gives the qualities of activity, motion, movement, assertiveness, stimulation, mobile, pain and action

rasas fluid essences of the body

rechaka controlled exhalation

rishi sage, Seer; the first mind-borne offspring of the Progenitor

sabija with seed

saccidananda existence–knowledge/consciousness–bliss; contraction of *sat chit ananda*

sadguru true, realized spiritual Master

sadhaka spiritual practitioner

sadhana spiritual practice

saguna with qualifications; limiting conditions of name and form

sahaja natural, spontaneous

sahasa courage

sahasrara thousand petaled lotus: seventh *chakra* at the crown of the head

sakshat-kara realization, Self-realization; direct experience

sakshi bhava awareness with the ability to witness; witnessing attitude or stance

sakshi witness

sakshi-chaitanya Witness consciousness; *cit*; absolute, unbounded or universal consciousness

samadhana power of concentration of the mind

samadhi absorption

samadhi-bhavana producing, developing, cultivating and nurturing *samadhi*

samahita harmonized

sambhogakaya "body of enjoyment;" the psychic, subtle or inner dimension of the Mahayana doctrine of the triple body of the Buddha

samhara withdrawal

Samkhya one of the six classical Hindu schools of thought concerned with the classification of categories of existence

samprajnata the lower (*sabija*) *samadhi* of wisdom in which wisdom comes to its most perfect expansion

samsara the world, cycle of birth and death, earthly existence

samshaya doubt

samskaras residues, seeds, subtle causes from past action in the unconscious mind; subtle unconscious residues; personality traits conditioned over one or many lives

samskrita Sanskrit

samtosha, santosha contentment

samvit universal or supreme consciousness

samyama unified concentration; *dharana* (concentration), *dhyana* (meditation) and *samadhi* (absorption) used together

sanchita karma dormant *karma*

sandhi euphony in Sanskrit

sandhya the wedding of the sun and moon

sankalpas desires; resolve

sankalpa-shakti will power, determination, strength of will

sankoca of *shakti* to withdraw the consciousness from going outward through the senses, turning it inwards towards the Self, the Centre of Consciousness – in other words, *pratyahara* or sensory withdrawal.

sarva hinsa vinirmukta abstention from violence

sarva prani hitata concern for universal welfare

sat existence, truth, being; experience of profound Existence or Being

sati (Pali) mindfulness; (Sanskrit *smriti*)

sati-patthana Buddhist mindfulness practice

satsang the spiritual practice of associating with the good company of saints, sages and Self-realized adepts

sat-tarka training the mind to being harmoniously one with the truth of the essential Self being *Shiva*, which will culminate in *bhavana*

sattva purity, illumination; principle of purity, luminosity, lightness, illumination; light which is buoyant, light, illuminating; knowledge and happiness

satya truthfulness

satyagraha truth force; Gandhi's term for non-violent, moral struggle

satyam jnanam anantam truth, knowledge, limitlessness

saumanasya good-mindedness

sa-vitarka with thought

shabdabrahman Brahman in the form of sound; see *nada*

shakti energy, potentia, potency, power, force; Shakti – Shiva's creative energy

shaktipata bestowing the energy, lighting the lamp or the descent of power as higher spiritual initiation

shama calmness, tranquility, quietude

shanta pacific, calm

shantih peace; Peace that passes all understanding

shastra kripa grace of the scriptures

shat-sampat six treasures of Vedanta

shauca, shaucha purity

shavasana corpse posture used for relaxation

shavayatra 61 point exercise; traveling through the body; part of *yoga nidra*

sheva, seva service

shishya student

shithali karana point to point breathing; part of *yoga nidra*

Shiva consciousness in Tantra; a major deity in the Hindu pantheon and the third god of the Hindu Trinity (the destroyer). Consciousness as the male and passive aspect of God as opposed to *Shakti* his creative power and the feminine, active and manifesting aspect of God

shraddha faith, devotion

shruti that which is heard; Divine revelation

shuchi purity

shuddha pure

shuddha vidya pure knowledge

shunya void; empty

shunyata universal voidness or emptiness

shvasa involuntary inhalation

siddhas disembodied saints who are often seen at their abode in sacred places

siddhi accomplishment, perfection, achievement; advanced powers that unfold during the practice of Yoga

sloka verse

smrty-upa-sthana (Buddhist *sati-patthana*) mindfulness meditation

spanda, spandana "throb." The creative pulsation or vibration in the motionless Consciousness of *Shiva* which brings about the manifestation, maintenance and withdrawal of the universe

Sri Vidya Solar Science

srishti creation

sthita prajna stable wisdom or stabilized consciousness, equipoise, *aequanimitas*

sthiti maintenance; stillness, stability, settling down, coming to rest, or steadiness

sthiti-ni-bandhana stability and steadiness of mind and body in life and meditation

sthula gross dimension or body; *sthula-sharira* the physical body

stotra laudatory hymn

styana procrastination

sukshma subtle dimension or body; individual memory and mind; *sukshma-sharira* the subtle body

sumeru mountain; referring to the spine; *sumeru* breathing – special breathing technique up and down the spine

sushumna the central *nadi* running along the spinal column from its base to the crown of the head (and in some systems, curving forward down to *nasagra*); when dominant both nostrils flow equally and the mind becomes quiet and pleasant, and can attain deep meditation

sushumna-nadi central subtle channel in the spine

sushupti dreamless sleep

sutra aphorism, verse

Sutratma the "thread-soul;" in Vedanta, the soul that passes like a thread through the universe

sva-bhava essence

svadhisthana "her own abode;" the second *chakra*

svadhyaya self-study

svapna dreaming state

sva-stha good health

taijasa see *svapna*

tamas inertia; brings inertia, stability, solidity, stagnation, stasis, torpor, stupor, and is heavy, enveloping, indifferent, and lazy

tapas ascetic endeavor (ascesis); intense practice, austerity

Tat tvam asi "That thou art." One of the *mahavakyas* for contemplation in Vedanta

tathata suchness

tattvas elements, principles

tejas splendor

theoria conceptual map, theory

titiksha fortitude, forbearance

turiya (*turya*) fourth; the fourth state of consciousness; supreme consciousness; absolute reality

turiyatita beyond *turiya*

unmani transition state between waking and dreaming

uparati a spirit of renunciation; withdrawal from worldly interests

upaya method

urdhva-kundalini restraint of the *kundalini* at the *ajna chakra*

utsaha persevering; enthusiasm, perseverance, fortitude, firmness, exertion

vachaka, that which enunciates or signifies

vachya meaning; that which is enunciated or signified

vaikhari articulate speech; third stage of descent of Divine Truth as sound

vairagya dispassion, detachment, non-attachment

vaishvanara see *jagrat*

vanaprastha forest dweller; the third *ashrama* or period of life corresponding to early retirement

vasanas propensities, deep desires in the unconscious mind

vashikara mastery or control; fourth stage in *vairagya*

Vasudeva one of the manifestations of *Ishvara*

veda body of knowledge; the most ancient revealed Sanskrit scriptures

via negativa see *neti neti*

vibhava incarnations

vidya knowledge, wisdom; science or branch of study

vijnana the intellect or cognition; applied knowledge

vijnanamayakosha see *buddhi*; intellectual or intuitive sheath or body; buddhi

vikalpakshaya the dissolution of all *vikalpas* or thoughts

vikalpas fancies and imaginations

vikasa of *shakti* concentration on the inner reality even while the senses are active

vikshepas distractions; nine obstacles or disturbances in the path of meditation

vikshipta distracted – away from meditation; state of mind distracted by thoughts; distracted

viparyaya perversive cognition; false cognition or perception; false beliefs and misunderstanding about the tradition

vipassana Buddhist insight meditation

virya vigorous, heroic, enthusiastic; virility, vigor, strength, energy, potency

Vishnu the preserver of the Hindu Trinity

vishranti see *sankoca*

vishuddha the throat center; the space center; the fifth *chakra*

vishva see *jagrat*

vitarka gross thought; worry, concern

viveka discrimination

viveka-khyati discriminative wisdom

vritti operations, activities, fluctuations, modifications, thoughts

vyadhi illness

vyakta manifest

vyatireka ascertainment, the second level in *vairagya*

vyuha various emanations

vyutthana-samskaras worldly involvements, worldly residues

weltanschauung model of the world, world view

yamas restraints of Yoga

yantras geometrical diagrams

yatamana initial effort in detachment

yoga nidra yogic (conscious) sleep

yoga union; union with God; a path or discipline leading to complete integration of consciousness or Self-realization

yoga-brahshta one who has fallen from the path of Yoga

yoga-samskaras residues laid down by the practice of Yoga

Yoga-Sutra manual on Raja, Classical or Ashtanga Yoga written by the sage, Patanjali, around 200 B.C.E.

Bibliography

Ajaya, Swami (1983). *Psychotherapy East and West: A Unifying Paradigm.* Himalayan Institute Press, Honesdale PA.

Alarius (1988). *The Force of Wisdom: Three Radical Shifts into Divine Expression.* Earth Mission Publishing, Sedona AZ (audiotapes).

Alper, Harvey P (Ed) (1989). *Mantra.* State University of New York Press, Albany.

Andreas, Steve & Andreas, Connirae (1987). *Change Your Mind and Keep the Change.* Real People Press, Moab, Utah.

Aranya, Swami Hariharananda (1981). *Yoga Philosophy of Patanjali.* University of Calcutta, Calcutta, India.

Aurobindo, Sri (1953). *Sri Aurobindo on Himself and on The Mother.* Sri Aurobindo Ashram, Pondicherry, India.

Austin JH (1999). *Zen and the Brain: Toward an Understanding of Meditation and Consciousness.* The MIT Press, Cambridge MA.

Austin JH (2006). *Zen-Brain Reflections.* The MIT Press, Cambridge MA.

Ballentine, RM (1987). *Transition to Vegetarianism: An Evolutionary Step.* Himalayan Institute Press, Honesdale PA.

Ballentine, RM (1999). *Radical Healing: Integrating the World's Great Therapeutic Traditions to Create a New Transformative Medicine.* Harmony Books, New York.

Benson H (1975). *The Relaxation Response.* William Morrow, New York.

Berendt, Joachim-Ernst (1983). *The World is Sound – Nada Brahma: Music and the Landscape of Consciousness.* Destiny Books, Rochester, Vermont.

Bhikkhu Nanamoli (1999). *Vishuddhimagga: The Path of Purification.* BPS Pariyatti Editions, Seattle, WA.

Bishop JP (2003). "Prayer, Science and the Moral Life of Medicine." *Archives of Internal Medicine,* 163: 1405–1408.

Blackmore, Susan (2004). *Consciousness: An Introduction.* Oxford University Press, New York.

Bohm D (1983). *Wholeness and the Implicate Order.* Routledge, Chapman & Hall, New York.

Boorstein S (Ed) (1996). *Transpersonal Psychotherapy.* (SUNY Series in the Philosophy of Psychology). State University of New York, Albany, New York.

Borba, Michele (2002). *Building Moral Intelligence: The Seven Essential Virtues that Teach Kids to Do the Right Thing.* Jossey-Bass, New York.

Boyd D (1976). *Swami.* Random House, New York.

Boynton, Robert S (2004). "The Tyranny of Copyright?" *The New York Times,* January 25.

Bragdon E (1990). *The Call of Spiritual Emergency: From Personal Crisis to Personal Transformation.* Jeremy Tarcher, Los Angeles.

Brennan BA (1987). *Hands of Light: A Guide to Healing Through the Human Energy Field.* Bantam Books, New York.

Brunton P (1935). *The Secret Path.* EP Dutton, New York.

Brunton P (1988). *The Notebooks of Paul Brunton (Vol. 15): Advanced Contemplation: The Peace Within You.* Larson Publications, Burdett, New York.

Buddhaghosa, Bhadantacariya (1975). *Visuddhimagga: The Path of Purification.* BPS Pariyatti Editions, Seattle.

Cameron-Bandler L (1985). *Solutions.* FuturePace Inc. San Rafael, CA.

Cheethan, Eric (1994). *Fundamentals of Mainstream Buddhism.* Charles E. Tuttle Co., Boston.

Chibnall JT, Jeral JM, Cerullo MA (2001). "Experiments on Distant Intercessory Prayer: God, Science, and the Lesson of Massah." *Archives of Internal Medicine* 161:2529–2536.

Chidananda, Swami (1998). *The Role of Celibacy in the Spiritual Life.* The Divine Life Society. Shivananda Nagar, Uttaranchal, India.

Chodron, Pema (1995). *Awakening Compassion.* Sounds True. Audiobook.

Clifford T (1994). *Tibetan Buddhist Medicine and Psychiatry.* The Diamond Healing. Motilal Banarsidass, Delhi.

Cohen CB, Wheeler SE, Scott DA; Anglican Working Group in Bioethics (2001). "Walking a Fine Line: Physician Inquiries into Patients' Religious and Spiritual Beliefs." *Hastings Center Report*, 31:29–39.

Collins, Francis S (2006). *The Language of God: A Scientist Presents Evidence for Belief.* Free Press, Simon & Schuster, Roseburg OR.

Collins M (1976). *Light on the Path: Through the Gates of Gold.* Theosophical University Press, Pasadena CA.

Coloroso, Barbara (2003). *The Bully, The Bullied, and the Bystander: From Preschool to High School, How Parents and Teachers Can Help Break the Cycle of Violence.* HarperResource, New York.

Combs A (1995). *The Radiance of Being: Complexity, Chaos and the Evolution of Consciousness.* Paragon House, St. Paul, Minnesota.

Coomaraswamy, Ananda (1948). *The Dance of Shiva: Fourteen Indian Essays.* Asia Publishing House, Bombay, India.

Cortright B (1997). *Psychotherapy and Spirit: Theory and Practice in Transpersonal Psychotherapy.* (SUNY Series in the Philosophy of Psychology). State University of New York, Albany, New York.

Crane L (1998). *The Abundance Course.* Audiotapes. Lawrence Crane Enterprises, Los Angeles.

Dalai Lama (2005). *The Universe in a Single Atom: The Convergence of Science and Spirituality.* Morgan Road Books, New York.

Damasio, Antonio (1999). *The Feeling of What Happens: Body and Emotion in the Making of Consciousness.* Harcourt Brace, New York.

Damon, William (1999). "The Moral Development of Children." *Scientific American*, August, pp 73–78.

Delmonte MM (1990). "The Relevance of Meditation to Clinical Practice: An Overview." *Applied Psychology: An International Review*, 39(3):331–354.

Dossey L (1997a). *Healing Words.* HarperSanFrancisco, San Francisco CA.

Dossey L (1997b). *Prayer Is Good Medicine: Reap the Healing Benefits of Prayer.* HarperSanFrancisco, San Francisco CA.

Dwoskin H (1991). *Freedom Now: The Sedona Method Basic Course.* Audiotapes. Sedona. Training Associates, Sedona AZ.

Dwoskin H (1999a). *Absolute Freedom: Uncovering Your Natural State of Being.* Audiotapes. Sedona Training Associates, Sedona AZ.

Dwoskin H (1999b). *Practical Freedom. Unlease Your Power to Have It All.* Audiotapes. Sedona Training Associates, Sedona AZ.

Dwoskin H (2003). *The Sedona Method.* Sedona Press, Sedona AZ.

Dwoskin H & Levenson L (2001). *Happiness Is Forever.* Books 1 through 5. Sedona Training Associates, Sedona AZ.

Dyczkowski MSG (1987). *The Doctrine of Vibration: An Analysis of the Doctrines and Practices of Kashmir Shaivism.* SUNY Press, Albany.

Easwaren, Eknath (1979). *Like a Thousand Suns: The Bhagavad Gita for Daily Living, Volume 2.* Nilgiri Press, Petaluma, CA.

Easwaren, Eknath (1984). *To Love Is to Know Me: The Bhagavad Gita for Daily Living, Volume 3.* Nilgiri Press, Petaluma, CA.

Ecklund, Elaine Howard (2005). "Spirituality Soars Among Scientists, Study Says." *Science and Theology News.* http://www.stnews.org/Research-1951.htm . Last visited Sept 12, 2005.

Edwards, Paul & Pap, Arthur (Eds) (1973). *A Modern Introduction to Philosophy: Readings from Classical and Contemporary Sources.* Ed 3. The Free Press, New York.

Elgin, Duane (1998). *Voluntary Simplicity: Toward a Way of Life That Is Outwardly Simple, Inwardly Rich.* Quill. Revised edition.

Ellis MR (2002). "Challenges Posed by a Scientific Approach to Spiritual Issues." *The Journal of Family Practice,* 51:259–260.

Essex, Christopher & McKitrick, Ross (2003). *Taken By Storm: The Troubled Science, Policy and Politics of Global Warming.* Key Porter Books.

Falk, Darrel R & Collins, Francis (2004). *Coming to Peace with Science: Bridging the Worlds Between Faith and Biology.* InterVarsity Press, Westmount IL.

Feuerstein Georg (1979). *Yoga-Sutra: An Exercise in the Methodology of Textual Analysis.* Motilal Banarsidass, New Delhi.

Feuerstein Georg (1989). *The Yoga-Sutra of Patanjali: A New Translation and Commentary.* Inner Traditions, Rochester, New York.

Feuerstein, Georg (1998). *Tantra: The Path of Ecstasy.* Shambhala, Boston.

Feuerstein, Georg (2001). *The Yoga Tradition: Its History, Literature, Philosophy and Practice.* Hohm Press, Prescott, AZ.

Feuerstein, Georg (2003) *The Deeper Dimension of Yoga: Theory and Practice.* Shambhala, Boston.

Fort AO (1990). *The Self and Its States: A States of Consciousness Doctrine in Advaita Vedanta.* Motilal Banarsidass, Delhi.

French, AP (1968). *Special Relativity.* W.W. Norton & Company, New York.

Freedman O, Orenstein S, Boston P, Amour T, Seely J, Mount BM (2002). "Spirituality, Religion and Health: A Critical Appraisal of the Larson Reports." *Annals (Royal College of Physicians and Surgeons of Canada)*, 35(2):90–93.

Furman ME & Gallo FP. (2000). *The Neurophysics of Human Behaviour: Explorations at the Interface of Brain, Mind, Behaviour, and Information.* CRC Press, Boca Raton.

Gach MR & Marco C (1981). *Acu-Yoga.* Japan Publications, Inc., Tokyo.

Gach MR & Henning BA (2004). *Acupressure for Emotional Healing.* Bantam Books, New York.

Gallo FP (1999). *Energy Psychology: Explorations at the Interface of Energy, Cognition, Behavior and Health.* CRC Press, Boca Raton FL.

Gallo FP (2000). *Energy Diagnostic and Treatment Methods.* W W Norton, New York.

Gallo FP & Vincenzi H (2000). *Energy Tapping.* New Harbinger Publications, Oakland, CA.

Gallop (2005). "Americans on the Paranormal." http://www.heartheissues.com/americanson-paranormal-g.html Last visited Aug 7, 2005.

Galton F (1874). "Statistical Inquiries into the Efficacy of Prayer." *Fortnightly Review* 12: 125–136.

Gandhi, Mohandas Karamchand (1983). *Autobiography: The Story of My Experiments with Truth.* Dover Publications, Mineola, N.Y., reprint.

Garrison AW (2005). "Religion, Health, and Questions of Meaning." *Medscape General Medicine* 7:(3). http://www.medscape.com/viewarticle/511714 .

Gazzaley A, Cooney JW, Rissman J, D'Esposito M (2005). "Top-down suppression deficit underlies working memory impairment in normal aging." *Nature Neuroscience*, 8(10):1298–1300.

Gazzaniga MS, Ivry RB, Mangun GR (1998). *Cognitive Neuroscience: The Biology of the Mind.* WW Norton, New York.

Gethin, Rupert (1998). *The Foundations of Buddhism.* Oxford University Press, Oxford.

Goleman D (1977). *The Varieties of the Meditative Experience.* EP Dutton, New York.

Goleman D (Ed) (2003). *Destructive Emotions: How Can We Overcome Them? A Scientific Dialogue with the Dali Lama.* Bantam Books, New York.

Goswami, Amit (1993). *The Self-Aware Universe: How Consciousness Creates the Material World.* Putnam, New York.

Goswami, Shyam Sundar (1999). *Layayoga: The Definitive Guide to the Chakras and Kundalini.* Inner Traditions, Rochester, VT.

Govindan M (2000). *Kriya Yoga Sutras of Patanjali and the Siddhas.* Kriya Yoga Publications, St. Etienne de Bolton, Quebec, Canada.

Greeley A (1975). "The Society of the Paranormal: A Reconnaissance." *Sage Research Paper*, Vol 3, series 90–023, Beverley Hills, CA.

Greene, Robert (2000). *The 48 Laws of Power.* Penguin, USA.

Griffiths, David J. (1995). *Introduction to Quantum Mechanics.* Prentice Hall, Englewood Cliffs, New Jersey.

Grigsby, Mary (2004). *Buying Time and Getting By: The Voluntary Simplicity Movement.* State University of New York Press, Albany, New York.

Grimes J (1989). *A Concise Dictionary of Indian Philosophy: Sanskrit Terms Defined in English.* State University of New York Press, Albany, New York.

Grinder J & Bandler R (1976). *The Structure of Magic, Volumes I and II.* Science and Behavior Books, Palo Alto, CA.

Grof S (2000). *Psychology of the Future: Lessons from Modern Consciousness Research.* (SUNY Series in Transpersonal and Humanistic Psychology). State University of New York Press, Albany, New York.

Grof C & Grof S (1989). *Spiritual Emergency: When Personal Transformation Becomes a Crisis.* Jeremy P Tarcher, Los Angeles.

Gunaratana, Bhante Henepola (2002). *Mindfulness in Plain English.* Wisdom Publications, Boston.

Hall LM & Belnap BP (2000). *The Sourcebook of Magic: A Comprehensive Guide to the Technology of NLP.* Crown House Pub Ltd, Bancyfelin, Wales.

Hall DE (2006). "Religious Attendance: More Cost-Effective Than Lipitor?" *Journal of the American Board of Family Medicine,* 19(2):103–109.

Hardy Sir A (1979). *The Spiritual Nature of Man: A Study of Contemporary Religious Experience.* Oxford University Press, Oxford, p 127.

Harrigan, Joan Shivarpita (1996). *Kundalini Vidya.* Patanjali Kundalini Yoga Care, Knoxville, TN.

Hart T, Nelson PL, Puhakka K (Eds) (2000). *Transpersonal Knowing: Exploring the Horizon of Consciousness* (SUNY Series in Transpersonal and Humanistic Psychology). State University of New York, Albany, New York.

Hawkins DR (1995). *Power vs Force: An Anatomy of Consciousness: The Hidden Determinants of Human Behavior.* Veritas Publishing, Sedona AZ.

Hawkins DR (2001). *The Eye of the I from Which Nothing Is Hidden.* Veritas Publishing, Sedona AZ.

Hawkins DR (2003). *I: Relativity and Subjectivity.* Veritas Publishing, Sedona AZ.

Hawkins DR (2005). *Truth vs Falsehood: How to Tell the Difference.* Axial Publishing Company, Toronto.

Hawkins DR (2006). *Transcending the Levels of Consciousness: The Stairway to Enlightenment.* Veritas Publishing, Sedona AZ.

Hey T & Walters P (2003). *The New Quantum Universe.* Cambridge University Press, Cambridge.

Hicks, E & J (2004). *Ask and It Is Given: Learning to Manifest Your Desires.* Hay House, Carlsbad, CA.

Hicks, E & J (2006). *The Amazing Power of Deliberate Intent: Living the Art of Allowing.* Hay House, Carlsbad, CA.

Humphreys, Christmas (1968). *Concentration and Meditation. A Manual of Mind Development.* Element, Rockport, MA.

Huxley A (1944). *The Perennial Philosophy.* Harper and Row, New York.

Jacobson E (1929). *Progressive Relaxation.* University of Chicago Press, Chicago.

James T & Woodsmall W (1988). *Time Line Therapy and the Basis of Personality.* Meta Publications, Cupertino CA.

Jennings, Charles (1999). *Brain: The Neurobiology of Morals*. Nature, Science Update, October 19.

Jerry, LM (1985). "Paradigm Shifts in Clinical Research: The Tomato Effect Revisited." *Clinical and Investigative Medicine*. 8:249–50.

Jerry LM (1996). "Psychoneuroimmunology." Chapter 87 in R Greger & U Windhorst (eds). *Comprehensive Human Physiology*, Vol 2. Springer-Verlag, Berlin.

Jerry LM & Jerry MB (2001). *Sutras of the Inner Teacher: The Yoga of the Centre of Consciousness*. Unlimited Publishing, Bloomington, Indiana.

Johari, Harish (1986). *Tools for Tantra*. Destiny Books, Vermont.

Johnsen, Linda (2000). *Meditation Is Boring? Putting Life in Your Spiritual Practice*. Himalayan Institute Press, Honesdale, PA.

Jnaneshvara Bharati, Swami (2004). http://swamij.com/maranatha.htm . Last visited August, 2005.

Jung CG (1975). *Psychological Commentary on Kundalini Yoga*, Lecture I. Spring 1975: 8.

Kabat-Zinn, Jon (2002). *Guided Mindfulness Meditation, Series 1*. Sounds True, Boulder, CO.

Kafatos M & Nadeau R (1999). *The Conscious Universe: Parts and Wholes in Physical Reality*. Ed.2. Springer, Berlin.

Kaji DS (2001). *Common Sense About Uncommon Wisdon: Ancient Teachings of Vedanta*. Himalayan Institute Press, Honesdale PA.

Kennedy, Mark (2004). "Gloomy Fear of Terrorism Cloaks Globe." *Calgary Herald*, Monday, January 19, pA1.

Koenig HG (2000). "Religion, Spirituality and Medicine: Application to Clinical Practice." *The Journal of the American Medical Association*, 284:1708.

Koenig HG, McCullough ME, Larson DB (2000). *Handbook of Religion and Health*. Oxford University Press, New York.

Korzybski A (1980). *Science and Sanity. An Introduction to Non-Aristotelian Systems and General Semantics*. Ed 4. The International Non-Aristotelian Library Pub. Co.

Kristof, Aziz (1999). *Transmission of Awakening, The Teaching of Aziz: A New Initiation into the Path of Self-Realization*. Motilal Banarsidass, New Delhi.

Kristof, Aziz (2000). *The Human Buddha: Enlightenment for the New Millennium*. Motilal Banarsidass Publishers Private, Delhi.

Kristof, Aziz & Emami, Houman (1999). *Enlightenment Beyond Traditions: The Complete Inner Map of Spiritual Awakening*. Motilal Banarsidass, Delhi.

Kutz I, Borysenko JZ, Benson H (1985). "Meditation and Psychotherapy: A rationale for the integration of dynamic psychotherapy, the relaxation response and mindfulness meditation." *The American Journal of Psychiatry*, 142: 1–8.

Lakshmanjoo, Swami (2000). *Kashmir Shaivism: The Secret Supreme*. Universal Shaiva Fellowship, Culver City, CA.

Larson GJ (1979). *Classical Samkhya*. Ed 2. Motilal Banarsidass, Delhi.

Larson DB, Swyers JP, McCullough ME (1997). *Scientific Research on Spirituality and Health: A Consensus Report*. National Institute for HealthCare Research, Rockville MD.

LeDoux, Joseph (2002). *Synaptic Self: How Our Brains Become Who We Are*. Viking Penguin, New York.

Lele A, Ranade A and Frawley D (1999). *Secrets of Marma.* International Academy of Ayurveda. Atrey Rugnalaya, Erandawana, Pune, India.

Levenson, L (1998). *No Attachments, No Aversions: The Autobiography of a Master.* Lawrence Crane Enterprises, Los Angeles.

Lincoln, YS & Guba, EG (1985). *Naturalistic Inquiry.* Sage Publications, Newbury Park, CA.

Lo B, Quill T, Tulsky J (1999). "Discussing Palliative Care with Patients." *Annals of Internal Medicine,* 130:744–749.

Lovejoy A (1936). *The Great Chain of Being.* Harvard University Press, Cambridge, Mass.

Lozanov, Georgi (1978). *Suggestology and Outlines of Suggestopedy.* Gordon and Breach, New York.

MacLean, Paul D (1984). "Psychosomatic Disease and the Visceral Brain: Recent Developments Bearing on the Papez Theory of Emotions." In *Basic Readings in Neurophysiology.* RL Isaacson (Ed.) Harper and Row, New York, pp 181–211.

Matthews DA, McCullough ME, Larson DB, Koenig HG, Swyers JP, Milano MG (1998). "Religious Commitment and Health Status: A Review of the Research and Implications for Family Medicine." *Archives of Family Medicine,* 7:188–124.

McFetridge G, Aldana J, Hardt J, Slavinski Z (2004a). *Peak States of Consciousness: Theory and Applications, Volume 1: Breakthrough Techniques for Exceptional Quality of Life.* Institute for the Study of Peak States, Hornby Island, BC.

McFetridge G, Pellicer M, Waisel A (2004b). *Peak States of Consciousness: Theory and Applications, Volume 2: Extraordinary Spiritual and Shamanic States.* Institute for the Study of Peak States, Hornby Island, BC.

Merrell-Wolff F (1994). *Experience and Philosophy: A Personal Record of Transformation and a Discussion of Transcendental Consciousness.* State University of New York Press, Albany.

Miller R (2000). *The Principles and Practice of Yoga Nidra.* The Advaitayana Yoga Tape Series, Volume 1. http://members.aol.com/millerYoga Last visited July, 2005.

Mitchell S (1988). *Tao Te Ching.* HarperCollinsPublishers, New York.

Mizuno, Kogen (1996). *Essentials of Buddhism.* Kosei Publishing, Tokyo.

Muktananda, Swami (1992). *I Am That: The Science of Hamsa from the Vijnana Bhairava.* SYDA Foundation, South Fallsburg, New York.

Nadeau, R & Kafatos, M (1999). *The Non-Local Universe. The New Physics and Matters of the Mind.* Oxford University Press, New York.

Nelson JE (1994a). *Healing the Spirit: A New Understanding of the Crisis and Treatment of the Mentally Ill.* Jeremy P Tarcher, Los Angeles.

Nelson JE (1994b). *Healing the Split: Integrating Spirit into Our Understanding of the Mentally Ill.* State University of New York Press, Albany.

Nikhilananda, Swami (1977a). Ed. 4. *The Upanishads: A New Translation.* 4 Volumes. Ramakrishna-Vivekananda Center, New York.

Nikhilananda, Swami (1977b). *The Upanishads: A New Translation.* Volume 1. Ramakrishna-Vivekananda Center, New York.

Nikhilananda, Swami (1987a). *The Mandukyopanishad with Gaudapada's Karika and Shankara's Commentary.* Advaita Ashram, Calcutta.

Nikhilananda, Swami (1987b). Ed 5. *The Mandukya Upanishad.* Advaita Ashrama, Calcutta.

Niranjanananda, Paramahamsa (1992). *Prashnopanishad (Yoga Siddhanta Bhashya).* Sri Panchdashnam Paramahamsa Alakh Bara, Deoghar, Bihar, India.

Niranjanananda, Paramahamsa (1993a). *Yoga Darshan: Vision of the Yoga Upanishads.* Sri Panchdashnam Paramahamsa Alakh Bara, Deoghar, Bihar, India.

Niranjanananda, Paramahamsa (1993b). *Dharana Darshan.* Sri Panchdashnam Paramahamsa Alakh Bara, Deoghar, Bihar, India.

Niranjanananda, Paramahamsa (1993c). *Sannyasa Darshan.* Sri Panchdashnam Paramahamsa Alakh Bara, Deoghar, Bihar, India.

Niranjanananda Saraswati, Swami (1995). *Yoga Sadhana Panorama, Volume I.* Bihar School of Yoga, Munger, Bihar, India.

Norbu, Namkhai (1992). *Dream Yoga and the Practice of Natural Light.* Snow Lion Publications, Ithaca, New York.

O'Connor, Joseph & Seymour, John (1990). *Introductory Neuro-Linguistic Programming.* Aquarian Press, Cornwall, England.

Olson, Lisa Darlene (2004). "Lesbian Chic." *Calgary Herald,* Friday, January 30, pA17.

Osho (1974). *The Book of Secrets: 112 Keys to the Mystery Within: A Comprehensive Guide to Meditation Techniques Described in the Vigyan Bhairav Tantra.* St. Martin's Griffin, New York.

Palmer H (1988). *The Enneagram.* Harper & Row, San Francisco.

Papez, JW (1937). "A Proposed Mechanism of Emotion." *Archives of Neurology and Psychiatry,* 38:725–743.

Payne RA (1995). *Relaxation Techniques: A Practical Handbook for the Health Care Professional.* Churchill Livingston, NY.

Post SG, Puchalski CM, Larson DB (2000). "Physicians and Patient Spirituality: Professional Boundaries, Competency, and Ethics." *Annals of Internal Medicine* 132:578–583.

Prakash P (1998). *The Yoga of Spiritual Devotion: A Modern Translation of the Narada Bhakti Sutras.* Inner Traditions International, Rochester, VT.

Purves D, Augustin, GJ, Fitzpatrick D, Katz LC, LaMantia AS, McNamara JO, Williams SM Eds. (2001). *Neuroscience.* Second Edition. Sinauer Associates, Sunderland, Mass.

Rama, Swami, Ballentine R, Ajaya S (1976). *Yoga and Psychotherapy: The Evolution of Consciousness.* Himalayan Institute Press, Honesdale PA.

Rama, Swami (1978). *Living with the Himalayan Masters.* Himalayan Institute Press, Honesdale, PA.

Rama, Swami (1980). *A Practical Guide to Holistic Health.* Himalayan Institute Press, Honesdale PA.

Rama, Swami (1982a). *Choosing a Path.* Himalayan Institute Press, Honesdale PA.

Rama, Swami (1982b). *Enlightenment Without God: Mandukya Upanishad.* Himalayan Institute Press, Honesdale PA.

Rama, Swami (1985). *Perennial Psychology of the Bhagavad Gita.* Himalayan Institute Press, Honesdale PA.

Rama, Swami (1988). *Path of Fire and Light, Volume II.* Himalayan Inst Press, Honesdale PA.

Rama, Swami (1989). *The Art of Joyful Living.* Himalayan Institute Press, Honesdale, PA.

Rama, Swami (1992a). *Meditation and Its Practice.* Himalayan Institute Press, Honesdale PA.

Rama. Swami (1992b). *Love and Family Life.* Himalayan Institute Press, Honesdale, PA.

Rama, Swami (1996). *Sacred Journey: Living Purposefully and Dying Gracefully.* Himalayan International Institute, New Delhi.

Rama, Swami (1999a). *Guru Purnima* Talk Reprinted by the Himalayan Institute Hospital Trust, Jolly Grant, Dehradun, Uttaranchal, India.

Rama, Swami (1999b). "Mastery Over Death." *Himalayan Institute Hospital Trust Bulletin,* VII(I):1–3, June.

Rama, Swami (2002a). *Calendar 2002.* Swami Rama Centre, Himalayan Institute Hospital Trust, Jolly Grant, Dehradun, Uttaranchal, India.

Rama, Swami (2002b). *A Personal Philosophy of Life.* Himalayan Institute Hospital Trust, Jolly Grant, Dehradun, Uttaranchal, India.

Rama. Swami (2002c). "Purifying the Chakras: The Practice of Bhuta Shuddhi." *Yoga International,* April/May, pp 71–79.

Rama, Swami (2002d). *Samadhi: The Highest State of Wisdom.* Himalayan Institute Hospital Trust, Jolly Grant, Dehradun, Uttaranchal, India.

Rama, Swami (2002e). *Conscious Living: A Guidebook for Spiritual Transformation.* Himalayan Institute Hospital Trust, Doiwala, Uttaranchal, India.

Rama, Swami (2005). *Happiness Is Your Creation.* Himalayan Institute Press. Honesdale, PA.

Ramana Maharshi, Bhagavan Sri (1974). *Spiritual Instruction of Bhagavan Sri Ramana Maharshi.* Sri Ramanasramam, Tiruvannamalai, India.

Ramana Maharshi, Bhagavan Sri (1988). *Who Am I? (Nan Yar?)* Sri Ramanasramam, Tiruvannamalai, India.

Rosenfeld, Richard (2004). "The Case of the Unsolved Crime Decline." *Scientific American,* 290(2):82–89, February.

Rossi, Ernest L (1991). *The 20 Minute Break: Using the New Science of Ultradian Rhythms.* Jeremy P. Tarcher, Los Angeles.

Rothberg DJ, Kelly S, Krippner S (Eds) (1998). *Ken Wilber in Dialogue: Conversations with Leading Transpersonal Thinkers.* 1st Quest Edition. Theosophical Publishing House, Pasadena CA.

Sagan, Nick (2003). *Idlewild.* Putnam, New York.

Salzberg S & Goldstein J (2001). *Insight Meditation: A Step-By-Step Course on How to Meditate.* Sounds True, Boulder, Colorado.

Sannella L (1992). *The Kundalini Experience: Psychosis or Transcendence?* Integral Publishing, Lower Lake, CA.

Satyananda Saraswati, Swami (1981). *A Systematic Course in the Ancient Tantric Techniques of Yoga and Kriya.* Bihar School of Yoga, Monghyr, Bihar, India.

Satyananda Saraswati, Swami (1984). *Yoga Nidra.* Bihar School of Yoga, Munger, Bihar, India.

Satyananda Saraswati, Swami (1997). *Bhakti Yoga Sagar.* Vol. 3. Sivananda Math, Fort, Munger, Bihar.

Satyasangananda Saraswati, Swami (1984). *Tattva Shuddhi: The Tantric Practice of Inner Purification.* Bihar School of Yoga. Munger, Bihar, India.

Satyasanganananda Saraswati, Swami (2003). *Sri Vijnana Bhairava Tantra: The Ascent.* Yoga Publications Trust, Munger, Bihar, India.

Schultze, Quentin J (2002). *Habits of the High-Tech Heart: Living Virtuously in the Information Age.* Baker Academic, Grand Rapids, MI.

Schwabl, Franz (1995). *Quantum Mechanics.* Springer-Verlag, New York.

Scotton BW, Chinen AB, Battista RJ, Chinen A, Chunen A (Eds) (1996). *Textbook of Transpersonal Psychiatry and Psychology.* Basic Books, New York, NY.

Shapiro DH Jr (1980). *Scientific/Personal Exploration of Meditation: Self-Regulatory and Altered State of Consciousness.* Aldine, New York.

Shapiro, Francine (1995). *Eye Movement Desensitization and Reprocessing.* Guilford Press, New York.

Shuman JJ & Meador KG (2003). *Heal Thyself: Spirituality, Medicine, and the Distortion of Christianity.* Oxford University Press, New York.

Singh, Jaideva (1979). *Siva Sutras: The Yoga of Supreme Identity.* Motilal Banarsidass, Delhi.

Singh, Jaideva (1980). *Spanda Karikas: The Divine Creative Pulsation.* Motilal Banarsidass, Delhi.

Singh, Jaideva (1987). *Pratyabhijnahridayam: The Secret of Self-Recognition.* Motilal Banarsidass, Delhi.

Singh, Jaideva (2003). *Vijnana Bhairava or Divine Consciousness: A Treasury of 112 Types of Yoga.* Motilal Banarsidass, Delhi.

Sivananda, Swami (1986a). *Tantra Yoga, Nada Yoga and Kriya Yoga.* The Divine Life Society, Rishikesh, Utaranchal, India.

Sivananda, Swami (1986b). *Concentration and Meditation.* The Divine Life Society, Shivanandanagar, Uttaranchal, India.

Sloan RP, Bagiella E, Powell T (1999). "Religion, Spirituality and Medicine." *Lancet,* 353:664–667.

Sloan RP, Bagiella E, VandeCreek L et al (2000). "Should Physicians Prescribe Religious Activities?" *The New England Journal of Medicine,* 342:1913–1916.

Sovik, Rolf (2005). *Moving Inward: The Journey to Meditation.* Himalayan Institute Press, Honesdale, PA.

Sri Ramananananda Saraswathi, Swami (1980). *Tripura Rahasya.* Sri Ramanasramam, Tiruvannamalai, India.

St-Onge, MP, Keller, KL, Heymsfield, SB (2003). "Changes in Childhood Food Consumption Patterns: A Cause for Concern in Light of Increasing Body Weights." *The American Journal of Clinical Nutrition,* 78(6):1068–73, Dec.

Teixeira, Bryan (1987). "Comments on Ahimsa (Nonviolence)." *The Journal of Transpersonal Psychology,* 19:1–17.

The Mother (1972). *Questions and Answers: 1950–1951.* Sri Aurobindo Ashram Press, Pondicherry, India.

Tigunait, Pandit Rajmani (1991). *Yoga on War and Peace.* Himalayan Institute Press, Honesdale, PA.

Tigunait, Pandit Rajmani (1996). *The Power of Mantra and the Mystery of Initiation.* Yoga International Books, Honesdale, PA.

Tigunait, Pandit Rajmani (1997). *From Death to Birth: Understanding Karma and Reincarnation.* Himalayan Institute Press, Honesdale, PA.

Tigunait, Pandit Rajmani (1998a). *Swami Rama of the Himalayas: His Life and Mission.* Himalayan Institute Press, Honesdale.

Tigunait, Pandit Rajmani (1998b). *Shakti, The Power in Tantra: A Scholarly Approach.* Himalayan Institute Press, Honesdale PA.

Tigunait, Pandit Rajmani (1999). *Tantra Unveiled. Seducing the Forces of Matter and Spirit.* Himalayan Institute Press, Honesdale PA.

Tigunait, Pandit Rajmani (2002). *The Himalayan Masters: A Living Tradition.* Himalayan Institute Press, Honesdale PA.

Tolle, Eckhart (2005). *A New Earth. Awakening to Your Life's Purpose.* Dutton, New York.

Tweedie I (1986). *Daughter of Fire. A Diary of a Spiritual Training with a Sufi Master.* Blue Dolphin Publishing, Nevada City, CA.

Vandenbroek, Goldian & Schumacher, E.F. (Eds) (1996). *Less Is More: The Art of Voluntary Poverty: An Anthology of Ancient and Modern Voices Raised in Praise of Simplicity.* Inner Traditions International. Ltd.

Vaughan F, Walsh R, Mack J (Eds) (1993). *Paths Beyond Ego: The Transpersonal Vision.* (A New Consciousness Reader). JP Tarcher, New York NY.

Veda Bharati, Swami (1974). *Superconscious Meditation.* Himalayan Institute Press, Honesdale, PA.

Veda Bharati, Swami (1979a). *God.* Himalayan Institute Press, Honesdale PA.

Veda Bharati, Swami (1979b). *Meditation and the Art of Dying.* Himalayan Institute Press. Honesdale PA.

Veda Bharati, Swami (1981). *Mantra and Meditation.* Himalayan Institute Press, Honesdale, PA.

Veda Bharati, Swami (1982). *Yamas and Niyamas.* Dawn, Winter. pp 27–33.

Veda Bharati, Swami (1985). *Philosophy of Hatha Yoga.* Ed 2. Himalayan Institute Press, Honesdale, PA.

Veda Bharati, Swami (1986). *Yoga-Sutras of Patanjali with the Exposition of Vyasa.* Volume I. Himalayan Institute Press, Honesdale, PA.

Veda Bharati, Swami (1997). *Five Pillars of Sadhana.* Sadhana Mandir Trust, Rishikesh, India.

Veda Bharati, Swami (1998). *The Himalayan Tradition of Yoga Meditation.* Sadhana Mandir Trust, Rishikesh, India.

Veda Bharati, Swami (1999). *Silence.* Sadhana Mandir Trust, Rishikesh, India.

Veda Bharati, Swami (2000). *Contemplative Walking.* Sadhana Mandir Trust, Rishikesh, India.

Veda Bharati, Swami (2001). *Yoga Sutras of Patanjali with the Exposition of Vyasa.* Volume II. Motilal Banarsidass, Delhi.

Veda Bharati, Swami (2004). *The Song of Silence: Subtleties in Sadhana.* The Meditation Center, Minneaplis MN.

Venkatesananda, Swami (1993). *Vasishtha's Yoga.* State University of New York Press, Albany.

Walker, Brian (1992). *Hua Hu Ching: The Unknown teachings of LaoTzu.* HarperSanFrancisco, New York, p 90.

Wangyal Rinpoche, Tenzin (1998). *The Tibetan Yogas of Dream and Sleep.* Snow Lion Publications, Ithaca, New York.

West M (1979). "Physiological effects of meditation: A longitudinal study." *British Journal of Social and Clinical Psychology,* 18:119–127.

Whicher, Ian (1998). *The Integrity of the Yoga Darshana: A Reconsideration of Classical Yoga.* State University of New York Press, Albany.

White J (Ed) (1972). *The Highest State of Consciousness.* Anchor, Garden City NY. pp 352–364.

WHO (1990). *Global Burden of Disease Publication Series.* http://www.hsph.harvard.edu/organizations/bdu/GBDseries.html . Last visited January, 2004.

Wilber K (1996). *A Brief History of Everything.* Shambala, Boston.

Willoughby D (2000). "The Long Journey Home: How mantra found its way back to Christianity." *Yoga International,* April/May 2000: 26–33.

Wilson W (1972). "Mental Health Benefits of Religious Salvation." *Diseases of the Nervous System,* 33:382–386.

Winter RE (Ed) (1983). *Coping with Executive Stress.* Executive Health Examiners. McGraw-Hill, New York.

World Community for Christian Meditation (2004). http://www.wccm.org . Last visited August, 2005.

Yogananda, Paramahamsa (1995). *The Bhagavad Gita.* Self-Realization Fellowship, Los Angeles CA.

Yogananda Paramahamsa (2004). *The Second Coming of Christ. The Resurrection of the Christ Within You.* Vols I and II. Self-Realization Fellowship, Los Angeles CA.

Ziegler, Gene (2004). http://www.people.cornell.edu/pages/elz1/clocktower/Highwayman.html . Last visited January, 2004.

Index

About the Authors

Born in the Province of Ontario, Canada, **Martin and Marian Jerry** have pursued parallel careers as health care professionals. Dr. Martin is a physician-scientist with over 30 years of experience as a university professor in teaching, research, administration and clinical care in internal medicine, oncology and immunology. Dr. Marian is a clinical psychologist with a background in nursing who has had over 30 years of experience in teaching, research, clinical and administrative aspects of health psychology as well as psychosocial oncology and palliative care. Both have published extensively and lectured internationally in their fields of expertise. The Jerrys have enjoyed an eight-year career in international development as consultants to the World Health Organization.

The Jerrys have been students of Yoga since 1971. They began their studies with Vishnudevananda at the Sivananda Ashram in Montreal, and subsequently studied Transcendental Meditation, and then with the Self-Realization Fellowship (tradition of Paramahansa Yogananda). In 1982 they met their spiritual teacher, Swami Veda Bharati (premonastic name: Dr. Usharbudh Arya), who initiated them and their two sons into the Tradition of the Himalayan Masters. He introduced them in 1985 to their Spiritual Master, H.H. Sri Swami Rama of the Himalayas, who initiated them further. The Jerrys studied with their spiritual preceptors at the Himalayan Institute in Honesdale, PA, USA, and in 1988 they hosted an international Yoga Congress for the Tradition in Calgary, Canada. At that time they established the Foothills Yoga Society in Calgary under the guidance of Swami Rama and Dr. Arya for which they have served as founding directors.

Under the guidance of Swami Rama the Jerrys initiated the Himalayan Rural Health Development Project through the Division of International Development at the University of Calgary. This was a Canadian International Development Agency (CIDA) sponsored primary health development project in villages in the Himalayan foothills in partnership with the Himalayan Institute Hospital Trust founded by Swami Rama in Rishikesh, India. This experience has been the source of their interests in medical applications of Yoga philosophy, psychology and practice and their clinical and laboratory research on the effects of meditation in cancer patients. The Jerrys are authors of the book *Sutras of the Inner Teacher: The Yoga of the Centre of Consciousness.*

Mahamandaleshvara Swami Veda Bharati, current Spiritual Director and Preceptor of Sadhana Mandir, Swami Rama's Ashram, and of Swami Rama Sadhaka Grama in Rishikesh, India, has spent the past 60 years teaching and providing spiritual guidance around the world. He was raised in the five-thousand-year-old tradition of Sanskrit-speaking scholar-philosophers of India, and has taught the *Yoga-Sutra* of Patanjali from the age of nine and the Vedas from the age of eleven. Author of the most comprehensive commentary on Patanjali's *Yoga-Sutra* and many other books, Swami Veda is a poet, scholar, research guide and international speaker par excellence.

All of his knowledge has come intuitively, and he has attained the highest academic degrees, B.A. (Honors) (London), M.A. (London), Dr. Litt. (Holland), all between June 1965 and 1967. In

1969, he met his Spiritual Master, Swami Rama, and was initiated into one of the highest paths of Dhyana-yoga.

He has studied and is well-versed in the scriptures of all religions, understands 17 languages with varying degrees of fluency, which allows him to teach meditation to people of different faiths – Hindus, Buddhists, Muslims, Christians, Sikhs – from within their own scriptural and meditative traditions, as he is familiar with all known meditative traditions and the different schools of eastern and western philosophies.

Before taking his vows of Swamihood in 1992, he was known as Dr. Usharbudh Arya. A prolific writer and speaker, he is the author of numerous books, including *Superconscious Meditation, Mantra and Meditation, Meditation and the Art of Dying, Philosophy of Hatha Yoga, God, Sayings,* and *Yoga-Sutra of Patanjali.*

Printed in the United States
88622LV00006B/143/A

9 781588 321732